PιιA 16

£3.50

COMPARATIVE
ANIMAL CYTOLOGY
& HISTOLOGY

WASPS *by* J. Philip Spradbery

RESEARCH METHODS IN MARINE BIOLOGY *edited by* Carl Schlieper

DESCRIPTION AND CLASSIFICATION OF VEGETATION *by* David W. Shimwell

MARINE BIOLOGY *by* Hermann Friedrich

MOLECULAR BIOLOGY AND THE ORIGIN OF SPECIES *by* Clyde Manwell
and C. M. Ann Baker

PRACTICAL INVERTEBRATE ZOOLOGY *by* F. E. Cox, R. P. Dales, J. Green
J. E. Morton, D. Nichols, D. Wakelin

ANIMAL MECHANICS *by* R. McNeill Alexander

THE BIOLOGY OF ESTUARINE ANIMALS *by* J. Green

STRUCTURE AND HABIT IN VERTEBRATE EVOLUTION *by* G. S. Carter

ANIMAL ECOLOGY *by* Charles Elton, FRS

A GENERAL ZOOLOGY OF THE INVERTEBRATES *by* G. S. Carter

ZOOGEOGRAPHY OF THE SEA *by* S. Ekman

THE NATURE OF ANIMAL COLOURS *by* H. Munro Fox, FRS,
and H. Gwynne Vevers

VERTEBRATE ZOOLOGY *by* Sir Gavin de Beer, FRS

THE FEATHERS AND PLUMAGE OF BIRDS *by* A. A. Voitkevich

In Preparation

THE INVESTIGATION OF NATURAL PIGMENTS *by* G. Y. Kennedy

ANIMAL DISTRIBUTION *by* Gustaf de Lattin (transl. from German)

MECHANISMS OF INSECT BEHAVIOUR *by* R. L. Miller and P. F. Howse

DIFFERENTIATION AND MORPHOGENESIS IN PLANTS *by* D. Brett

COMPARATIVE ANIMAL CYTOLOGY & HISTOLOGY

by

ULRICH WELSCH

Institute of Anatomy in the University of Kiel

and

VOLKER STORCH

Institute of Zoology in the University of Kiel

SIDGWICK & JACKSON

LONDON

First published in Great Britain 1976
by Sidgwick and Jackson Limited

Copyright © 1976 by Gustav Fischer Verlag, Stuttgart

Copyright © this translation 1976
Ulrich Welsch and Volker Storch

Originally published in Germany by
Gustav Fischer Verlag under the title
'Einführung in Cytologie und Histologie der Tiere'

ISBN 0.283.98255.1 (Hard)
0.283,98256.X (Paper)

Typeset by Malvern Typesetting Services Ltd
Malvern, Worcestershire
and Printed in Great Britain by
Biddles Ltd. Guildford, Surrey
for Sidgwick and Jackson Limited
1 Tavistock Chambers, Bloomsbury Way
London, WC1A 2SG

Preface

The present book is a revised and enlarged translation from our *Einführung in Cytologie und Histologie der Tiere,* which had been written because no modern comparative histology exists, at least in the German language.

More than half of the illustrations are electromicrographs or drawings based on electron micrographs. We feel that in comparison with light micrographs these illustrations have the advantage of greater clarity so that the essential details of the microscopic structure of the animals are easier to understand for the beginner.

In the present English version we could give consideration to advice of numerous colleagues and our teaching experience. Furthermore new results, which in the comparative field are coming up in great quantities, have been added to the text.

At the end of each chapter a brief list of literature has been added. This of necessity is incomplete and comprises mainly new important papers or review articles in which further literature can be found.

The present translation has been done by the authors in collaboration with Prof. Dr R. P. Dales, London, for whose advice and patience we are particularly grateful. Sincere thanks are also due to Prof. Dr Drs h.c. W. Bargmann who critically read the German text. We gratefully acknowledge the help of Mrs G. Kleber and Miss W. Röhe-Hansen, who prepared the majority of the accurate line drawings, and of Miss K. Jacob, who helped in the production of the light micrographs; furthermore we wish to express our appreciation to Mrs L. Trappe, Miss K. Hilbers, Mrs A. Löwe, and Mr H. Mrohs, all of Kiel, Western Germany.

London, late spring 1975

ULRICH WELSCH
VOLKER STORCH

Contents

Preface   v

Introduction   x

1. THE CELL   1
    Membranes   2
    Nucleus   4
        Nuclear division   9
        Structure of chromosomes   11
    Endoplasmic reticulum (ER) and ribosomes   12
    Golgi apparatus   17
    Lysosomes   22
    Peroxisomes (microbodies)   26
    Mitochondria   26
    Microtubules and microfilaments   30
    Glycogen   32
    Lipid inclusions   32
    Crystalline inclusions   33
    Pigments   33
    Specializations of the cellular surface   34
    Specializations for cell attachment   38
    Centrioles and cilia   41

2. TISSUES   48
    Epithelia   48
    Connective tissue   53
        Loose connective tissue   61
        Dense connective tissue   69
        Cartilage and bone   69
        Vesicular tissue and notochord   77
        Reticular connective tissue   80
        Lymphatic tissue (mammals)   80
        Blood-forming tissue (myeloid tissue)   82
        Mesenchyme   84
        Mesogloea   85

	Muscular tissue	85
	Nervous tissue	98
	Neurons	98
	Neuroglial cells	108
3.	INTEGUMENT	117
4.	RECEPTOR CELLS (SENSORY CELLS)	154
	Chemoreceptors	156
	Thermoreceptors	163
	Electroreceptors	164
	Mechanoreceptors	166
	Photoreceptors	177
5.	NERVOUS SYSTEM	189
6.	ENDOCRINE ORGANS	205
	Pituitary gland	208
	Endostyle and thyroid gland	212
	Ultimobranchial gland	219
	Parathyroid gland	219
	Islets of Langerhans	220
	Gastrointestinal tract	223
	Adrenals, interrenal and suprarenal bodies, chromaffin tissue	224
	Corpuscles of Stannius	226
	Gonads	226
	Placenta	227
	Pineal organ	227
7.	DIGESTIVE TRACT	230
	Invertebrates	230
	Vertebrates	247
	Mucous membranes	247
	Oral cavity	248
	Oesophagus	251
	Stomach	251
	Midgut	253
	Large intestine	254
	Liver	255
8.	RESPIRATORY ORGANS	263
	Tracheae	263
	Lungs	265
	Gills	269
9.	LYMPHATIC ORGANS, BLOOD CELLS AND BLOOD VESSELS	274
	Lymphoepithelial organs	274

Lymph nodes   275
Thymus   277
Spleen   279
Blood cells   282
    Vertebrates   282
    Invertebrates   286
Blood vessels   288
    Vertebrates   288
    Invertebrates   292

10. ORGANS OF EXCRETION, OSMO- AND IONIC
    REGULATION   295
    Pulsating vacuoles   295
    Protonephridia   295
    H-shaped systems   300
    Malpighian tubules   303
    Metanephridia   303
    Vertebrate kidney   311
    Salt glands   319

11. REPRODUCTIVE ORGANS AND CELLS   321
    Male animals   321
    Female animals   332

Index   339

INTRODUCTION

It is the aim of histological and cytological studies to understand structures of living cells, tissues and organs. The main tool for such investigations is the microscope, of which several species exist ranging from a simple light microscope to a high power electron microscope. Living cells, because of their relative thickness and transparency, are, however, unsuitable objects for such studies (Fig. 1). Therefore, normally it is necessary to work with chemically fixed material, of which thin sections can be prepared, which are stained by various dyes in order to distinguish the individual components of a tissue or cell. A good fixation causes relatively few structural changes in comparison with the living cell. The fixative hardens the tissue and prevents its postmortem decomposition. Some fixatives improve the stainability of certain structures with particular dyes.

Fixatives most frequently used are: formalin, potassium dichromate, acetic acid, picric acid, osmic acid, glutaraldehyde and ethanol. Many fixatives are mixtures, which occasionally are termed after their inventors, e.g. Bouin's fluid is composed of picric acid, formalin and acetic acid.

Usually material is simply immersed in a bath of fixative, which means that the peripheral parts of this piece of tissue will be better preserved than the centrally located parts, particularly so in bigger blocks of tissue. Better results can be obtained by fixative methods in which the fixative fluid is perfused through the blood vascular system of the animal.

After fixation the material is embedded in a medium, e.g. paraffin wax, which can be cut into thin sections. Before embedding, the tissue is dehydrated in alcohol and afterwards transferred to a bath of xylene or toluene. These two steps are necessary for the complete penetration of the paraffin into the tissue. The wax is initially fluid and warm and later hardens. Now the material, which is soaked with the embedding medium, is cut with a special knife into 4-10 μm-thick sections, which are attached to glass slides. Here the embedding medium is removed again and the sections can be stained.

It is important to note here that the material has been treated so far by fixative reagents, lipid solvents (alcohol, xylene), and warm paraffin. This means that lipid inclusions are dissolved out of the cytoplasm or that possibly other distortions may have been caused. In any case one has to consider to what extent artifacts have been introduced into the section. The dehydration in alcohol leads to a considerable shrinkage of the tissue, which is particularly obvious in nervous tissue (up to 50 per cent) and in many invertebrates the tissues of which contain much watery fluid.

Frequently sections are stained with the routine stain haematoxylin and eosin (H and E). Haematoxylin is a dark bluish basic dye, which stains acid components of a cell, e.g. nucleic acids. Structures stained by haematoxylin are termed basophilic (e.g. nuclei of cells). Eosin is a red acid dye, structures stained by it are termed acidophilic or eosinophilic. The H and E stain gives a good general picture but ordinarily does not show details of the cellular cytoplasm. Therefore, often it is useful to apply special stains in order to recognize as many details as possible in a section. A great variety of such special stains exist, which make it possible to demonstrate all important components of the cell, e.g. mitochondria, Golgi-apparatus and endoplasmic reticulum, in the light microscope (Fig. 2).

Often in routine preparations the connective tissue components are stained selectively. In the commonly used Azan stain the collagen fibres are stained blue, in the Goldner stain green, in van Gieson's stain red. Elastic fibres are best demonstrated with resorcin fuchsin or orcein.

Since in the following text structures are now and then referred to which can be demonstrated by silver-methods, these will also be mentioned briefly:

(a) By the argentaffin reaction, ammoniated silver hydroxide is reduced to metallic silver. The reaction is given by structures containing polyphenols, aminophenols and polyamines in ortho- and paraposition. Cells containing such substances, e.g. the endocrine enterochromaffin (=argentaffin) cells of the gastrointestinal tract, are stained black in the preparation.

(b) Argyrophil structures reduce silver salts only after addition of a reducing agent (e.g. hydrochinon). Also in this silver procedure structures are stained black (argyrophil structures); examples are reticular fibres and argyrophil cells of the gastrointestinal tract.

Histochemical staining methods allow recognition of particular chemical components of a tissue or cell, e.g. lipids, mucopolysacchaarides or enzymes. For this purpose frozen sections are often used (cut in a cryotome), thus avoiding preparatory steps introducing artefacts and the denaturation of proteins. Today it is known, that the histochemical demonstration of many enzymes also marks the presence of certain cell organelles: e.g. acid phosphatase is localized in lysosomes, the Gogi apparatus and less frequently also in the rough endoplasmic reticulum; alkaline phosphatase usually marks brush borders and other transport-active cell membranes; cytochromoxidase is localized in mitochondria, acetyl cholinesterase in the rough ER, the Golgi apparatus and on the plasma-membrane of nerve cells and many polypeptide producing endocrine cells, and thyamin pyrophosphatase in the Golgi apparatus and on the brush border.

Histochemical demonstrations may also be carried out in paraffin embedded material. An example is the PAS-reaction (periodic acid-schiff). This method depends on a selective oxidation by periodic acid, which attacks 1,2-glycols and 1,2-amino alcohols, oxidizing the adjacent groups to aldehydes and breaking the carbon chain at these sites. The aldehydes are then detected *in situ* by their reaction with Schiff's reagent to form a reddish purple colour. Structures rich in polysaccharides, mucopolysaccharides, glycoproteins or glycolipids are the principal ones stained.

If particular lipids are to be studied the fixed material also has to be cut in the cryostat (to avoid the alcohol step in the paraffin embedding).

In order to prevent a shrinkage of the tissues and to retain particular components in the cells, the water can also be withdrawn from it by the relatively gentle freeze drying techniques. Blocks of tissue are rapidly frozen, e.g. in liquid nitrogen, and afterwards dehydrated in a vacuum at low temperatures; the dehydrated tissue is fixed in formalin vapour and finally embedded in paraffin. This method allows numerous histochemical demonstrations, e.g. of biogenic amines and various mucoproteins.

The biogenic amines can be demonstrated after freeze drying and treatment with formalin vapour in the fluorescence microscope; examples are: 5-hydroxytryptamine (5-HT), dopamine, noradrenaline, adrenaline, histamine (see Figs. 102, 117). This method is particularly useful in studies on nervous tissue since even very small ramifications of nerves can still be visualized by it. Usually the fluorescent perikarya or nerve fibres have to be analysed in a microspectrofluorimeter in order to determine the specific spectra of their biogenic amines.

With the aid of the fluorescence microscope among others also antigen-antibody reactions can be demonstrated in a section (immuno-histochemistry). This technique has given valuable results, e.g. in detecting specific hormone-producing cells.

The short above-mentioned remarks refer to light microscopical preparations. For ordinary electron microscopical preparations the pieces of tissue are processed in a basically similar way. Fixation has to be done particularly carefully since the structure of the cell must be preserved down to a macromolecular level. During fixation weak intermolecular bondages should be replaced by tighter bondages, which prevent destruction caused by the solutions of the embedding media, by mechanical forces during sectioning and by the beam of electrons. Usually a double fixation is employed at physiological pH; initially in glutaraldehyde and/or formaldehyde and afterwards in osmic acid. The osmium combines with the lipoprotein membranes of the cell and because of its electron-density enhances the contrast of the preparation. Embedding medium is a resin (araldite or epon). Sections, 50–100 mμ thick, usually are cut with glass or diamond knives. The contrast in the section is further enhanced by treating the preparations with salts of heavy metals (lead citrate, uranyl acetate). Such sectioned material is looked at in the transmission electron microscope.

With the aid of relatively new methods also the surface of cells can be viewed in the electron microscope. In freeze-etched preparations (Fig. 4) small blocks of tissue are frozen, then the upper part of it is chopped off and the free surface is covered by a thin layer of metal (platinum, tungsten). The tissue under this metal film is removed and the surface replica is viewed in the ordinary electron microscope.

While in this type of preparation fractured surfaces of cells are observed, in the scanning electron microscope natural surfaces, e.g. of inner epithelia or of the body surface (Fig. 76) are viewed. It is useful to fix the preparations before coating them with a film of metal.

Autoradiography is a technique devised to define the localization of radioactive substances within light- or electron microscopic sections. A radioactive compound, e.g. triturated thymidine for the localization of nuclear DNA or radioactive aminoacids, is injected into an animal. After defined times the animal is sacrificed and histological sections are prepared, covered by a photographic emulsion, exposed for a suitable time-interval and subsequently developed as in ordinary photography.

The rays emitted by the radioisotope furnish the energy necessary to transform the silver bromide of the emulsion into photolytic silver, which may then be developed into visible black silver grains. Such grains overlie the sites of deposition of the radioactive

xiv   INTRODUCTION

substance in the histological section (Fig. 7).

By this method it is possible to see a labelled element in a cell or tissue. The fate of that element in the cell body may be detected by following the element through from structure to structure. The metabolism of any labelled compound can thus theoretically be traced throughout the animal body, provided that the labelled material is retained in its original site in a tissue during processing for autoradiography. The advantage of this method for the progress of histology and cytology is apparent, since the significance of known structures will often be revealed by the substance which they incorporate.

LITERATURE

ADAM, H., and CZIHAK, G. 'Arbeitsmethoden der makroskopischen und mikroskopischen Anatomie.' *Großes Zool. Praktikum.* Teil I. G. Fischer, Stuttgart (1964). 583 pp.

BARKA, T., and ANDERSON, P. J. *Histochemistry - theory, practice and bibliography,* Harper and Row, New York (1963), 660 pp.

EMMEL, V. M., and COWDRY, E. V. *Laboratory tecnnique in biology and medicine.* William and Wilkins Company, Baltimore (1964), 549 pp.

LILLIE, R. D. *Histopathologic technic and practical histochemistry.* Blackinston Company, Philadelphia (1954), 786 pp.

PEARSE, A. G. E. *Histochemistry theoretical and applied* 3rd ed. J. & A. Churchill, London, Vol. I (1968), Vol. II (1972), 1518 pp.

ROMEIS, B. *Taschenbuch der mikroskopischen Technik.* 16th ed. Oldenbourg, München (1968), 757 pp.

Chapter 1
THE CELL

The cells of all animals are delimited by a plasma membrane and contain the nucleus and the cytoplasm (Figs. 1, 2, 3).

The cytoplasm, which often forms the most voluminous part of the cell, consists of the cytoplasmic matrix (= groundplasm), the organelles and various inclusions. In light- and electron-microscopical preparations the cytoplasmic matrix generally shows little or no structural organization and often appears to be 'empty'. It serves for transport and numerous other metabolic processes, plays a role in morphogenetic phenomena and – according to studies in amoebae – by its contractility can take part in movements. The morphogenetic function of the groundplasm is particularly evident in some amoebae, the cytoplasm of which is divided into an outer

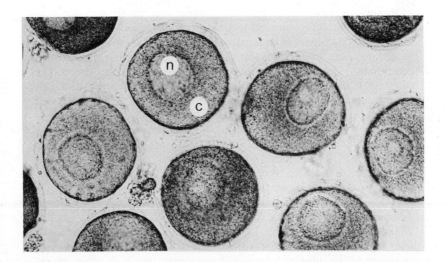

Figure 1.   Unstained living egg cells of the sea urchin *Psammechinus*; n: nucleus, c: cytoplasm

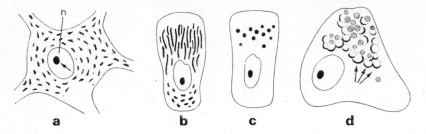

a   b   c   d

Figure 2.   Various cell organelles as seen in the light microscope; **a:** nervous cell with Nissl-bodies which correspond to stacks of rough ER cisternae; n: nucleus with nucleolus (arrow). **b, c:** intestinal epithelial cells from the mammalian midgut; **b:** with mitochondria; **c:** with lysosomes; **d:** exocrine cell from the pancreas with Golgi apparatus (arrows) and round secretory granules

part (ectoplasm, consisting of groundplasm exclusively) and an inner part (endoplasm, consisting of groundplasm, organelles and inclusions). After application of certain ions, e.g. SCN⁻, ectoplasm is transformed into endoplasm. Analysis of this process with the electron microscope shows that within a few minutes various membranous structures make their appearance by transformation of ecto- into endoplasm. Filamentous structures also can be formed by the groundplasm. On the other hand such membranes and filaments can be dissolved again in the cytoplasmic matrix.

Organelles are embedded in the cytoplasmic matrix and occur in almost all cells. They correspond to specific, generally membrane-delimited structures with their own metabolic functions. The membranes of the organelles divide the cytoplasm into several spaces and segregate the interior of the organelles from the cytoplasmic matrix. Thus different compartments are created which are characterized by specific concentrations of substrates and enzymes. Well-known organelles are, for example, the endoplasmic reticulum, the Golgi apparatus, and the mitochondria.

The term inclusions comprises several accumulations of metabolic products which are excluded temporarily from the active metabolism of the cell, such as lipid droplets, glycogen particles, protein crystals, and pigment granules.

Membranes

The plasma membrane (= cell membrane, plasmalemma) is generally 7-10 nm (70-100 Å) thick. Its diameter is below the resolving power of the light microscope. Frequently, however, other structures are apposed to its inner and outer surfaces which absorb stains and can often be seen in the light microscope. In ordinary electron microscopic preparations it can be seen to consist of three layers (leaflets), an inner and outer electron-dense dark layer and a central lighter one. This type of membrane has been found to be of universal occurrence and has been called the unit membrane. Also most intracellular membranes are such unit membranes the thickness of which, however, varies considerably. It is generally assumed that the dark layers correspond to protein components; the lighter zone in the middle consists of two layers of polar phospholipid molecules, the hydrophobic regions of which form the common border between the two lipid layers, the hydrophilic groups extend to the exterior and are connected with the proteins. The double layer of phospholipids is essentially responsible for the structural qualities of the membrane and forms a permeability barrier. The chemical composition of the lipids varies in different kinds of membranes. The fatty acids do not form a rigid crystalline lattice but under physiological temperatures have the nature of liquid crystals. This condition is dependent on the number of unsaturated fatty acids and is of great importance for transport processes through the membranes, which is particularly rapid in the presence of a large number of unsaturated fatty acids. Organisms living in a cold climate generally have a relatively high percentage of unsaturated fatty acids in their membranes.

The proteins comprise 10-20 per cent of the membrane volume. According to more recent investigations they do not form homogeneous layers. Their arrangement can be very irregular. On the inside and on the outside of the membrane they can be connected individually or in groups with the hydrophilic pole of the lipid molecules; they can be included in one of the lipid layers or can fill the whole membrane from inside to outside. The proteins are e.g. enzymes building up the lipid layers or carrier molecules transporting material through the membrane. Particularly rich in protein is the inner mitochondrial membrane. From it extend into the mitochondrial matrix toadstool-like particles 9nm (90 Å) in diameter called inner membrane sub-units, which can be visualized by a special electron microscopic method (negative staining). The plasma membrane is a barrier, the properties of which determine which substances are transported into or out of the cell (selective permeability). The transport is either a passive process through tiny hypothetical pores or is mediated by carriers and enzymes, the activity of which is energy-dependent. An active transport can be achieved against concentration-gradients.

Specific activities of a cell often are correlated with special molecules of their plasma membrane. Examples are the receptor molecules in the cell membrane of nerve and muscle cells which bind transmitter molecules released from the nerve terminals, and the adenyl cyclase which is regarded to mediate the effect of some hormones.

Substances can also be transported into cells by being incorporated into vacuolar or vesicular elements which are pinched off from the plasma membrane (Fig. 3). In the course of this process the plasma membrane envelops small particles like bacteria (phagocytosis) or molecules (pinocytosis) which have become adherent to its outer surface. When the particles or molecules are completely surrounded by the plasmalemma, the membrane-covered particles or substances detach from the cell membrane and move into the cytoplasm, where they are called phagocytotic vacuoles and pinocytotic vesicles. Pinocytotic vesicles can be smooth surfaced or covered by fine filamentous material (coated or spined vesicles). The latter comprise many different types and are thought to transport proteins or glycoproteins. They are particularly frequent in the epidermis of gutless parasites and in the epidermis of moulting insects. Pinocytotic vesicles are always much smaller than phagocytotic ones (see also page 24).

The plasmalemma of almost all cells is covered by a carbohydrate containing cell coat (glycocalyx), which forms a film of variable thickness which can be demonstrated in the light microscope by the PAS technique and also by similar methods in the electron microscope. This coat is particularly prominent on the surface of free and moist epithelia where it constitutes a fine filamentous fuzz (Fig. 16). It has been shown to consist of glycoproteins containing sialic acid groups. It acts as an adhesive, plays a role in immunological phenomena and is responsible for many other characteristics of the cell surface. The material of this coat probably originates in the Golgi apparatus and is transported to the surface by coated vesicles.

Nucleus

The nucleus contains the genetic code which has its chemical basis in deoxyribonucleic acid (DNA) and which controls the metabolism of the cytoplasm. Most cells possess one nucleus which is of spherical or ellipsoidal shape. Often its surface is indented, occasionally it possesses branching processes as in the muscle cells of appendicularians, nutritive cells in the ovary of some insects (*Forficula*), and macronuclei of some ciliates. Infrequently, two nuclei occur in a cell: e.g. in the club-shaped cells in the epidermis of lampreys and occasionally in hepatocytes and epithelial cells of the urinary bladder (Fig. 25). More often several nuclei per cell can be observed (e.g. osteoclasts, mammalian skeletal musculature).

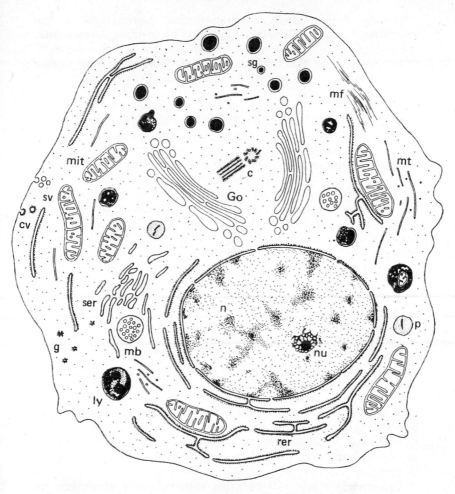

Figure 3. Fine structure of an animal cell. n: nucleus; nu: nucleolus: mt: microtubules, mf: microfilaments; sg: secretory granules; mit: mitochondrium; c: centrioles; Go: Golgi apparatus; sv: smooth surfaced micropinocytotic vesicles; cv: coated vessicles, ser: smooth endoplasmic reticulum; mb: multivesicular body, g: glycogen, ly: lysosome rer: rough endoplasmic reticulum, p: peroxisome. After REMANE, STORCH, WELSCH, 1974

The size of the nuclei varies a great deal, the smallest nuclei are 0.5 μm in diameter, the longest ones can surpass 1 mm in length. The nuclei of body cells usually contain two sets of chromosomes (diploid condition); often, however, more sets of chromosomes can be found (up to over 2000 in the water strider *Gerris lacustris*).

In fully differentiated cells the nucleus normally is in the interphase (interphase nucleus) and consists of three components: the nucleolo-chromosomal complex, the nuclear sap (karyolymph, nucleoplasm) and the nuclear envelope. Normally, only during nuclear divisions (see below) the individual chromosomes can be seen in the microscope.

The nucleolo-chromosomal complex corresponds to the genetic apparatus. DNA is combined with proteins which together form the so-called chromatin which in the interphase nucleus either is loosely distributed – euchromatin, or forms variously shaped dense clumps – heterochromatin (Fig. 4). The latter can be stained with basic dyes in light microscopic preparations. The areas containing euchromatin are pale and take up little or no dye. The distribution pattern of the heterochromatin is different in different cell types and can be used for the identification of a cell. Since heterochromatin is considered to represent inactive genetic material, its amount is an indicator of the metabolic activity of a cell, that is pale nuclei with little heterochromatin point to a high cellular activity and *vice versa*. In this respect the consecutive stages of maturation of the mammalian red blood cells are particularly illustrative. The nucleus of the erythroblasts displays a normal chromatin distribution with small irregularly scattered particles of heterochromatin. In the course of the proceeding differentiation haemoglobin synthesis comes to a standstill. This event is paralleled by nuclear changes: the amount of heterochromatin increases forming coarse clumps, which finally fill the whole nucleus which in addition becomes smaller. At the end of this process the inactive nucleus is extruded from the cell. An extreme concentration of heterochromatin can also be found in mature spermatozoa; here the DNA is so tightly coiled that it cannot be attacked by many reagents or by DNA-ase. In dead or degenerating cells the nuclei shrink and become a dense mass (karyolysis).

The nucleolus is a relatively big rounded body which can be stained with basic or less frequently also with acidic dyes. In living cells it is a light-refringent structure. The basophilia is explained by the contents of RNA in the nucleolus, which actually consists of ribosome precursors, which are produced at particular regions, the nucleolar organizers, of certain chromosomes. The number of nucleoli varies in different cell types and in individual cells. The most frequent numbers are one to three, in oocytes of amphibia up to 2000 nucleoli occur. In one cell their number can vary within a few hours. The somatic cells of man can contain five nucleoli, which, however, often fuse. Nucleoli generally disappear during cell division, only in a few protozoans (*Opalina*; some peridineans) they

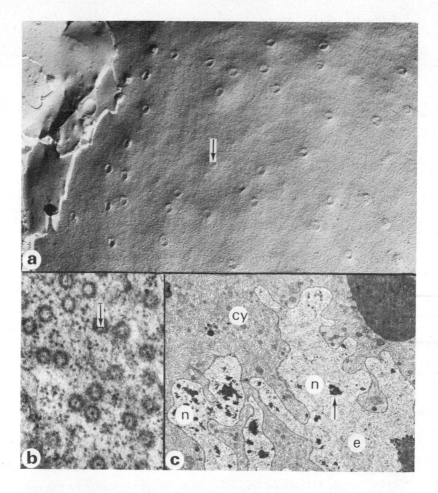

Figure 4.   Nuclear fine structure. **a:** freeze-etched preparation of the nuclear surface, arrow points to nuclear pore (preparation W. Buchheim) x 18 000; **b:** Nuclear pores (arrow), tangential section, midgut diverticulum, *Porcellio* (Crustacea) x 43 000; **c:** Multilobed nucleus (n), prosomal gland, *Bdella (Acari),* cy: cytoplasm, e: eucnromatin, arrow points to heterochromatin x 6000

remain intact throughout cell division. With the electron microscope three components of the nucleolus can be recognized:

1. Fibrillar parts, the fine filamentous elements of which are 3–10 nm (30–100 Å) in diameter and several hundred Å long; they consist of protein and rRNA.

2. Granular parts, which consist of particles of about 150 Å diameter, which closely resemble ribosomes and predominantly contain rRNA.
3. An amorphic matrix containing protein of low electron density.

The fibrillar components which are believed to be precursors of the granular ones may form a spongy network, the nucleolonema which under favourable conditions can also be seen in the light microscope. In other cells the nucleolus has a dense and compact structure; in this case it can contain a core of fibrillar material which is surrounded by the granular components (e.g. rat oocytes). Other nucleoli are ring-shaped.

In the nuclear sap many metabolic pathways have been demonstrated which also occur in the cytoplasm: glycolysis, hexosemonophosphate shunt, citric acid cycle, etc. The hexosemonophosphate shunt is important since it supplies the nucleus with pentoses. Further, in the nucleus NAD is synthesized, which is the coenzyme of numerous dehydrogenases. Characteristic enzymes of the nucleus are DNA- and RNA-polymerases.

The nucleus is surrounded by two unit membranes, between which is located a narrow space, the perinuclear cisterna. The whole complex is called nuclear envelope (nuclear membrane in light microscopy). This envelope is pierced by numerous pores (Fig. 4), around the edge of which outer and inner nuclear membrane fuse. Their diameter generally varies from 300-1000Å. Many pores are closed by thin diaphragms, others seem to be open. The pores provide a means for rapid passage of macromolecules between nucleus and cytoplasm. The perinuclear cisterna is in direct communication with the lumen of the rough endoplasmic reticulum. Since also the outer nuclear membrane often bears ribosomes, the whole envelope may be regarded as part of the rough endoplasmic reticulum.

Occasionally inclusions like crystals or microfilaments or microtubules or annulated lamellae may be observed in nuclei.

The nucleus of the protozoans frequently exhibits particularities, some of which are illustrated in Fig. 5. In some dinoflagellates the interphase nucleus contains typical chromosomes which in the electron microscope can be seen to consist of helically arranged thin filaments. Macronuclei of ciliates are often characterized by clumps of fine particles and fine filamentous material, the larger of which are interpreted as representing nucleoli, the smaller DNAcontaining structures. Occasionally, e.g. in the ciliate *Spirostomum*, bacteria live in the nucleus. In foraminiferans the nucleolar substance can form a thick shell in the periphery of the nucleus,

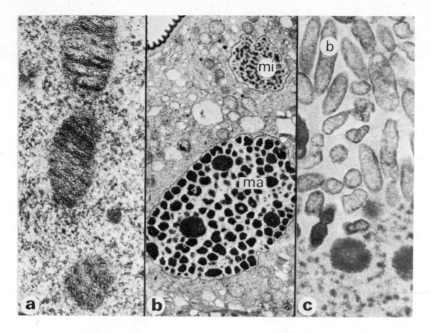

Figure 5. Fine structure of the nuclei of various protozoans. **a:** nucleus with fine helically coiled filaments in the chromosomes, dinoflagellate from the mesogloea of *Velella;* x 18 000 **b:** macro-(ma) and micronucleus (mi) of *Epistylis* (Ciliata) x 5000; **c:** nucleus with bacteria; *Spirostomum* (Ciliata) x 18 000

whereas its centre contains chromatin. Individually in ciliates (e.g. *Stylonychia*) the chromosomes may exhibit cross striations. In most protozoa the chromosomes of the interphase nucleus are almost exclusively present in the form of euchromatin.

Nuclear division

Mitosis. The life cycle of a normal cell is divided into interphase and the stages of the mitotic cell division: pro-, meta-, ana- and telophase. The cells spend most of their lives in the interphase. The nucleus of this phase is the interphase nucleus described in the previous section. It is characterized by an active metabolism and lies between two mitotic divisions. Before mitosis the DNA contents is duplicated which can be recognized by the formation of the chromatides (see below). The mechanism of mitosis ensures equal qualitative and quantitative distribution of DNA material to the daughter cells.

During prophase the chromosomes become visible, each of them being divided into two identical chromatids, which are only interconnected in one particular area of the chromosome, the kinetochor (= centromere, Fig. 6). In the cytoplasm the spindle apparatus is formed and the nucleolus and the nuclear envelope disappear.

The spindle apparatus consists of centrioles and microtubules. In the prophase the pair of centrioles duplicates, each pair moving to opposite poles of the cell. The microtubules may be classified into spindle and central continuous tubules. The spindle tubules extend from the centriolar pairs to the chromosomes; the central continuous tubules pass from one pair of centrioles to the other, without being attached to chromosomes.

In the following metaphase the chromosomes condense, thus becoming shorter and thicker, and arrange themselves in the equatorial plane of the spindle. The spindle tubules become attached to the kinetochors. Now the chromatids of the individual chromosomes begin to separate. After this separation the chromatids are considered as chromosomes and move to opposite

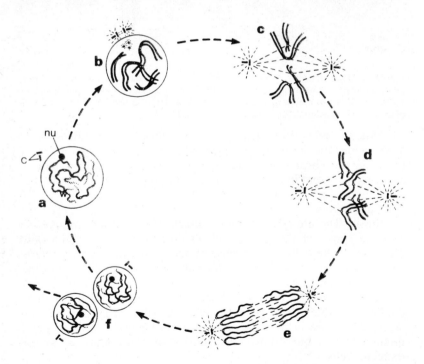

Figure 6. Mitosis. **a:** early; **b:** late prophase; **c:** metaphase; **d:** anaphase; **e:** telophase; **f:** newly formed daughter cells; nu: nucleolus; c: centrioles. After Dobszhansky from Remane, Storch & Welsch, 1974

sides of the cell (anaphase). The speed of the wandering chromosomes is 1 to several μm/min.

In many cells the chromosomes approach the spindle pole, the spindle tubules possibly shortening by loss of their globular subunits. In other cells the spindle becomes elongated, the poles moving in opposite directions, so that the distance between chromosomes and spindle pole remains constant.

In the final telophase the movement of the chromosomes ends. The cell forms a cleavage furrow in the area of the equatorial plane and divides into two daughter cells (cytokinesis). The chromosomes lose their visible individuality, a new nuclear envelope forms and the nucleoli reappear.

Endomitosis is characterized by a separation of the chromatids without dissolution of the nuclear envelope and without spindle formation.

Occasionally not only two but several or numerous chromatids arise during prophase. These do not separate but form thick bundles and constitute the so-called giant- or polytene chromosomes (see below).

Amitosis. During amitosis a ring-shaped bundle of microtubules surrounds the nucleus and divides it into two. The chromatin apparently remains in the interphase condition.

Structure of chromosomes

Chromosomes are elongated or oval elements which may be normally seen individually only during cell division. During interphase they exist in a dispersed condition and form the chromatin mentioned above but also in this phase they maintain their individuality. They can possess a cross striation (dark stripes: chromomeres) and regularly exhibit a constriction in a fixed localization which is called kinetochor or centromere. The centromere divides the chromosome into two arms. The area of the nucleolus organizator has already been referred to. During mitosis one can see that the chromosomes consist of two strings (chromatids), which are held together only at the centromere.

Until recently two theories tried to explain the molecular make up of the chromosomes. According to the first hypothesis one chromosome in anaphase consists of several threads of DNA molecules, according to the second such a chromosome consists only of one DNA molecule. Recently it was found that the latter hypothesis is correct. The general structural plan presumably is a series of DNA-protein loops extending laterally from a core protein held together by disulphide bond linkages. It was furthermore established that chromosome duplication is semiconservative: each daughter-chromatid - which is the chromosome of the interphase - receives half of the DNA contents from the longitudinally split mother-chromosome which means that it consists of one DNA double helix. At the beginning of cell division a second double helix is synthesized. From the nuclei of some somatic cells of *Drosophila* complete DNA double helices have been isolated which were exactly of the length which was to be expected according to the DNA-contents of the corresponding chromosome and also according to the above-mentioned hypothesis. Molecular weights up to 80×10^9 daltons have been measured which corresponds to a length of one DNA double helix of 40 mm.

A favourable object for the study of chromosomes are the giant or polytene chromosomes, which have been found in several animals and which have been analysed in particular in the salivary glands of Diptera. They are relatively thick cords consisting of numerous chromatids which may be ten times longer than normal chromosomes. They exhibit a clear cross striation. The strongly stained dark lines are of different breadth and are particularly rich in DNA, whereas the pale intercalated discs contain less DNA. The giant chromosomes of different cells exhibit an identical pattern of these cross striations; however, in the individual organs the regular sequence of dark and pale lines is interrupted in a characteristic way by chromosomal inflations which originate from dark cross-striations. If the inflations are of small dimensions they are called puffs, if they are bigger they are called Balbiani rings. They indicate strong genetic activity (RNA synthesis) and consist of DNA sections which can protrude up to 5 μm from the rest of the chromosome (Fig. 7). Chromosomes with numbers of large laterally protruding loops often occur in oocytes, they are called lampbrush chromosomes.

Endoplasmic reticulum (ER) and ribosomes

In almost all cells of animals a network of cisternae, vesicles and tubules occurs termed endoplasmic reticulum (ER) which is delimited by a unit membrane. The latter separates an inner compartment (reticuloplasm) from an outer one (groundplasm). Both differ in chemical composition and concentration of ions so that electrical potentials occur along this ER-membrane. Often parts of the ER become isolated from the rest of the system and lie as roundish or flattened vesicles within the groundplasm.

Formerly it was believed erroneously that this system only occurs in the inner parts of the cytoplasm, in the endoplasm, as opposed to the outer ectoplasm, hence the name 'endoplasmic reticulum'. In cells in which the endoplasmic reticulum is particularly well developed forming stacks of parallel cisternae (Fig. 8), it can also be

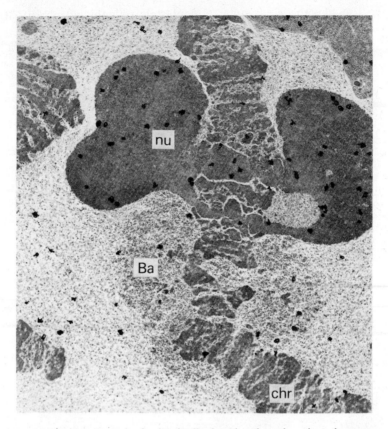

Figure 7. Radioautograph of a longitudinal section through a giant chromosome (chr) of *Chironomus* (Diptera) with its attached nucleolus (nu) and an adjacent Balbiani ring (Ba). Nucleolar processes extend into the chromosome. Twenty-seven hours after injection of tritiated uridine silver grains (dark spots) are distributed over the entire nucleolus and less abundantly over the Balbiani ring, indicating incorporation into RNA in these sites. Preparation B. v. GAUDECKER x 18 000

seen in the light microscope. In glandular and other cells it has been described as ergastoplasm, a name which was given to a basophilic area of the cytoplasm. In the cell bodies of nerve cells it forms the basophilic tigroid or Nissl bodies, in cross-striated muscle cells a reticular system.

According to its ultrastructure two forms of the endoplasmic reticulum can be distinguished (Fig. 8):

1. The rough or granular endoplasmic reticulum (rough ER)

2. The smooth or agranular endoplasmic reticulum (smooth ER)

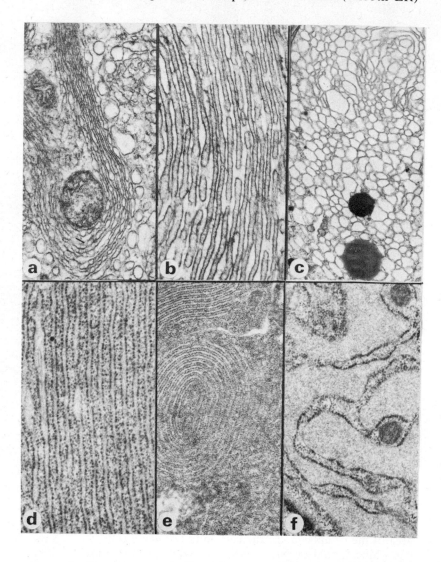

Figure 8. Fine structure of the endoplasmic reticulum; different types of arrangement. a–c: smooth ER; d–f: rough ER; **a:** *Cavia* (guinea pig) adrenal cortex; **b:** *Buccinum* (prosobranch snail), sensory cell in the osphradium; **c:** *Neptunea* (prosobranch snail), sensory cell in the osphradium; **d:** *Felis* (cat), exocrine pancreas, **e:** *Boophthora* (Diptera), salivary gland; **f:** *Cavia*, thyroid follicular epithelial cell. c x 5400, a,b,d–f x 20 000

Both categories of the ER may be considered to be parts of one system since they are often continuous with one another. In mammalian liver cells they are generally represented in almost equal proportions, but under certain conditions one type of ER can predominate. In rat liver cells before birth granular ER predominates, immediately after birth the smooth variety is prevalent. In the liver cells of man and other mammals the smooth ER increases in volume after application of drugs and toxic substances.

The outer aspects of membranes of the granulated ER are studded with ribosomes. These small electron dense particles have a diameter of 12–30 nm (120–300 Å) and consist of ribosomal RNA and proteins. The largely helical RNA is responsible for the light microscopical basophilia of ribosome-rich areas in the cytoplasm (e.g. ergastoplasm and Nissl bodies). Ribosomes consist of two subunits; the larger one is responsible for the attachment to the ER membranes.

The ribosomes are the site of protein synthesis the programme of which is encoded in the mRNA which associates with several ribosomes. Such complexes consisting of one molecule of mRNA and several ribosomes are called polysomes. The size of the polysomes is dependent on the size of the protein to be synthesized: the polysomes of reticulocytes elaborating the α-chain of haemoglobin consist of four ribosomes; myosin producing polysomes in muscle cells are composed of 60–80 ribosomes. Corresponding with the function of the ribosomes the granular ER is particularly well developed in cells producing proteins.

Individual ribosomes and polysomes also often occur freely in the cytoplasm and less frequently in mitochondria. In undifferentiated cells predominantly free ribosomes are to be found, whereas in differentiated cells, which secrete proteins, the ribosomes mainly are bound to ER membranes. The number of ribosomes in one liver cell has been calculated to be about 6×10^6.

The rough ER does not only synthesize substances but also concentrates, transports and stores them.

Sites of protein synthesis and paths of transport can be studied by autoradiography. The injected labelled amino acids can be demonstrated initially at the ribosomes, where they are built together to constitute proteins. The proteins then enter the lumen of the ER cisternae whence they are transported to the Golgi apparatus. In this organelle they are further modified, concentrated and finally transported in smaller or larger vesicles or granules which migrate to the cellular surface. Here the membrane of the vesicles or granules fuses with the plasma membrane and the contents are given off into the intercellular space (exocytosis, Fig. 11).

Specific proteins may be demonstrated in the rough ER system as follows. The enzyme peroxidase - which is a protein - can normally be demonstrated with histochemical techniques in the rough ER and the perinuclear cisterna of various cells, e.g. white blood cells. If this enzyme of one animal species, e.g. a cow, is injected into the blood stream of another animal, e.g. a rabbit, the plasma cells of the latter will produce antibodies (immunoglobulins) which specifically react with the injected foreign protein, which is called antigen - in our case peroxidase. If after two days the spleen of the rabbit is removed, fixed, cut into sections, and exposed to an antigen (peroxidase) solution, then in all those places in which antibodies have been produced, an antigen-antibody-reaction will take place. After removal of the free and unbound peroxidase by washing, a histochemical demonstration of peroxidase shows that it is localized in the rough ER cisternae of the spleenic plasma cells, where the newly synthesized specific antibody against the peroxidase was stored. Thus the histochemically demonstrable enzyme marks the site of the occurrence of a specific protein.

The membranes of the rough ER additionally have been found to contain enzymes of the lipid metabolism and enzymes catalysing the formation of glycoproteins.

Lipid metabolism also has been demonstrated to occur in the groundplasm, at mitochondrial membranes and in the smooth ER. In the epithelial cells of the holocrine sebaceous glands the smooth ER is closely connected with lipid metabolism, in the resorptive epithelial cells of the intestine smooth and rough ER have been found in association with lipid droplets, whereas in the mammary gland the lipid droplets arise in areas of the rough ER.

The membranes of the smooth ER are devoid of ribosomes and are not in connection with the nuclear envelope. In vertebrates the smooth ER rarely forms extensive cisternae but predominantly a variable system of tubules. It is particularly prominent in steroid producing cells (adrenal cortex, ovaries, testes) where the tubules generally are of equal diameter and not branched. In liver cells where the smooth ER is thought to be in connection with glycogen metabolism, the tubules are branched and of variable diameter.

The smooth ER is also prominent, e.g. in sensory cells, the chloride cells of fish epidermis and gills, and in cross-striated muscle cells.

The annulated lamellae are also often considered to be part of the ER system. They often make their appearance in cells which are rapidly developing, e.g. in germinal cells or pathologically differentiated tissues (cancer cells). Their structure resembles that of the nuclear envelope, corresponding to flat cisternae perforated by numerous pores. They occur - in part in stacks - in the cytoplasm and in the nucleus (Fig. 12). In some cells they presumably originate in the Golgi apparatus, in others they may be derived from the nuclear envelope. Their function is unknown; after application of drugs their number can increase. In the nuclei of the giant cells of the rat placenta intranuclear annulated lamellae occur, which are in association with the inner nuclear membrane and with the nucleolus; possibly they here serve the transport of material from the nucleus to the cytoplasm or *vice versa*. A number of observations gave rise to the assumption that annulated lamellae are also a regular constituent of mature cells with an active metabolism, e.g. neurons and pinealocytes of some mammals. On the other hand it is believed that this membrane system only occurs under special physiological conditions.

Golgi apparatus

The Golgi apparatus is an organelle which was discovered by C. Golgi in 1898 in nerve cells. Later it was shown to be present in almost all cell types which have been subjected to prolonged impregnation with silver salts or osmic acid. In such preparations it can be demonstrated as a blackened network (Figs. 2, 54) or compact field usually located in the perinuclear region. In ordinary light-microscopic preparations it may often be identified in negative image as an unstained juxtanuclear area.

In the electron microscope it was found to consist of one or several stacks of 3–12 flattened smooth-surfaced cisternae or saccules (Figs. 9, 10). One stack has two faces, a forming or immature face which is usually convex, and a mature face, which is usually concave. The forming face is directed towards the endoplasmic reticulum and generally points to the base of the cell. The mature face frequently faces the apex of the cell. The saccules of the mature face, especially in their periphery, exhibit swellings, which are caused by accumulation of material in their lumina. These swollen portions become pinched off. As they become free they are relatively large and their contents are rather light. Soon, however, the density of the contents increases; so that these vesicles are called condensing vacuoles. As they move away from the Golgi apparatus towards the apex of the cell they are termed secretion granules. As they reach the apical plasma membrane their membrane fuses with the plasmalemma and their contents are delivered into the intercellular space. Part of the contents can form the coat covering the plasma membrane (see p. 4).

This process of the formation of secretion granules constantly uses up membranous material of the Golgi apparatus and this organelle

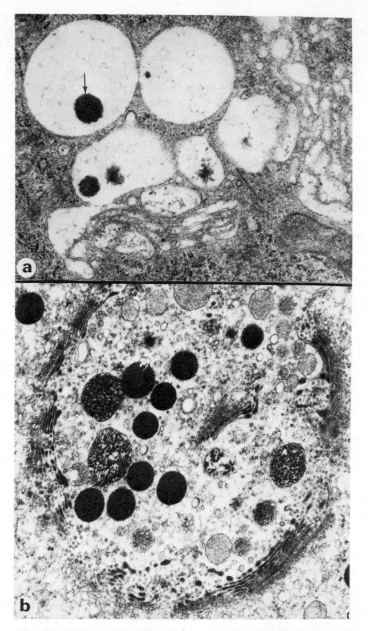

Figure 9.   Fine structure of the Golgi apparatus. **a:** rat, mammary gland, note the voluminous Golgi vacuoles containing condensed electron dense material (casein, arrow) x 25 000; **b:** *Lineus* (nemertean), cerebral organ, extensive circularly arranged Golgi apparatus, the cisternae of which contain dense material; in the centre secretory granaules of increasing electron density x 18 000

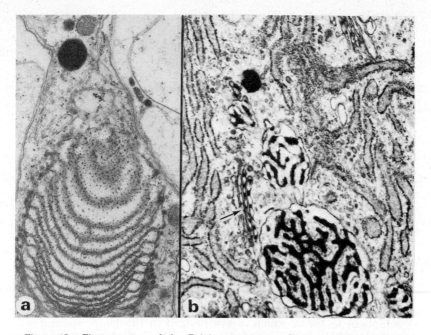

Figure 10. Fine structure of the Golgi apparatus. **a:** *Ceratonereis* (Polychaeta), epidermal mucus cell x 18 000; **b:** *Halicryptus* (Priapulida), epidermal mucus cell, note the striking 'zebra' pattern of the secretory granules, which can already be recognized in the Golgi cisternae (arrow); preparation K. MORITZ x 18 000

would rapidly disappear unless constantly new membranous material is added to it at the immature face. Thus, the stack remains of constant size since new saccules form as rapidly on the forming face of the stacks as saccules are used up for secretory vesicles on the maturing face.

The new membranous material originates from the transfer vesicles (microvesicles) which pinch off from the rough ER close to the immature face of the Golgi apparatus. As they bud off they lose their ribosomes. They approach the Golgi stack and fuse with the first saccule they reach. Thus, the transfer vesicle provides membrane that enables this saccule to increase in size. An extremely rapid turnover of saccules is observed in the goblet cells of the rat colon. There is a complete turnover of a whole stack in about forty minutes. A new saccule is assembled from transfer vesicles on the forming face about every two minutes. The transfer vesicles have a second important function: they transport protein material from the rough ER to the Golgi apparatus. As can be seen on Figs. 9, 10, not only the saccules of the mature face but almost all of the saccules of one stack can be filled with secretory material.

It is generally assumed that the Golgi apparatus originates from the endoplasmic reticulum. The chemical analysis of the cisternae of the immature face of the Golgi stack has shown that they are of almost identical composition as the membranes of the ER. Also their dimensions closely agree: both are about 2.5–4 nm (25–40 Å) thick. At the mature face the membranes are thicker (75 Å) and closely resemble the plasma membrane. Within the Golgi stack evidently the ER membranes are transformed, a process which is considered to be irreversible. The analysis of Golgi stacks of the rat liver has shown that the contents of unsaturated fatty acids of the membranes decreases from ER via Golgi apparatus to plasma membrane. Similar differences exist in respect of the protein components.

If the nucleus is removed from an amoeba, the Golgi apparatus degenerates. If the nucleus is again transferred into the cell, new Golgi saccules arise from the granulated ER after 30–60 minutes.

The Golgi apparatus fulfils a central role in the secretion process. It accumulates and concentrates the protein components from the ER and very often modifies them by adding a carbohydrate component to them, which is synthesized in the Golgi apparatus itself. Also lipids can be added to the carbohydrate component in the Golgi apparatus. Thus the secretory product leaving the Golgi apparatus is either a glycoprotein or glycolipid. The mucopolysaccharides forming the extracellular coat of the cell are also synthesized in this way: the protein component is produced in the rough ER and is combined with a carbohydrate component in the Golgi apparatus.

Lipid droplets have been observed in the Golgi apparatus of sebaceous and sweat glands. In the liver cells it plays a role in the formation of the bile. In all mucus-producing cells it is particularly well developed (Fig. 10). In mucus cells and chondrocytes the Golgi apparatus is the site of sulphate substitution of the carbohydrates of glycoproteins. Apart from forming secretory products the Golgi apparatus can also store material, e.g. in the epithelial cells of the intestine it can store lipids.

In melanocytes the pigment granules arise in the Golgi apparatus. The synthesis of melanin, however, occurs in the rough ER. In spermatocytes the Golgi apparatus produces small vesicles, which in the spermatids fuse to form the acrosome (Fig. 172). It is often believed that the Golgi apparatus also plays a role in the regulation of the intracellular water metabolism. Lysosomes also originate from the Golgi apparatus (see below).

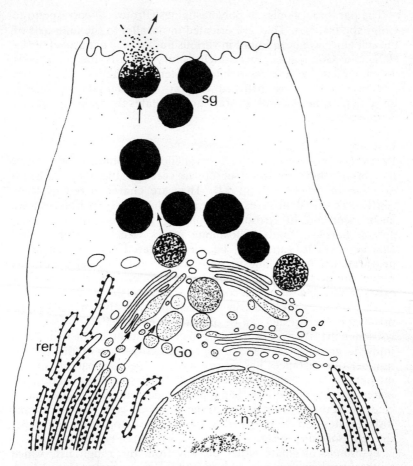

Figure 11. Formation of secretory products in an exocrine glandular cell. Arrows indicate the passage from the rough ER *via* the Golgi apparatus to the cell surface. n: nucleus, rer: rough ER; Go: Golgi apparatus, sg: secretory granule. After REMANE, STORCH, WELSCH, 1974

According to the various functions of the Golgi apparatus, it is endowed with numerous enzymes. Two groups of enzymes can be distinguished: (1) those which take part in the formation of lipoprotein-membranes, of polysaccharides and the combination of carbohydrates with other components; (2) those which are only concentrated in the Golgi apparatus and transported in small vesicles into the cytoplasm, e.g. the lysosomal enzymes. Characteristic enzymes are thiamine pyrophosphatase and N-acetyl-glucosamingalactosyltransferase.

The parabasal bodies of polymastigines (Protozoa) correspond to Golgi apparatuses. They are oriented in parallel to the long axis of the cell and have been found in various numbers. That aspect of the elongated Golgi apparatus which points towards the nucleus is accompanied by a cross-striated protein containing fibre. The parabasal bodies are believed to play an essential role in the formation of the cell wall. In starving flagellates the Golgi apparatus degenerates.

Lysosomes

Lysosomes are spherical cell organelles surrounded by a unit membrane; their size and structure are very variable, they can be up to 5 μm in diameter (Fig. 12). They are characterized by their contents of acid hydrolases. So far more than thirty hydrolases have been identified in lysosomes, splitting proteins, nucleic acids, polysaccharides, lipids, phosphate esters, etc. A characteristic enzyme, which can also be demonstrated in histochemical preparations, is acid phosphatase. Under pathological conditions which are due to genetic defects lysosomes devoid of their enzymes exist. In addition they often contain heavy metals.

All lysosomes take part in intracellular digestive processes; the material to be digested can be of intra- or extra-cellular origin. The lysosomal membrane normally prevents a diffusion of the hydrolases into the groundplasm and thus a self-destruction of the cell. A number of substances has an influence of the permeability of this membrane, e.g. cortisone has a stabilizing effect; vitamin A increases its permeability. Some pathological alterations are due to changes of the lysosomal membrane. In dying cells this membrane disintegrates and the enzymes escape into the cytoplasm and destroy the cell. Normally the enzymes act only within the lysosomes.

Lysosomes originate either directly from the rough ER, which synthesizes their enzymes, or from the Golgi apparatus (Fig. 13). A lysosome budding off from a Golgi saccule is called a primary lysosome or dense body or inactive lysosome. As soon as the primary lysosome interacts with material from inside or outside the cell, it is called a secondary lysosome. The digestion of exogenous material is called heterophagy, that of endogenous material, autophagy.

Primary lysosomes are of different appearance in different cell types and often also in one cell type during different stages of development, e.g. in young monocytes of the rat they correspond to electron-dense granules, in mature monocytes to light vesicles. In many cells they appear in the form of spined vesicles.

Secondary lysosomes are called phago-lysosomes if they interact with material which is of extracellular origin (e.g. bacteria, viruses

THE CELL 23

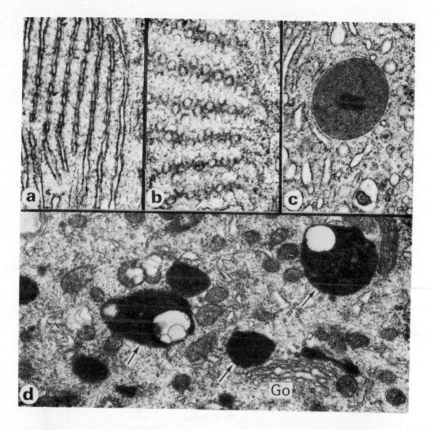

Figure 12. **a, b:** annulated lamellae, longitudinal (a) and tangential (b) section, note continuity with rough ER on fig. a, midgut diverticulum, *Neomysis* (Crustacea) a x 32 000, b x 30 000; **c:** peroxisome with nucleoid, midgut diverticulum, *Coenobita* (hermit crab) x 18 000; **d:** lysosomes (arrows), nerve cell, trigeminal ganglion *Triturus* (Urodela). The lysosomes originate from the Golgi apparatus (Go) x 18 000

or macromolecules). This material first adheres to the cell membrane, which then invaginates and envelops the foreign particle forming a vesicle which sinks into the cytoplasm. This vesicle is termed a phagosome, the process of its formation, phagocytosis. When a phagosome meets a primary lysosome, the two fuse to form a phagolysosome. Further primary lysosomes may meet with and fuse with this phagolysosome, their enzymes digesting the foreign particle. If there remains indigestible material in this secondary lysosome it is called a residual body (or tertiary lysosome). Such bodies may finally be extruded from the cell.

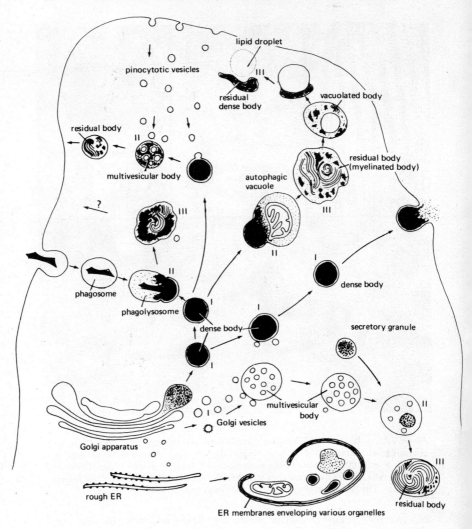

Figure 13.   Various types of lysosomes, I different types of primary lysosomes (dense bodies, smooth surfaced and spined Golgi vesicles), II secondary lysosomes, III residual bodies. Note that different types of multivesicular bodies exist containing either Golgi or pinocytotic vesicles. The extrusion of lysosomal enzymes has been described e.g. in molluscs and the epidermis of land-living vertebrates. After HAM and FARQUHAR.

If foreign material enters the cell in small light vesicles (pinocytotic vesicles), these can be incorporated into primary lysosomes. In this case seemingly intact vesicles appear within the lysosome, which thereupon is called a multivesicular body, which of course is also a secondary lysosome. Protein can be absorbed in special spined or coated vesicles which are incorporated into the multivesicular bodies. Apparently a different type of multivesicular bodies exists: a number of small light primary lysosomes is enveloped by a common membrane.

If primary lysosomes digest material originating in the cytoplasm, i.e. of endogenous origin, the resulting secondary lysosomes are termed autophagic lysosomes or autophagic vacuoles or cytolysosomes. They e.g. enclose worn out mitochondria, parts of the ER, glycogen and other functionless material of the cell. Indigestible residues may accumulate in these lysosomes in the form of lipofuscin pigment, which is a 'wear and tear' pigment and is particularly prominent in heart muscle cells, neurons and liver cells. How the lysosomes recognize the material which is to be destroyed is unknown. Observations on insects seem to show that they have an ability to select certain material, since at a given period they predominantly contain one type of cell organelle to be digested. Occasionally ER cisternae having lost their ribosomes and containing lysosomal enzymes envelop worn-out intracellular material in order to digest it.

All terminal stages of lysosomes which contain indigestible material are ocasionally also termed telolysosomes.

In the thyroid gland of vertebrates the lysosomes fulfil a special task in liberating the thyroid hormone into the bloodstream or lymph. They fuse with vesicles transporting the thyroglobulin-containing colloid into the cytoplasm. Their enzymes split the thyroglobulin, liberating thyroxine or triiodothyronine.

* In some animals, e.g. mussels, the primary lysosomes seem to liberate their enzymes on to the surface of epithelia. Here they may serve extracellular digestive processes.

Lysosomes also occur in protozoans. Here they typically occur as digestive vacuoles. Within primary lysosomes enzymes produced in the rough ER are transported to the ingestive vacuole which has accumulated food from the environment. The two bodies fuse forming a phagolysosome or digestive vacuole. During final stages of this process the vacuole is termed egestive vacuole. It liberates indigestible material into the surrounding medium. If a mechanism of defecation does not exist as in some suctorians the food residues are stored within residual bodies. In these animals excessive feeding shortens the life span and favours the rapid occurrence of death.

Peroxisomes (microbodies)

Peroxisomes are spherical cell organelles surrounded by a unit membrane and characterized by a fine granular matrix (Fig. 12). Often this matrix contains a crystalline core (nucleoid). The individual elements of the core consist of minute tubules often of two sizes: 10 nm (100 Å) and 4.5 nm (45 Å) in diameter. In some animals, e.g. hamster and hedgehog, the core forms a thin sheet. In liver cells the core is assumed to be the site of urate oxidase.

Peroxisomes are often located in the vicinity of the rough ER and arise by budding off from this system. They have been demonstrated in many cell types and have already been classified, e.g. on the basis of their diameter.

In mammalian liver and kidney cells peroxisomes contain enzymes which are associated with hydrogen peroxide metabolism, three of these enzymes synthesizing, one (catalase) splitting it. Catalase corresponds to 40 per cent of the protein contents of the peroxisomes and is located in their matrix. In mammals and the protozoan *Tetrahymena* peroxisomes have been demonstrated to play a role in the transformation of lipid to carbohydrate (gluconeogenesis). In the peroxisomes of mammalian liver and kidney presumably purines also are degraded. In the kidney they occur abundantly in the proximal convoluted tubule.

Occasionally peroxisomes in respect of their function are regarded as primitive mitochondria. Often there is a correlation in the numbers of peroxisomes and mitochondria per cell: in liver cells it was found that high numbers of mitochondria are correlated with low numbers of peroxisomes and vice versa.

Mitochondria

Mitochondria are roundish to rod-shaped organelles which are known since the latter half of the 19th century. After fixation in an osmium mixture they can be visualized in almost all cells by staining with acid fuchsin. In fresh tissue they can be demonstrated by the supravital staining method with Janus green.

As other cell organelles they are absent in mature erythrocytes of mammals, in the other cells they are of variable number: in protozoans more than 500,000 in certain species, in endothelial cells of vertebrate blood vessels less than 100 have been counted; in metabolically active cells, e.g. muscle cells, they can correspond to more than 50 per cent of the cell volume. The mitochondrial number in one cell is not constant, e.g. during starvation their number decreases. Normally their size is 1-5 μm, in many cells, however, bigger ones have been described, e.g. in muscle cells of insects, chaetognaths, birds and mammals they may reach a length of 50 µm. In muscle cells they are often of an elongated shape. In tissue cultures they can be observed in living cells and it was found that they can move, alter their shape and undergo fission.

The electron microscope has shown that mitochondria have two membranes, an outer and an inner one, and that these two are separated by a space, the outer matrix or intracristae-space, which is 4–8 nm (40–80 Å) wide (Fig. 14). The inner membrane is thrown into folds (*cristae mitochondriales*) or forms tubules (*tubuli mitochondriales*), or saccules (*sacculi mitochondriales*), prisms or other structures which extend into the inner parts of the mitochondria. Outer and inner membranes differ in structure and function, thus creating different compartments. Typical enzymes are monoaminoxidase (outer membrane) and cytochromoxidase (inner membrane). Both membranes can actively transport substances.

The interior space, which is surrounded by the inner membrane, is termed the mitochondrial matrix (or inner matrix). It is particularly rich in enzymes, whereas the intracristae space presumably is a site for dissolved low molecular compounds.

Often the mitochondrial matrix contains electron dense small granules (*granula intramitochondrialia*). They are of 300–500 Å in diameter and composed of 75 Å sub-units. These granules are particularly prominent in cells transporting ions and water. Calcium, iron and other bivalent cations presumably constitute these granules. Their presence testifies to the ability of the mitochondria to concentrate cations to a point where they precipitate. The intramitochondrial granules also show a relation to the lipid contents of the cell; if the lipid contents are increased their number decreases, if there is less lipid their number increases.

Number and fine structure of the mitochondria usually are dependent on the cellular activities. In metabolically inert cells their numbers are low and they are of a simple structure. In active cells, in which material is produced or which transport substances or which transform chemical into mechanical energy (muscle cells), they occur in vast numbers and their cristae or tubules are close together. Generally they are randomly distributed in a cell; often, however, they occur in those places in which energy is used, e.g. in muscle cells they are closely attached to the muscle fibrils which ensures a rapid supply of energy from the mitochondria to the contractile apparatus. A comparable topographical arrangement is to be found in the proximal section of sperm tails, where mitochondria supply the energy for the movements of the sperm flagellum. Also in the basal labyrinth of transport-active epithelial cells mitochondria occur in an ordered arrangement (Fig. 158). In oocytes vast

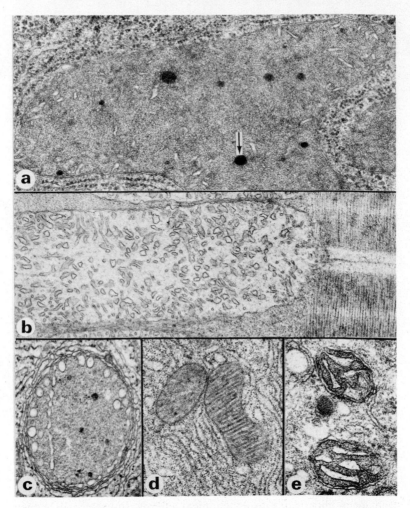

Figure 14.   Fine structure of mitochondria. **a:** *Ichthyophis* (Gymnophiona) liver cell, note well developed matrix, the mitochondrial granules (arrow) and the paucity of cristae and tubules x 30000; **b:** *Oikopleura* (Appendicularia) muscle cell from the tail, mitochondrium with variously shaped tubules, x 18 000. **c:** *Erinaceus* (hedgehog), adrenal cortex, mitochondrium with saccules x 30000; **d:** *Bdella* (Acari), prosomal gland, mitochondrium with cristae x 18 000; **e:** *Nephtys* (Polychaeta) epidermal ciliated cell, mitochondria with prismatic tubules, x 50 000

accumulations of mitochondria can be found in the juxtanuclear region, a phenomenon which has been seen in connection with the formation of yolk droplets. Often mitochondria are surrounding lipid droplets, e.g. in teleost liver, cells of midgut diverticula of crustacea and the mammary gland.

These topographical relations indicate the main functions of the mitochondria. Within the mitochondria those metabolic pathways take place which serve the oxygen dependent degradation of substrates. The energy of these processes is made available and stored in form of ATP, which is synthesized within the mitochondria from ADP and phosphate. Among the three fundamental food stuffs, lipid and protein can be broken down in the presence of oxygen exclusively; β-oxidation and amino acid oxidation thus occur within the mitochondria. In addition they house the enzymes of the common final oxidation of substrates (citric acid cycle, respiratory chain). Thus the close relation between mitochondria and sites of energy consumption and their high numbers in certain cells can be explained.

Mitochondria of a simple structure can contain enzymes catalysing synthetic reactions. This explains the occurrence of mitochondria in cells the metabolism of which is of anaerobic nature, as can be found, e.g. in certain intestinal parasites.

Mitochondria contain DNA and RNA; whether these nucleic acids function in self-reproducing and protein-synthesizing processes is not yet definitely proved, but can be assumed.

The life-span of mitochondria is shorter than that of a cell. Therefore there must be constant new formation of these organelles. In respect of this process two possibilities are discussed: division of old mitochondria or de novo formation. The first possibility is supported by cinematographic observations of living cells and electron microscopic observations which indicate fission, budding and new formation in the matrix space. In respect of the de novo formation almost all cell organelles have been thought to be able to give rise to new mitochondria, e.g. nucleus, nuclear envelope, ER, Golgi apparatus, etc. It has only been proved by autoradiographic studies in the mould Saccharomyces mitochondrifer.

There is an old theory which considers the mitochondria originally to have been intracellular parasites which became symbionts of cells. This theory is largely based on speculation on early evolutionary events.

Protozoans frequently contain mitochondria of the usual structure. Specialized protozoan mitochondria are the kinetoplasts, which singularly occur in some flagellates (bodonids, trypanosomatids) being localized proximally of the basal corpuscle of the cilia. These mitochondria contain cristae and are of variable size. The extracellular Leptomonas form of *Leishmania donovani* contains a big kinetoplast with numerous cristae, the intracellular

Leishmania form contains a small kinetoplast with few cristae. The matrix contains fibrillar material, presumably corresponding to DNA. Trypanosomes of vertebrate blood, the kinetoplasts of which have been artificially removed, reproduce in unlimited numbers; however, can no longer be transferred to insects.

Microtubules and microfilaments

Microtubules are presumably part of the cytoplasm of all cells. Their diameter is 20–30 nm (200–300 Å), their length is difficult to determine. Their wall consists of globular sub-units, a dozen of which can be recognized per cross-section. It is believed that they are helically arranged at the same time forming longitudinal rows. Microtubules are to be found abundantly in cellular processes, e.g. those of neurons and protozoans. In erythrocytes they form a bundle which runs in parallel to the edge of these disk-shaped cells. Furthermore they constitute the mitotic spindle. The microtubules of cilia show a definite arrangement (Fig. 20). Two main functions are believed to be performed by these tubules: (1) maintenance or control of the cellular shape; (2) participation in movement phenomena. In addition they may serve the transport of material. Microtubules can be destroyed by high pressure, low temperature and a number of chemicals (e.g. colchicine). Such destruction is frequently reversible.

Many cells contain fine filaments (microfilaments), which presumably are composed of proteins. Their thickness and probably also their function and chemical composition vary in different cell types. Their chief functions are providing skeletal support to the cell and taking part in movement phenomena; e.g. in the microvilli of the epithelial cells of many animals microfilaments occur which render rigidity to these processes (Figs. 16, 19). In the same and other cells they form a horizontally arranged web of filaments in the apical zone (terminal web). In epidermal cells they usually form bundles which are called tonofibrils, and which often terminate in the neighbourhood of desmosomes or hemidesmosomes (Fig. 19). Other cells with well-developed bundles of microfilaments are the cells of the vertebrate notochord, some glia and endocrine cells. The relation of these filamentous structures to movement is particularly clear in muscle cells (p. 85). Their contractibility in chordal and epidermal cells has also been held responsible for the changes during metamorphosis in tunicates.

Microfilamentous and microtubular systems are particularly well developed in protozoans. Filaments often form an intracellular framework, which can be distributed throughout the cytoplasm or concentrated in the cellular periphery (Fig. 17). Often the basal corpuscles of cilia are interconnected by bundles of filaments.

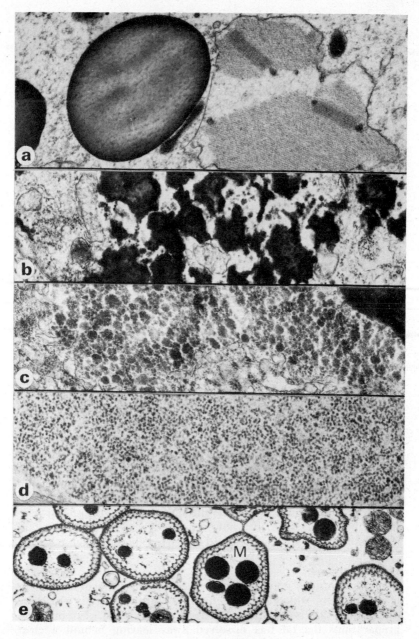

Figure 15. Fine structure of various cellular inclusions and organelles.
a: *Echinorhynchus* (Acanthocephala), epidermis, lipid-(left) and crystalline (right)
inclusions; **b:** *Nephtys* (Polychaeta), intestinal epithelium, irregularly shaped lipid
inclusions; **c:** *Nephtys* (Polychaeta) intestinal epithelium, glycogen rosettes (α-
particles); **d:** *Columba* (pigeon) glial cell from the glycogen body, glycogen particles
(β-particles); **e:** *Magelona* (Polychaeta), cross-section through the neck of mucous
cells (M) with microtubules in the cellular periphery, all x 20 000

Axostyles, which are characteristic for many polymastigines and which can perform undulating movements, consist of microtubules. Also the axonemata in the axopodia of Heliozoa consist of microtubules which in cross-section exhibit a spiral arrangement. Organelles facilitating the uptake of food, e.g. the pharyngeal apparatus of some ciliates, also contain complicated systems of microtubules. In the tentacles of suctorians they are considered to be part of a contractile apparatus and have been called already by light microscopists myonemata; here, they additionally form guide lines for transport processes. In *Stentor* a special filament and tubule system are to be distinguished. Both alter length and shape of the body during contractions. The microtubule system consists of individual, vertically arranged bundles, each of which is connected with one pair of basal corpuscles (kinetosomes). Each bundle contains twenty-one microtubules. The individual bundles slide past each other during changes of the body length. Also the highly contractile ciliate *Spirostomum* possesses bundles of microtubules which run longitudinally under the pellicle. However, bundles of microfilaments are responsible for the retraction of the ciliated corona of *Epistylis*.

Glycogen

Carbohydrates are stored in the cells of animals in form of the polysaccharide glycogen. In the cells of different tissues of flatworms and in liver cells of well-fed vertebrates it is particularly prominent and can fill large areas of the cytoplasm. In the electron microscope it is of variable appearance (Fig. 15). Often it can be seen in the form of isodiametrical particles of 15–30 nm (150–300 Å) in diameter. These are called β-particles. If such β-particles form bigger aggregates, the latter are called α-particles or rosettes. They can be up to $0 \cdot 1$ µm in diameter. The structure of glycogen particles often differs in different organs of one animal and in one organ in different species. In the liver cells of amphibia for example, the glycogen particles are markedly smaller than those of mammalian liver cells. Occasionally it can be difficult to distinguish β-particles from ribosomes. Normally, however, the glycogen particles stain more intensively with lead ions and are bigger than ribosomes.

Lipid inclusions

Lipid inclusions appear in many cells in the form of smaller or larger droplets, which are particularly big in the fat cells which are specialized in synthesizing and storing lipids. In ordinary preparations the fat has dissolved away leaving behind a clear vacuole. It can be fixed by osmic acid which prevents its dissolution in alcohol and the clearing agents which are used in the process of embedding the tissue. It can also be demonstrated in frozen sections stained with special fat stains, e.g. oil red O or Sudan black, which colour the fat droplet red or brown-black. In the electron microscope lipid droplets are either pale or to various degrees electron dense. The density reflects the number of unsaturated fatty acids which combine preferentially with osmic acid. The construction of fat droplets can be particularly well demonstrated in freeze-etched preparations. In these the lipid either forms randomly distributed crystals or concentric monomolecular layers of triglycerides. Occasionally fat is stored in the form of irregularly shaped bodies (Fig. 15). Fat globules are not surrounded by a unit membrane. A layer of microfilaments may occasionally occur at the surface.

Ordinarily monoglycerides and fatty acids are resorbed into cells where they are resynthesized to form triglycerides. Occasionally, however, also small droplets, being composed of triglycerides, can be incorporated into a cell. In resorbing intestinal epithelial cells the newly synthesized or the resorbed triglycerides can often be found in the membrane delimited cisternae of the ER and the Golgi apparatus. If much lipid is resorbed it can also be found in the cytoplasm often forming irregularly shaped bodies. After resorption and resynthesis in the intestinal epithelium the lipid material is extruded into the intercellular space between the epithelial cells, whence in tetrapods it is transported into the lymph vessels.

Crystalline inclusions

Crystalline inclusions have been known for a long time to be a typical constituent of certain cell types, e.g. of the cytoplasm of the Sertoli and the Leydigs cells in the testes of man, of the epidermal cells of *Branchiostoma* and of the liver cells of some canids, in which they lie in the nucleus. The electron microscope has shown that such crystals occur in many more cells (Fig. 15). They can occur in the nucleus, in mitochondria, in the ER, in the Golgi apparatus, in secretory granules and free in the cytoplasm. Usually they are thought to represent aggregated proteins, their significance normally is unknown.

Pigments

The colour of tissues and organs can be either due to exogenous material (exogenous pigments) taken into the body like carotenoids, dust particles, mineral salts and colour crystals artificially driven into the skin (tattoo marks) or to endogenous substances (endogenous pigments) generated inside the body from non-pigmented precursors.

Among the endogenous pigments various groups can be distinguished which usually are confined to a special cell type each, which in general are called chromatophores (chromocytes). Melanin is the brown pigment in skin, hairs, eyes, certain areas of the vertebrate brain, etc. In lower vertebrates it is even of a wider distribution and occurs in the serous linings of the body cavities and in the connective tissue of many other organs. Melanin is produced in the irregularly shaped melanocytes, which in vertebrates have their origin in the neural crest. The pigment is concentrated in ellipsoidal electron dense granules, the melanosomes, which arise in the Golgi apparatus. In early stages of its formation the melanosome is limited by a membrane and contains longitudinally oriented lamellae. In the course of maturation melanin is deposited upon these lamellae until it completely obscures the internal structure. In the epidermis of vertebrates melanosomes can be transferred from the melanocytes to epidermal epithelial cells (see p. 146).

Specializations of the cellular surface

The electron microscope has shown that the surface of numerous cell types possesses delicate finger-shaped processes which are called microvilli and the main function of which is to increase the surface area of the cell. At the free surface of resorbing cells (intestine, kidney, nephridia and others) the microvilli are of uniform length, stand erect and are in close parallel array. Together they form the striated or brush border which can also be seen in the light microscope in different groups of animals as a refractile apical border exhibiting vertical striations. The microvilli of such brush borders are of different height and of different diameter (Fig. 16). The cytoplasm in the interior of the microvilli contains a bundle of parallel microfilaments which extend to some extent into the apical cytoplasm of the cell where they usually are anchored in the terminal web, which consists of horizontally arranged filaments in the apical cytoplasm. The microvilli are covered by a fine filamentous coat which is rich in mucopolysaccharides. In the intestine the region of the microvilli contains numerous enzymes having a function in the resorption of food molecules (peptidases, disaccharases, alkaline phosphatase and others).

In contrast to the microvilli of such brush borders which are constant structures, those of other cells are of irregular number and height according to different physiological states of the cell. In the inactive epithelial cell of the thyroid gland they are e.g. low and rare, in the activated gland they in contrast are high and numerous.

Occasionally microvilli may be extremely long and in this case they normally lack the supporting internal filaments. In some

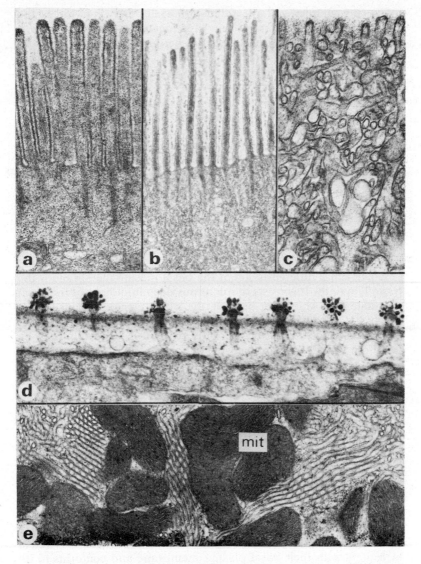

Figure 16. Surface specializations, **a-d:** microvilli; **a:** *Erinaceus* (hedgehog) intestinal epithelium, note the microfilaments in the core of the microvilli; **b:** *Podura* (Collembola) intestinal epithelium; **c:** *Buccinum* (prosobranch snail) surface epithelium of the osphradium; **d:** *Synchaeta* (Rotatoria) epidermis, due to oblique sectioning the basal parts of the microvilli are not to be seen, note extra-cellular material on and between the microvilli. a–d x 20 000. **e:** *Bryobia* (spider mite), tubular apical infoldings, mit: mitochondrium x 18 000

molluscs such microvilli are coiled with each other (Fig. 16); in the epididymal duct of mammals they glue together forming a long tuft on the cells. The individual processes here are as long as cilia and have also been called stereocilia (cilia that do not move). In other cells (sensory cells of the inner ear) plump and stout microvilli containing numerous microfilaments are also called stereocilia (Figs. 86, 91).

Sometimes microvilli are branched, e.g. on the surface of some developmental stages of trematodes and on the gill epithelium of crabs (Fig. 137). In cestodes they possess long pointed tips (Fig. 68), in other cells they are clavate or club-shaped (choroid plexus). In insects they frequently contain mitochondria (salivary glands, Malpighian tubules, Fig. 156). A specialization similar to the microvilli are thin apical folds of the plasmalemma which can be clearly distinguished from microvilli only in surface view. Such folds e.g. occur on the endothelial cells of the capillaries of the *pecten oculi* (Fig. 147) in the eye of birds and on special resorbing cells in the intestine of some insects.

A particular differentiation of the basal plasma membrane is the basal labyrinth. It consists of numerous deep infoldings of the basal plasmalemma which can pervade the whole cytoplasm and almost reach the apical surface. In close apposition to these infoldings elongated mitochondria occur. This type of specialization can be found in epithelial cells transporting ions and fluids; thus it is present (1) in various excretory and osmoregulatory organs like nephridia, kidneys, Malpighian tubules, salt glands of reptiles and birds; (2) in certain parts of the duct system of various salivary glands; (3) in most parts of the intestine of insects; (4) the *stria vascularis* of the vertebrate inner ear, etc.

The basal surface of epithelial cells usually rests upon an extra-cellular thin fibrous layer, which in the light microscope usually is termed basement membrane; it can be demonstrated particularly clearly by the PAS reaction. In the electron microscope this membrane was found to be of complex structure. Immediately below the epithelial cells a fine filamentous dense layer of 50-80 nm (500-800 Å) diameter occurs, which is termed the basement lamina or basal lamina. It is produced by the overlying epithelial cells and is in contact with their basal plasma membrane and conforms to its contours. However, in a space of 30-40 nm (300-400 Å) the density of this lamina is low and often only the deeper rather dense zone of the lamina is called the basal lamina (Fig. 28). Outside the basal lamina reticular fibres occur embedded in an amorphous ground substance. All these components contribute to the 'basement membrane' seen in a light microscope. The thickness of the individual components

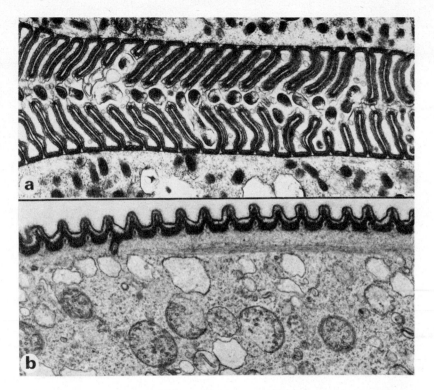

Figure 17. Surface of protozoans **a:** gregarine (*Lankesteria*) from the intestine of *Dendrodoa* (Ascidia); surface of two animals with densely arranged folds x 18 000. **b:** *Epistylis* (Ciliata) pellicula of the body exhibiting folds which run circularly around the animal. Under the plasmalemma a zone with electron dense material and layer of microfilaments x 18 000

mentioned varies considerably, e.g. at the inner surface of the vertebrate cornea the basal lamina can attain a height of 5 to 10 μm (Descemet's membrane).

Particular surface specializations can often be met within protozoans, in particular in ciliates (Fig. 17). In these animals below the plasma membrane often flattened membrane-delimited saccules occur which are called pellicular alveoles. Together with the plasma membrane they form the surface zone of the cell, the pellicula. Many flagellates and ciliates contain in their apical cytoplasm structures which are extruded when the animals are irritated (extrusomes). In some ciliates these are known as trichocysts, which are to be found over the whole surface of the animals. They consist of a shaft and an apical tip, which is surrounded by a cap. Extrusion is initiated by swelling of the proximal part. Within milli-seconds the length of the trichocysts extends about tenfold. The shaft transforms into a long cross-striated tube at the front of which the unchanged tip is located (Fig. 18). These organelles mainly serve to defend the animal. In some predacious holotrich ciliates so called toxicysts occur in the neighbourhood of the cytostome, which paralyse their prey. Of a simpler structure are the mucocysts which extrude mucous substances (Fig. 18).

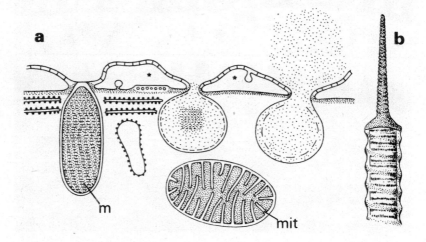

Figure 18. **a:** Pellicle and mucus cyst (m) of *Tetrahymena* (Ciliata), various stages of the extrusion of the mucus are shown from left to right. Below the plasma membrane, flattened membrane delimited vesicles (asterisks) or alveoli occur which are arranged in pairs around the base of each cilium. The outer vesicle membrane lies close to the cell membrane, often the two are interconnected by electron dense material; the inner vesicle membrane is underlain by a dense layer of cytoplasm (epiplasm), mit = mitochondrium. After TOKUYASU and SCHERBAUM, 1965. **b:** tip of extruded trichocyst of *Paramecium*

Specializations for cell attachment

Between neighbouring cells special areas of cell attachment are frequently formed. These are particularly well developed in epithelia but can also be found in other tissues. They help to maintain cell to cell cohesion and contribute to the structural integrity of the epithelia or other tissues.

In invertebrates and vertebrates the following types can be distinguished with the electron microscope:
1. The *macula adhaerens* (=desmosome), a bipartite plaque-like or

discoid structure consisting of local specializations of the opposing plasma membranes. The intercellular space is of normal dimensions (200Å) and can contain dense extracellular material which is thought to be a cementing substance. Though the plasma membranes are of normal dimensions, apposed to the inner aspect of the membrane is a thin layer of electron dense material making it appear to be thickened. Immediately below this membrane lies an electron-dense layer of fine filamentous material into which microfilaments from the cytoplasm normally converge. These form narrow loops in this dense layer and turn back into the cytoplasm. Desmosome-like formations at the basal part of an epithelial cell which do not face another cell are called half desmosomes (hemidesmosomes) since they actually consist only of one half of a normal desmosome.

2. The *zonula adhaerens*, the intercellular space again is of normal dimensions, but the plasma membranes are strengthened by moderately dense fine filamentous material. In contrast to the desmosome the *zonula adhaerens* forms a continuous band surrounding the whole cell.

3. The *zonula occludens* (tight junction), the cell membranes of the neighbouring cells converge and the outer leaflets of their unit membranes seem to fuse. The intercellular space becomes completely obliterated. No concentration of filamentous material occurs at the tight junctions. Since the zone extends around the whole cell this type of contact seals off the intercellular space of an organ or epithelium against a free surface. In respect of electrical conductivity they also offer low resistance connections.

The three types of cell attachment mentioned so far in many epithelia and in the mammalian heart muscle occur together forming a junctional complex, which in the light microscope appears to be a single structure: the terminal bar. The arrangement of the individual components normally is (from apical to basal): *zonula occludens, zonula adhaerens, macula adhaerens* (Figs. 19, 49).

4. The gap junctions are similar to tight junctions, the intercellular space, however, is not completely obliterated. Gap junctions and tight junctions between smooth muscle cells or endothelial cells often are called nexuses. In many tissues gap junctions have been found to correspond to a site of lowered intercellular ionic resistance (e.g. in vertebrate smooth muscle and myocardial cells, axons of crustaceans). The gap normally is 20–40Å wide; in freeze-etched preparations the gap junction extracellular surface displays a polygonal lattice of particles.

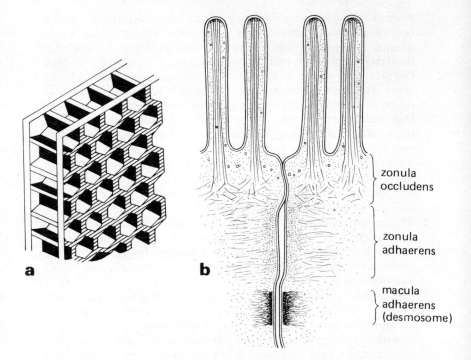

zonula
occludens

zonula
adhaerens

macula
adhaerens
(desmosome)

a   b

Figure 19. Fine structure of the junctional complex between epithelial cells **a:** comb desmosome. The membranes of two neighbouring cells (transparent) are interconnected by hexagonal structures. After DANILOVA, ROKHLENKO & BODRYAGINA 1969. **b:** junctional complex of two intestinal epithelial cells of a mammal. Plasma membrane: double line. After BLOOM & FAWCETT, 1968

The following types have been found only in invertebrates:

5. Septate desmosomes, the epithelial cells are interconnected by thin septa running perpendicularly between the neighbouring plasma membranes. The septa are highly probably differentiations of the intercellular space.

6. Honey comb desmosomes. The epithelial cells are interconnected by hexagonal structures which are presumably also composed of extracellular material (Fig. 19). It can be distinguished from the septate desmosome only in tangential sections.

7. In stenoglossan gastropods cell junctions have been described which superficially resemble septate desmosomes. Here the connecting septa consist of fused areas of the plasma membrane of the neighbouring epithelial cells.

Centrioles and cilia

Centrioles are cylindrical bodies of polar structure which usually occur in pairs (diplosome). The long axes of the individual centrioles, which often are 0.3–0.4 μm long, are normally perpendicular. The wall of each centriole is composed of nine groups of parallel and longitudinally arranged sub-units each of which consists of one to three microtubules, which are fused together (Fig. 21). In vertebrates usually three microtubules are to be found forming a so-called triplet. The typical orientation of the groups of microtubules can be seen in Fig. 21. Occasionally the centre of the centriole contains two additional tubules. One end of the centriole is open, the other is closed by a wheel-like structure. At their outsides centrioles often bear clubshaped appendages (satellites).

Centrioles are self duplicating bodies, which contain DNA and possibly also RNA. Replication occurs in many different modes at the closed pole of the centrioles. Centrioles also give rise to cilia and flagella, which originate at the open pole of the centrioles. The base of a typical cilium, the basal body (=basal corpuscle, kinetosome, blepharoplast) corresponds to the centriole which gave rise to a cilium. During cell division they are the centres for the organization of the spindle.

Centrioles often lie in a clear zone of cytoplasm near the nucleus and often partially surrounded by the Golgi apparatus: the centrosome.

Many varieties of centrioles exist, e.g. in the germinal cells of male neuropterans up to 8 μm long giant centrioles occur one end of which is covered by a balloon-like cap.

Cilia are long and usually motile cell processes. They are delimited by the plasma membrane. Their inner structure consists of longitudinally arranged systems of microtubules (often called fibrils).

That part of the cilium extending over the surface of the cell, the ciliary shaft, contains in its periphery nine pairs of fused microtubules (doublets) and in its centre two microtubules which are separated by a narrow interspace (9+2 pattern). The central tubules frequently terminate at the level of the cellular surface in a basal plate or an axial granule (axosome). The peripheral tubules extend without interruption into the basal body which corresponds to a transformed centriole in the apical cytoplasm. In most vertebrate cells at the transition between shaft and basal body a third microtubule appears so that the wall of the basal body consists of nine groups of three microtubules each (triplets). The triplets can be interconnected by filamentous material. They also can extend thin septa into the interior of the basal body where they terminate at a tubule-like structure.

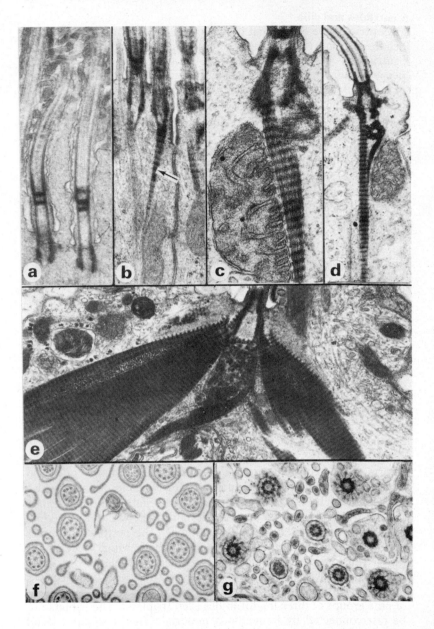

Figure 20—see legend opposite.

The walls of the microtubules in the ciliary shaft in general consist of about thirteen rows of globular protein molecules. The doublets of the ciliary periphery consist of two microtubules which share one part of their wall in common. In these double structures the protein molecules are arranged in about twenty-three rows. The protein, which is called tubulin, resembles the muscle protein actin. The arm-like processes at the peripheral doublets are quite striking (Figs. 20, 21). One tubule (the A-tubule) bears two rows of these processes, which point clockwise towards the next doublet, when the ciliary shaft is looked at from the base. These arms are absent in the extreme tip and base of the shaft. Each arm consists of one molecule of the protein dynein which, in common with the muscle protein myosin, has the ability in the presence of certain concentrations of bivalent cations such as calcium and magnesium to act as an ATP-splitting enzyme and to liberate energy from the ATP molecule. The other tubule without arms is called the B-tubule. Often between peripheral and central tubules nine so-called secondary filaments occur.

Deviations from the 9+2 pattern mainly occur in cilia of sensory cells (Chapter 4) and spermatozoa (Chapter 11).

Variously structured rootlets can be attached to the basal bodies. They consist of groups of filaments exhibiting a cross striation (Fig. 20).

If cilia occur singly at one cell they often are called flagella. Their length varies between 1 μm and about 2 mm. Their terminal part can be a thin thread-like appendix containing only the two central microtubules. The surface of the flagella of some flagellates bears - as that of the cilia of some rotifers - a thick coat of fine filamentous material. Flattened flagella can form undulating membranes, which, however, do not fuse with the cell body, but are interconnected with it by extracellular material. Flagella serving the attachment of some flagellates (haptonemata) differ in their fine structure from that of ordinary flagella. In their interior they possess variously arranged groups of microtubules; on the outside they are delimited by three unit membranes, the outer two of which correspond to a duplication of the cell envelope.

Figure 20. Fine structure of cilia in various invertebrates. a–e: longitudinal sections; f–g: cross-sections. **a:** *Pomatias* (prosobranch snail) sensory cell x 24 000; **b:** *Clithon* (prosobranch snail) sensory cell x 18 000; **c:** *Branchiostoma* (Acrania) endostyle x 40 000; **d:** *Lingula* (Brachiopoda) intestinal epithelial cell x 18 000; **e:** *Priapulus* (Priapulida), sensory cell x 18 000. Note differences in respect of structure of the basal body and rootlets (arrow) and the associated mitochondria (in c); in a) rootlets are absent. **f:** *Lycastis* (Polychaeta) sensory cell, the cilia are surrounded by a cuticular sheath x 18 000; **g:** *Lycastis* basal bodies, cut at various levels x 18 000

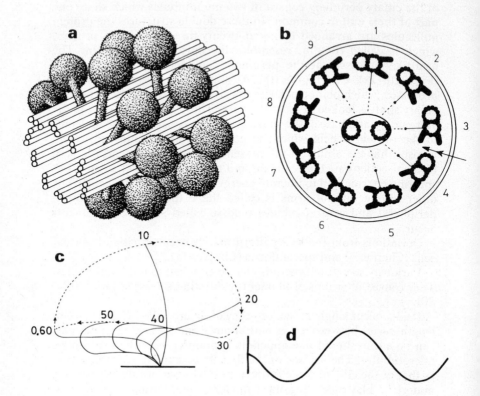

Figure 21. **a:** Fine structure of a centriole with two sets of satellites. After SCHNEIDER, 1973. **b:** Structure of a cilium as seen on a cross-section. Spherical tubulin molecules form the wall of the central and peripheral microtubules ('fibres'), large dynein molecules ('arms') extend from one of the peripheral tubules. In the planar ciliary beat the movement occurs in the plane of the vertical line at a right angle to the plane of the central microtubules. The double arrow indicates the site at which presumably cross-linkages are formed between the arms of doublet 3 and doublet 4. In the same way connections are formed between the other pairs of neighbouring doublets. **c:** A series of profiles showing an unspecialized example of a cycle of ciliary beating as viewed from the side (cilium on the gill of *Sabellaria*/Polychaeta). Numbers indicate the time in msec from the beginning of the effective stroke, during which the ciliary shaft moves from left to right and swings through a large arc. During the recovery stroke the bent cilium unrolls towards the left. **d:** Planar waves of a flagellum, amplitude and length of the wave frequently increase towards the tip. After SLEIGH, 1971

Several types of movement of cilia and flagella exist. Flagella move in an undulating manner. The movement may take place approximately in a single plane or the flagellum may move out of the plane to a greater or lesser extent, usually in helical form. Such movements are normally regular and symmetrical in a healthy flagellum and several complete waves of movement of the organelle may be seen within the length of the flagellar shaft. Helical or planar undulations may travel along the flagellar shaft in either direction, but the waves of movement originate at the flagellar base much more commonly than at the tip of the flagellum. Most flagella beat ten to forty times per second. The speed of the waves of movement is about 100-1000 μm per second.

The movement of cilia shows a rich diversity of patterns. Frequently the ciliary beat takes place more or less in a single plane and involves two phases, one in which the cilium moves towards one side while bending only in the basal region, and a second in which the region of bending is propagated up the ciliary shaft to the tip and returns the cilium to the starting position. The latter phase usually occupies much more than half of the beat cycle, and is referred to as the recovery stroke, while the rigid swing is referred to as the effective stroke in recognition of the fact that the movement of water achieved by this stroke is normally much greater than that in the recovery stroke. A simple 12 μm long cilium beats about thirty times per second with an angular velocity of about 12°/ms; the speed of the ciliary tip during the effective stroke is about 2.5 mm/s.

When a cilium moves it carries with it a surrounding layer of fluid, the extent of which depends on the viscosity of the fluid and the velocity of the cilium. Normally more water is propelled by the faster effective stroke than by the slower recovery stroke, so that a pulsed flow of water is caused from one side of the cilium towards the other. When two cilia lie close enough for their transported water layers to overlap, interference will occur between the movements of the two cilia, and the activity of the two cilia will probably become hydrodynamically linked. Such hydrodynamic linkage also accounts for the synchrony of beat seen in tufts of flagella and the co-ordination between the flagella of separate spermatozoa seen in packed suspensions. It is also assumed to be responsible for the waves of co-ordination of the flagella, which densely cover the body of the larger zooflagellates. Hydrodynamic linkage is also called viscous mechanical coupling.

The compound ciliary organelles of protozoa contain cilia, which are structurally separate but appear to beat as a single compound unit in life. The bases of the component cilia in cirri and membranelles lie so close together that there is tight viscous mechanical coupling between adjacent cilia, and the beat of all the units is normally synchronized. In ciliary undulating membranes the cilia are arranged in a long line; if a cilium at one end of the line beats, the motion of this cilium is coupled to the next and is passed to all members of the row in sequence, so that the cilia beat metachronally and waves of movement pass along the membrane. The patterns of metachronal co-ordination are diverse. The plane of the effective stroke of the beat is often at right angles to the row along which the metachronal waves pass (diaplectic metachronism, with dexioplectic pattern in which the beat is towards the right, and laeoplectic pattern in which the beat is towards the left). Rarely the metachronal waves of cilia pass over a field of cilia in the same direction as the effective stroke (symplectic metachronism) or in a direction opposite to the effective stroke (antiplectic metachronism). Usually the direction of the beat is fixed, but it can be altered, e.g. the flagellate *Opalina* and the ciliate *Paramecium* can change the direction of the ciliary beat. The co-ordination of beat direction depends upon membrane potential, depolarization of the membrane leading to reversed beating and hyperpolarization to enhanced forward beating. In many protozoans it has been demonstrated that neither the co-ordination of reversed beating nor ciliary-metachronism are dependent upon fibre systems associated with the ciliary bases. The significance of the rich innervation of ciliated epithelia is still unknown.

Particular macrocilia have been found in the comb jelly *Beroë*. They are about 60 μm long and 10 μm in diameter. Whereas the plasma membrane of a normal cilium encloses one typical set of 9+2 microtubules, in these macrocilia there are up to 3000 of such sets surrounded by a common unit membrane. The whole macrocilium beats like a normal cilium. Smaller but comparable cilia have been observed in tunicates and brachiopods.

In some ciliates so-called cirri or membranelles occur which consist of groups of cilia which are arranged in two to three rows. Their basal bodies are interconnected by filaments or electron dense material. Their shafts. however, exhibit no connecting structures.

In ctenophores thousands of uniformly oriented cilia are united to form the comb plates. The two central tubules of the individual cilia lie on a line perpendicular to the ciliary beat. The peripheral doublets lying on the same line are connected with the plasma-membrane by a band of electron dense material. The interconnection of the cilia, which can be observed in the living animal, has not yet been found to have a structural equivalent in the electron microscope.

A particular morphogenetic effect is exerted by the short ciliary shafts of peritrichs which extend into the extracellular space of the stalk. Material extruded from the cell is transformed in their vicinity into cross striated fibres extending through the complete stalk. If the stalk is contractile (*Vorticella, Zoothamnium*) in addition a cellular process extends into it; if it is not contractile (*Epistylis*) its complete cross-section is filled by such fibres.

LITERATURE

AFZELIUS, B. *Anatomy of the cell. Phoenix Science Series.* The University of Chicago Press, Chicago and London (1966), 127 pp.

BARDELE, CH. F. 'A microtubule model for ingestion and transport in the suctorian tentacle'. Z. Zellforsch. **126,** 116-134 (1972).

BIELKA, H. *Molekulare Biologie der Zelle.* G. Fischer Verlag. Jena, Stuttgart (1973). 725 pp.

DANILOVA, L. V., ROKHLENKO, K. D., BODRYAGINA, A. V. 'Electron microscopic study on the structure of septate and comb desmosomes.' Z. Zellforsch. **100,** 101-117 (1969).

DE DUVE, C., BAUDHUIN, P. 'Peroxisomes'. *Physiol. Rev.* **46,** 323-338 (1966).

DOUNCE, A. L., CHANDA, S. K., TOWNES, P. L. 'The structure of higher eukaryotic chromosomes.' *J. theor. Biol.* **42,** 275-285 (1973).

FARQUHAR, M. G., PALADE, G. E.: 'Cell junctions in Amphibian skin'. *J. Cell. Biol.* **26,** 263-291 (1965).

FOX, F. 'The structure of cell membranes.' *Scient. Am.* **226,** 2, 30-38 (1972).

FAWCETT, D. W. *An Atlas of fine structure: the cell.* W. B. Saunders Co., Philadelphia (1966), 448 pp.

FLOWER, N. E. 'Septate and gap junctions between the epithelial cells of an invertebrate, the mollusc *Cominella maculosa*'. *J. Ultrastruct. Res.* **37,** 259-268 (1971).

GRELL, K. G. *Protozoology.* Springer Verlag. Berlin, Heidelberg, New York (1973), 540 pp.

HIRSCH, G. C., RUSKA, H., SITTE, P. *Grundlagen der Cytologie.* G. Fischer Verlag. Jena, Stuttgart (1973). 790 pp.

HORRIDGE, G. A. 'Macrocilia with numerous shafts from the lips of the ctenophore Beroë'. *Proc. roy. Soc.* **B 162,** 351-364 (1965).

HUANG, A. H. C., BEEVERS, H. 'Localization of enzymes within microbodies.' *J. Cell Biol.* **58,** 379-389 (1973).

MUNN, E. A. *The structure of mitochondria.* Academic Press, London (1974). 465 pp.

NOVIKOFF, A., HOLTZMAN, E. *Cells and organelles.* Holt, Rinehart and Winston, Inc., New York, Chicago etc. 1970, 337 pp.

SLEIGH, M. A. *The biology of protozoa.* Edward Arnold, London (1973). 315 pp.

WISCHNITZER, S. 'The annulate lamellae. *Internat. review cytol.* G. H. Bourne and J. F. Danielli, ed. **27,** 65-100 (1970).

Chapter 2
TISSUES

Usually cells are assembled in coherent associations and interconnected by varying amounts of fibrous and amorphous intercellular substance to form tissues. There are only four basic types of
tissues: epithelium, connective tissue, muscular tissue and nervous
tissue. Cells of these basic tissues are in different ways combined to
form larger functional units which are termed organs. The
boundaries between the basic tissues are not always clear-cut, e.g. in
many epithelial cells of cnidarians, brachipods, bryozoans,
Branchiostoma and other invertebrates muscle-filaments occur (see
page 118). Connective tissue is also supporting tissue; however,
in many invertebrates products of epithelia, e.g. cuticles, have a
supporting function. Also muscle cells forming rod-shaped
structures, e.g. the notochord of *Branchiostoma,* or acting against
fluid-filled spaces (hydroskeleton), can exert a supporting function.

Epithelia
Closely aggregated cells with very little intercellular substances
constitute epithelia (Fig. 22). Very often they cover internal or
external surfaces, e.g. lining tubular structures of the body (blood
vessels, intestine, gonoducts, etc.) or forming the outer cover of the
body, the epidermis. Epithelial cells are frequently of a polar
organization and normally they are interconnected by prominent
junctional complexes. Blood vessels usually do not invade the
epithelia, and they generally rest upon a basement lamina. Because
of the relatively unprotected position, they are often rapidly worn
out, so epithelia usually contain embryonic replacement cells.
In invertebrates in particular there are exceptions to these
generalizations. In animals possessing intra-epithelial nervous
plexuses, the basal parts of epithelial cells may form slender
processes which are separated by wide intercellular spaces.
Occasionally in the basal parts of the epidermis the typical epithelial
cell aggregation can be completely dissolved: in this area processes
of nerve – glial – and epithelial cells freely intermingle (Fig. 23). A

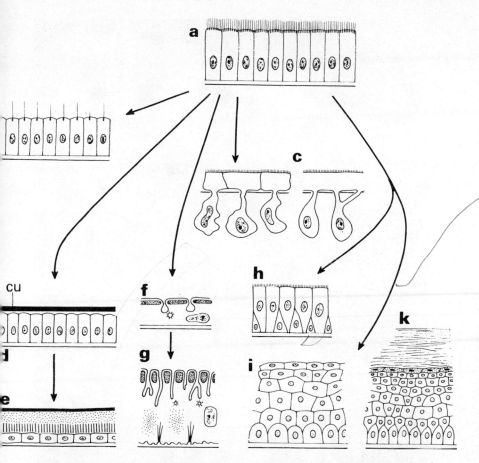

Figure 22. Different types of epithelia. **a:** simple prismatic ciliated epithelium; **b:** flagellated epithelium; **c:** submerged epithelium, cellular (left) and syncytial (right); **d,e:** epithelia with cuticle (cu); **d:** simple type; **e:** nematode; **f,g:** epithelia with intra-cellular armour (from electron microscope observations); **f:** rotifer; **g:** acanthocephala; **h:** pseudostratified epithelium; **i:** squamous stratified epithelium; **k:** cornified squamous epithelium. After REMANE, STORCH & WELSCH, 1974

basement lamina may be absent, even under the blood sinusoids of the liver of some mammals, In the enamel pulp of the developing teeth of mammals epithelial cells acquire a reticular appearance like that of connective tissue.

During ontogeny, cells may emigrate from sheet-like epithelia, forming special organs within the connective tissue. Thus in

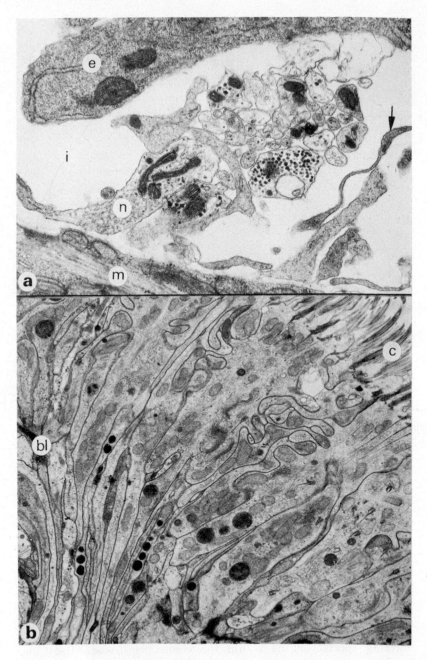

vertebrates the glands of the skin, the large glands of the intestine (pancreas, liver) and many endocrine glands consist of epithelial cells. The latter even lose their connection with the surface.

Epithelia are the first tissues formed during ontogeny. All three primary germ layers can produce epithelia. Those epithelia originating from the mesoderm, which line the coelomic cavities, are often called mesothelia or coelothelia. The linings of blood- and lymph-vessels, which are also of mesodermal origin, are usually called endothelia. Other epithelia of the mesoderm, e.g. in the kidney, have no special designation.

Epithelia have various functions. Often they exert a protective function by their superficial location and by secreting various substances. Epithelia often contain sensory cells or nerve endings. Further they are characterized by their ability to transport substances into or out of the body, thus many epithelia are specialized for absorption, secretion or excretion. Normally special functions depend on specially structured epithelia (Fig. 27): surface covering and protective epithelia are dealt with in Chapter 3, receptor cells in epithelia in Chapter 4, resorptive epithelia in Chapter 7, epithelia in excretory organs in Chapter 10.

Epithelia are classified and named according to the number of cell layers and the shape of the cells. One layer of cells constitutes a simple epithelium, two or more layers form stratified epithelia. The epithelial cells can be squamous, cuboidal or columnar (= prismatic) (Fig. 22). A single layer of flat cells forms a simple squamous epithelium. If there are several layers, it is the shape of the uppermost cells which is taken for the classification; e.g. a stratified columnar epithelium consists of several cell layers the uppermost of which is built up by columnar cells (the cells of the lower layers can be of different shape).

Simple squamous epithelia usually line blood and lymph vessels, coelomic cavities and alveoli of the lung. Simple cuboidal epithelia constitute large parts of the epidermis of amphioxus. Columnar epithelia can be found in the intestinal tract of almost all animals and in the epidermis of molluscs. If the epithelial cells bear apically cilia they are called ciliated squamous epithelial cells, ciliated columnar epithelial cell, etc., which together form e.g. a ciliated stratified columnar epithelium. If there is only one cilium per cell, such epithelia can be termed flagellate epithelia. Ciliated epithelia

Figure 23. Unusual types of epithelia. **a:** *Rhynchelmis* (Oligochaeta) epidermis; basal part of the epidermis contains bundles of nerve fibres (n), surrounded by wide intercellular spaces (i), arrow points to slender process of an epidermal cell (e); m: muscle cell x 18 000; **b:** *Lineus* (nemerteans) epidermis of the frontal head region, ciliated extensions of receptor neurons form an uninterrupted epithelium-like formation; (c) cilia; (bl) basal lamina, perforated by the receptor neurons x 6000

occur in most groups of animals, but are absent in nematodes and insects. Flagellate epithelia have been described from the intestine of echinoderms, amphioxus and brachiopods. In gnathostomulids the epidermis is a flagellate epithelium.

Simple epithelia are characteristic of invertebrates, stratified epithelia mainly occur at the body surface of vertebrates.

A special case of simple epithelium is the pseudostratified epithelium. Here the nuclei occur in two or more levels so that the epithelium appears to be stratified. However, close examination shows that all cells are in connection with the basement lamina.

In stratified epithelia the superficial cells can accumulate in their cytoplasm the fibrous protein keratin and change into dead scale-like structures without nucleus and organelles. These dead cells form the uppermost layer of these epithelia – called keratinized stratified squamous epithelia – which above all occur in the epidermis of land-living vertebrates. Unkeratinized stratified squamous epithelia constitute e.g. the epidermis of fishes, line the oral cavity and the oesophagus of many tetrapods, the vagina of many mammals, and the cornea of most mammals. The epidermis of Amphibia exhibits traits intermediate between keratinized and unkeratinized stratified epithelia, in so far as the superficial cells accumulate keratin but normally retain their nuclei.

The inner aspect of the nictitating membrane of many reptiles and birds is lined by a so-called feather epithelium (Fig. 24): the uppermost cells possess a feather-shaped cornified process which cleans the cornea. Such epithelia are particularly well developed in birds which take up their food on the ground, which may be dusty, e.g. pigeons and pheasants; it is absent or poorly developed in water birds and in many birds of prey.

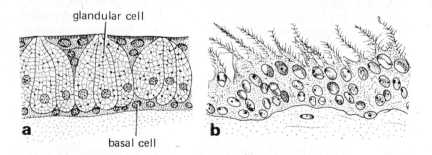

Figure 24. **a:** Endoepithelial groups of glandular cells in the epithelium of the pharynx of ammocoetes larvae. The basal cells correspond to replacement cells. After SCHAFFER, 1895. **b:** feathered epithelium at the inner aspect of nictitating membrane of a pigeon. After KOLMER, 1924

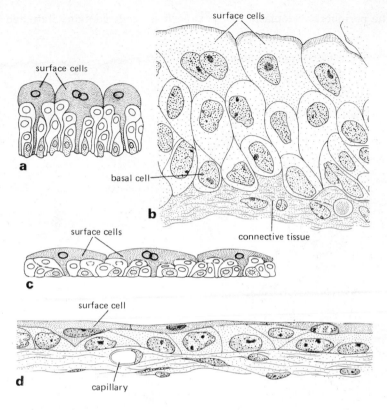

Figure 25. Transitory epithelium of the urinary bladder. **a,b:** empty bladder; **a:** schematic representation of the epithelial structure; **b:** light microscopical preparation (mouse); **c,d:** distended bladder; **c:** schematic drawing; **d:** typical light microscope preparation. a,c: after LEONHARDT, 1974; b,d: after SCHAFFER, 1927

The epithelia of the urinary tract of mammals have for long been thought to be stratified. Studies with the electron microscope have shown that it is pseudostratified (Fig. 25). It is called transitional epithelium, and can adapt to the varying extensions of the urinary bladder and the ureter. The lower cells are generally more or less cuboidal, the apical cells are relatively large, polyploid and often contain two nuclei (Fig. 25). They are of the shape of a mushroom covering the underlying cells and produce a mucoid protective substance. The electron microscope has shown that the cells of the transitory epithelium exhibit numerous specializations which presumably are adaptations towards the varying distensions of the bladder and ureter. The free surface shows numerous indentations, the peripheral cytoplasm of the superficial cells contains flattened

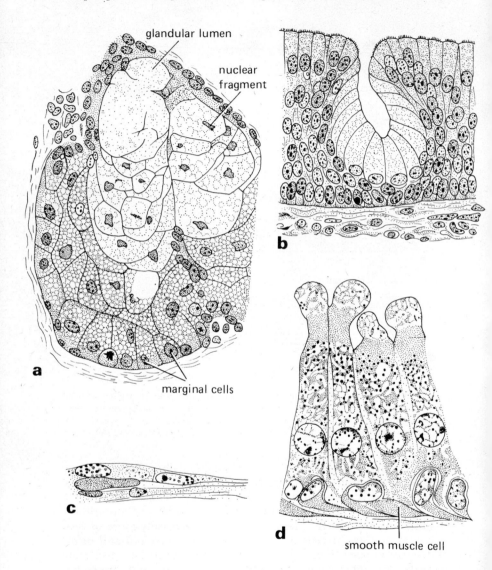

Figure 26.   **a:** Sebaceous gland of a bat; **b:** group of mucous cells in the epithelium of the epiglottis, man; c,d; different functional phases of the epithelium of odoriferous glands (man); **c:** flattened non-secreting cell; **d:** mature secretory cell with apical protrusions. The smooth muscle cells lie between the bases of the glandular cells; a,b, after PATZELT, 1923; c,d, after SCHAFFER, 1927

vesicles, the membrane of which is as thick as the plasma membrane. They may be structures in which surface membrane is stored and which may be mobilized if the bladder is distended and the epithelium becomes stretched out.

Special types of epithelia are (1) submerged or sunken epithelium (Figs. 22, 68): the pericarya, i.e. those parts of the cells containing the nucleus and the majority of cell organelles, are submerged into the underlying connective tissue but are interconnected with the apical strands of cytoplasm by thin cytoplasmic bridges; (2) epithelio-muscular cells (Figs. 64, 65): basal processes of epithelial cells contain myofilaments (in vertebrates the term myoepithelial cells often is inappropriately used for smooth muscle cells within exocrine glands); (3) syncytia: the plasma membranes running vertically in

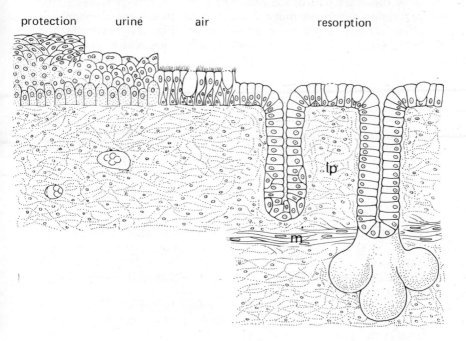

protection   urine   air   resorption

Figure 27. Different types of mucous membranes in vertebrates, serving different functions. From left to right: mucous membrane with squamous stratified epithelium, protective functions; with transitory epithelium (urinary passages); with respiratory epithelium, mucous and ciliated cells, air conducting passages, with simple columnar epithelium and tubular (left) and alveolar (right) gland (gastro-intestinal tract). In the gastrointestinal tract the mucous membrane usually is delimited against the underlying connective tissue by a layer of smooth muscle cells (m). The *lamina propria* (lp) among others contains numerous small blood vessels and free cells. After BRAUS & ELZE, 1956

relation to the epithelial surface and separating neighbouring cells disappear, thus giving rise to large masses of cytoplasm containing numerous nuclei.

Two types of secretory epithelial cells (= glandular cells) are to be distinguished, exocrine and endocrine cells. The first deliver their product to the free surface of the epithelia, the latter deliver it into the blood stream.

Exocrine cells frequently occur in columnar epithelia of numerous organs. According to their histological structure two types of secretory cells are often distinguished: mucous cells and serous cells. Mucous cells contain a basally located, flattened, relatively dark nucleus and (in routine stains) a pale, often foamy cytoplasm. Serous cells contain a roundish relatively light nucleus in the middle or in the lower half of the cell. The basal cytoplasm is basophilic containing numerous rough ER cisternae; in the apical cytoplasm often distinct secretory granules occur. Fig. 11 illustrates the formation of the secretory product, a process which basically is similar in the two cell types. Fig. 28 shows a typical serous cell, Fig. 77 various mucous cells.

Originally it was thought that these two cell types also produce fundamentally different types of secretions: the mucous cells (= mucocytes) a viscous mucous substance, the serous cells (= serocytes) a clear watery fluid rich in enzymes. Although this correlation is true in some exocrine glands of mammals, there are so many exceptions and transitory types of secretory cells that the distinction of serous and mucous cells now appears to be meaningful only on the morphological level. In the epidermis of soft skinned invertebrates frequently all glandular cells are called mucus cells, regardless of their structure and chemical composition of their products, which can fulfil numerous tasks: protection against desiccation in land-living turbellarians, nemertines, annelids, gastropods, etc. supplying the material for the construction of the tubes the animals live in, serving the transport of food particles, the formation of cocoons, etc.

It is also difficult to classify according to the above-mentioned scheme (mucous-serous), the numerous secretory cells of arthropods producing protective and defensive substances: e.g. chinones (Opilionida, Chilopoda, Coleoptera, Isoptera), phenols (Chilopoda, Coleoptera), aldehydes (Chilopoda, Coleoptera, Hemiptera), carbonic acids (Uropygi, Coleoptera, Lepidoptera, formicids), steroids (Coleoptera) etc.

Exceptionally the surface of exocrine cells can exhibit deep finger-shaped invaginations lined by microvilli, e.g. in the parietal cells of the mammalian stomach (Fig. 129). Exocrine glandular cells can occur individually in epithelia (= unicellular glands) or they can form groups which are called multicellular glands or simply 'glands'.

Unicellular glands are for example the mucus-producing goblet cells of the vertebrate intestinal tract (Fig. 128) or mucous cells in the epidermis of many worms and molluscs. The lower parts of such cells can be submerged into the underlying connective tissue and reach the epithelial surface only by a thin neck-like process (many turbellarians, nemertines, annelids and molluscs). Multicellular glands are of different complexity and structure. In their simplest form they correspond to a certain section within an epithelium producing secretory substance. Such glandular formations occur on the feeding tentacles of polychaetes or constitute the surface epithelium of the mammalian stomach and at certain stages the uterus epithelium of the higher primates. Fig. 24 shows such groups of exocrine cells in the pharyngeal area of *Petromyzon*. They are called intraepithelial glands if they form small bud-like groups which can be arranged around a small lumen of their own.

All other multicellular exocrine glands correspond to tubular invaginations extending into the underlying connective tissue. In this location they can be termed exoepithelial glands. Usually the glandular cells are confined to the secretory or terminal portions of the invagination, consisting of serous, mucous or other cells which must be classified by their own characteristics. If both serous and mucous cells occur within one gland, it is called a mixed gland. The secretory product normally reaches the surface through an excretory duct, generally consisting of less specialized cells.

Simple exocrine glands consist of a secretory unit connected to the surface directly or by an unbranched duct. Two subgroups exist: tubular (the terminal portion is of tubular shape) and acinar (= alveolar, the terminal portion forms a spherical or sac-like structure) glands, which can be straight, coiled, etc.

Compound exocrine glands possess repeatedly branched ducts and can have acinar, tubular or both types of terminal portions. Fig. 29 illustrates a compound gland of mammals.

A few examples will illustrate this classification. Simple tubular glands are e.g. the intestinal glands (crypts) of Lieberkühn of higher vertebrates, simple coiled tubular glands are the sweat glands of man. Compound tubular glands are the glands of Brunner in many mammals; to the category of the compound tubulo-alveolar glands belong the salivary glands of mammals; the mammary gland is a compound tubulo-alveolar gland. Among the countless exocrine glands of invertebrates are: defensive, salivary, midgut, genital, silk-spinning, and the odoriferous glands.

Glandular cells absorb substances from the blood stream which

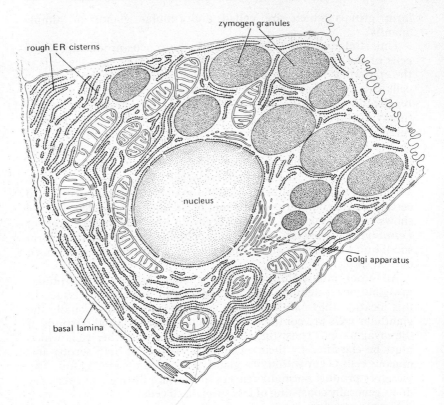

Figure 28.   Fine structure of a principal cell from a mammalian stomachal gland (fundus). Example for a typical protein producing cell. Note abundant rough ER, Golgi apparatus and secretory granules, here termed zymogen granules, containing precursors of the enzyme pepsin. After BLOOM & FAWCETT, 1970

are transformed to secretory products and extruded at the apical pole of the cytoplasm. Three different types of the process of extrusion can be distinguished:

1. Merocrine (= eccrine) extrusion. The glandular cells extrude only the contents of their secretory granules; there is apparently no loss of membranes (Fig. 28); for example, exocrine pancreas of vertebrates.
2. Apocrine extrusion. Part of the apical cytoplasm is lost in the process of the delivery of the secretory product. Frequently a number of secretory granules accumulate apically which then together with apical cytoplasm and membranes are pinched off. After the extrusion the height of the cell has markedly decreased.

Examples: odoriferous glands of mammals (Fig. 26), intestine of some insects, mucus glands of *Peripatus*.
3. Holocrine extrusion. The complete cell becomes filled with secretion granules and as a whole is extruded from the epithelium, examples are the sebaceous glands of mammals (Fig. 26) and facial glands of some bats.

Occasionally, different products of one cell may be extruded by a different mechanism, e.g. in the mammary gland the protein is extruded by merocrine, the lipid by the apocrine mechanism.

The term secretion is used in different ways. Here it includes both the intracellular formation of the secretory product and its extrusion.

Many glands, in particular those associated with sexual reproductive activities, exhibit a sexual dimorphism. Among those glands not immediately connected with the functions just mentioned, the lacrimal gland exhibits sexual dimorphism. In female rats it possesses small acini with a narrow lumen and vacuolated pigment containing glandular cells, in male rats the gland consists of big acini with a wide lumen and glandular cells with a marked polymorphism of the nuclei and particular Golgi areas.

Endocrine cells and glands are of diverse structure. The cells often form clusters or cords surrounded by blood capillaries (Fig. 114), occasionally they form follicles (Fig. 112). A primitive location is that of individual endocrine cells within a columnar epithelium (comparable to the unicellular exocrine glands). Such isolated endocrine cells occur in the intestinal tract of tunicates, amphioxus, vertebrates and presumably also in insects and other animals. Chapter 6 gives a short description of the main endocrine glands.

Polypeptide-, protein- or glycoprotein-producing endocrine cells possess a fine structure which is comparable to that of exocrine cells (well developed rough ER and Golgi apparatus, secretory granules). Those endocrine cells producing steroid hormones often contain many lipid droplets, smooth ER and tubular mitochondria.

Connective tissue
Connective tissue consists of fixed and wandering cells, which are embedded in a voluminous extracellular space containing an amorphous ground substance and different types of fibres. Vertebrates possess a particularly well developed connective tissue. Since our knowledge about the connective tissue of invertebrates and also of lower vertebrates is still imperfect, many of the following generalizations are based on findings in mammals, and also here exceptions exist as well as transitory types between the sub-groups

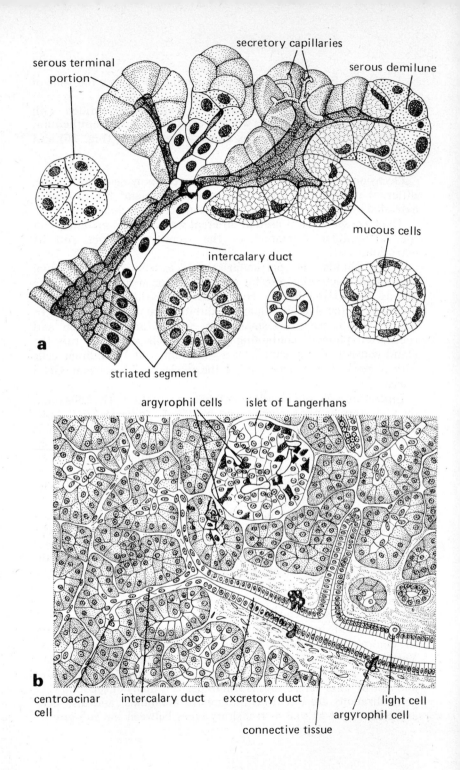

serous terminal portion

secretory capillaries

serous demilune

mucous cells

intercalary duct

striated segment

a

argyrophil cells

islet of Langerhans

centroacinar cell

intercalary duct

excretory duct

connective tissue

light cell

argyrophil cell

b

of this tissue as listed below.

Loose connective tissue
1. Extracellular components
   This type of connective tissue contains loosely woven fibrils
without a preferred orientation. The space occupied by the ground
substances is rather large and can vary according to its contents of
tissue fluid. The fibres are responsible for its tensile strength and
resilience, the ground substance is the medium between cells and
blood through which nutrients and wastes must pass.
   Three types of fibres are to be distinguished:

A. Collagenous fibres (Figs. 30, 32, 36). These fibres can be
   demonstrated clearly even· in routine light microscopic preparations, e.g. in the Azan and Goldner and also in haema-
   toxylin/eosin stain. They are usually randomly distributed and
   tend to have a slightly wavy course, if the tissue is not under
   tension. The electron-microscope shows that they are composed
   of individual fibrils 20-100 nm (200-1000 Å) in diameter and of
   indefinite length. These fibrils are cross-striated, i.e. they
   demonstrate along their lengths repeating structural units.
   Ordinarily a 64 nm (640 Å) periodicity can be found; by special
   staining procedures additional bands can be detected. The
   periodicity is probably due to the arrangement of tropocollagen
   molecules constituting the fibril. The tropocollagen consists of
   three helical polypeptide chains, which are coiled around each
   other. They contain two aminoacids otherwise rarely found in
   organisms: hydroxyproline and hydroxylysine. Collagen-fibrils
   under certain conditions can induce the formation of hydroxyapatite crystals, a property which is important for the calcification of the bone and tooth matrix. Collagen fibres are flexible but
   hardly extensible, they can be denatured by boiling yielding
   gelatin.
B. Reticular fibres. These fibres usually form fine networks, which
   appear early during ontogenesis and which later on often are
   replaced by collagen fibres. In adult organisms they occur rather

Figure 29. **a:** Schematic drawing of an exocrine gland (human salivary gland).
Formation of secretory product occurs in the serous terminal portion (end piece,
secretory units) and in the mucous cells of the intercalary duct. The serous demilunes
(crescents) correspond to serous terminal portions pushed apart by mucous cells.
Between the glandular cells widened intercellular spaces occur ('secretory
capillaries'). In the striated segments of the ducts, the basal parts of the cells show a
parallel striation, which is attributable to vertically arranged mitochondria and
infoldings of the basal plasma membrane. After VIERLING, BRAUS & ELIZE, 1956. **b:**
exocrine and endocrine pancreas (mammal) After FERNER, 1952

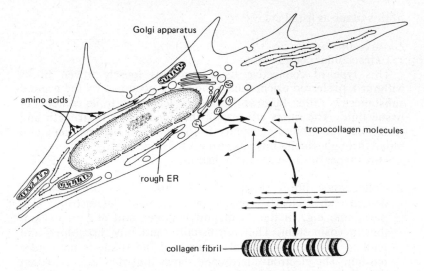

Figure 30. Schematic representation of the formation of a collagen fibril. Aminoacids are interconnected to polypeptides in the ribosomes of the fibroblast rough ER. The polypeptides are transported to the Golgi apparatus and extruded in the form of tropocollagen molecules into the extracellular space, where they polymerize to collagen fibrils. After BLOOM & FAWCETT, 1970

plentifully, e.g. in lymphatic organs (Fig. 142), around fat and muscle cells, in the *lamina propria* of the digestive tract, in the liver, etc. In the light microscope they may best be demonstrated by silver methods. In the electron microscope they closely resemble collagen fibres (with the same periodicity and chemical composition). Thus they appear to be just particularly delicate collagen fibres confined to certain organs.

C. Elastic fibres. This type of fibre is usually not plentiful in the loose connective tissue where it forms a wide meshed network. The fibres stretch easily and when released return to their original length. They can be demonstrated in the light microscope by special stains, e.g. by resorcin - fuchsin. The fibres are composed of the protein elastin, which does not only form fibres but in blood vessels also fenestrated membranes (e.g. the *elastica interna*). In the electron microscope elastic fibres appear rather homogeneous and are of low contrast (Fig. 148).

The ground substance normally is invisible in histological preparations. It mainly contains mucopolysaccharides, ions and water. The commonest mucopolysaccharides are hyaluronate and

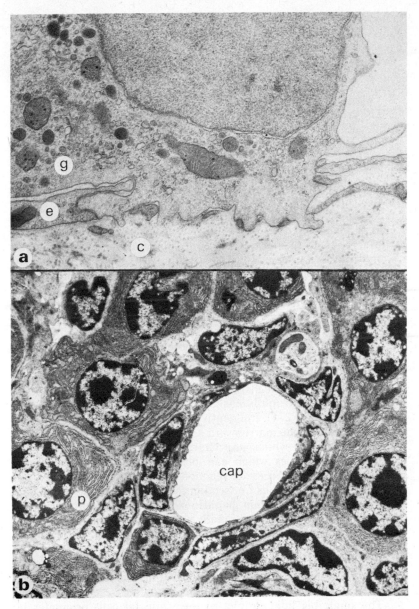

Figure 31. Free cells. **a:** Granulocyte (g) of *Rana*, penetrating the epithelium (e) of a venule and emigrating into the connective tissue (c), x 15 000; **b:** plasma cells (p) surrounding a blood capillary (cap) in the connective tissue of the testis of a sparrow (*Passer*) x 6000

chondroitin sulphates. Hyaluronate is of a high viscosity in aqueous solution, it exerts a certain supportive function, and hinders the spread of bacteria, which however can possess the enzyme hyaluronidase which depolymerizes the hyaluronate.

2. Cellular components

The majority of fibres are produced by one cell type, the fibroblast (Fig. 30). In the case of collagen they extrude tropocollagen molecules into the intercellular space where they polymerize to form the fibril. The shape of the fibroblasts varies according to their synthetic activities. They are usually spindle-shaped possessing long peripheral processes, occasionally they are star-shaped. In the light microscope often only the elliptical nucleus can be clearly recognized, especially in quiescent cells. The basophilia of active cells in due to well developed rough ER cisternae.

Macrophages (histiocytes) are large polymorphic cells which can wander and are characterized particularly by their ability to phagocytize foreign particles (e.g. bacteria) or cellular debris. Since they also ingest dye particles injected into an animal, they can be advantageously visualized by such a procedure. Their high contents of lysosomal enzymes clearly distinguishes them in histochemical preparations for acid phosphatase, β-glucosaminidase and other enzymes. The macrophages of the loose connective tissue normally represent transformed monocytes; in the reticular connective tissue (see below) also the reticular cells are called macrophages.

Often white blood cells can be found in the connective tissue (lymphocytes, neutrophils, eosinophils) (see page 282). Also plasma cells (Fig. 31 page 275), frequently occur in this situation. Mast cells originate in the bone marrow and are relatively large cells of various shapes (Fig. 32) which are characterized by their rather big cytoplasmic granules which can be stained by various methods (especially by metachromatic reactions, thus they also stand out in Richardson preparations i.e. sections stained in tolidine blue). The granules generally contain heparin and histamine and, in some mammals (mouse, rat) additionally serotonin. The fine structure of these granules varies in different vertebrate species. Occasionally they contain two nuclei.

Fat cells. In mammals unilocular (one big lipid inclusion, white fat) and plurilocular (numerous smaller lipid inclusions, brown fat) fat cells can be distinguished (Fig. 33).

The single big lipid droplet of the white fat cells originates by fusion of several smaller ones. It fills most of the cell, and the cytoplasm is confined to a narrow peripheral rim. In ordinary light microscopical preparations the fat droplet has been dissolved during

erythrocytes   elastic fibres
capillary   mast cell   collagen fibres

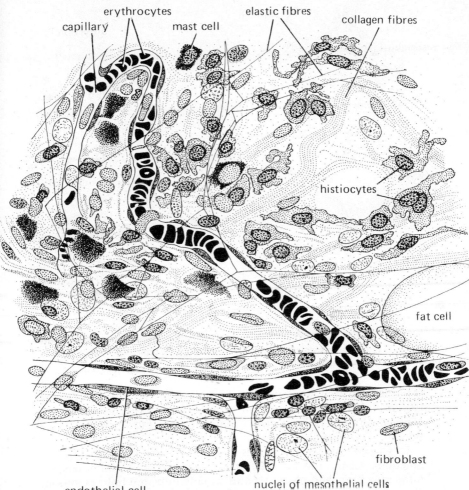

histiocytes

fat cell

fibroblast

endothelial cell   nuclei of mesothelial cells

Figure 32. Surface of a stretched piece of mesenterium (man), loose connective tissue with elastic and collagen fibres, fibroblasts, mast cells, histiocytes and blood vessels. Mesothelial cells form the surface of the mesenterium. After MAXIMOW, 1927

the embedding process, thus the cells appear to contain a huge vacuole. The cells of the brown fat apart from their relatively small lipid droplets contain crowds of mitochondria, the cytochromes of which are thought to be responsible for the brown colour of this type of fat. Brown fat occurs in embryos and young animals; in adults it

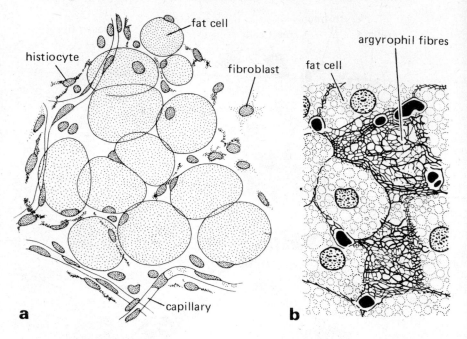

Figure 33. Mammalian fat cells. **a:** group of white fat cells in the loose connective tissue of the rabbit mesentery, after MAXIMOW, 1927; **b:** brown fat cells, argyrophil fibres = reticular fibres, after SINGH: 1970

is particularly well developed in hibernating species, above all in the region of the shoulder girdle, in which it is an important source of energy. Brown fat is richly supplied by blood vessels and sympathetic nerve fibres.

In various groups of animals particular fat organs of different functions occur. The fat cells of the amphibian fat body possess numerous branched processes and usually only one lipid inclusion. They are not surrounded by a basement lamina as are the cells of the white and brown fat in mammals. In starving animals the cells are of roundish shape. In some amphibians these fat cells have been shown to synthesize steroid hormones.

The fat body (*corpus adiposum*) of insects is usually located in the abdomen, but may extend into thorax and head. Ontogenetically it arises from ventral parts of the coelomic epithelium. Originally it is of metameric arrangement. Later it is mainly to be found around the intestine and the ventral nerve cord and under the epidermis, or it is loosely distributed in the abdominal cavity. Normally the fat body is composed of small lobules which are bathed within the haemolymph

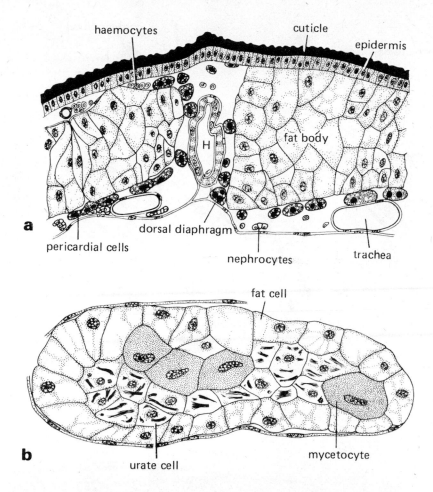

Figure 34. Fat body of insects. **a:** cross-section through the dorsal thorax of the stick insect *Carausius*, H: heart lined by a thin fibrous layer ('endocardium'). The sessile pericardial cells lie in groups or individually around the heart. They are characterized in the light microscope by vacuoles and granules; often they contain several nuclei. Since they are able to take up substances from the haemolymph (proteins, colour particles) they are considered to be phagocytizing elements. Presumably they also produce a heart accelerating factor. In the electron microscope these cells are characterized by numerous infoldings of the plasma membrane and peripheral spined vesicles. The whole cell is surrounded by a basement lamina. Nephrocytes are also sessile cells, which take up substances. **b:** lobule of the fat body of *Blaberus.* Three cell types occur: uni- and plurivacuolar fat cells, mycetocytes containing symbyontic microorganisms, and urate cells containing excretory products. After SEIFERT, 1970

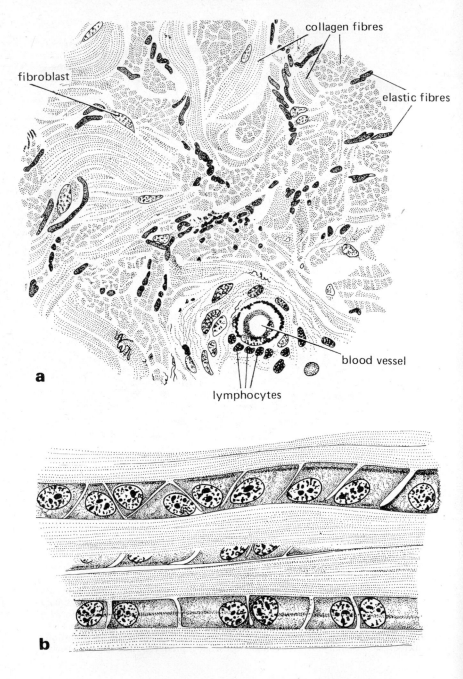

(Fig. 34). In many insects it contains three cell types: uni- and plurilocular fat cells which are interconnected by intermediate cells, mycetocytes, containing symbionts and urate cells which are filled with excretory products. The fat cells normally also contain considerable amounts of glycogen. The mycetocytes also contain lipid droplets and glycogen, their symbionts produce vitamins and occasionally are able to degrade excretions containing uric acid for their own protein synthesis.

The principal function of the insect fat body is the storage of lipids, glycogen and probably also of proteins. It is a centre of many metabolic pathways and in some respects resembles the liver of the vertebrates. Some of its cells have an excretory function, in collembolans these can replace the Malpighian tubules. The urate cells accumulate the majority of uric acid produced by these animals.

In some insects the fat body is transformed into a luminescent organ.

Dense connective tissue

In this type of connective tissue the fibrous components clearly predominate over the cellular components. The fibres, usually collagen fibres, are either of irregular arrangement (Fig. 35), e.g. in the capsules of many organs, or oriented in one direction, e.g. in tendons, ligaments, fasciae, etc. (Fig. 35). In tendons the fibroblasts form long rows of cells, which extend lamellar processes between the bundles of collagen fibrils. In the cornea of vertebrates and under the epidermis of many lower vertebrates and of amphioxus the collagen fibrils form layers in each of which the direction of the fibrils changes by 90 degrees (Fig. 36).

Cartilage and bone (structured connective tissue)

Both bone and cartilage are other types of connective tissue and consist of cells, fibres and ground substance; their distinguishing feature is that their ground substances either are calcified (bone) or transformed into an elastic, relatively stiff, homogeneous mass (cartilage). Both tissues provide internal support for the body. Cartilage grows by interstitial deposition of new material, bone by apposition of new material on its surface. The ground substance (matrix) always contains collagen fibres.

Figure 35. **a:** dense connective tissue in which the collagen fibres are of random distribution (human skin). Between the bundles of collagen fibres, elastic fibres occur. **b:** tendon in the tail of a rat, example for a dense connective tissue with an ordered arrangement of the collagen fibres between which rows of fibroblasts occur. After MAXIMOW, 1927

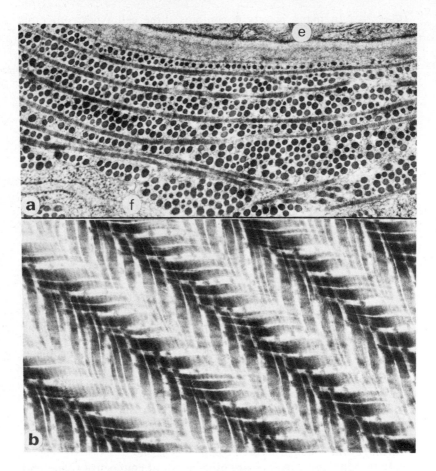

Figure 36. Regularly arranged collagen fibrils under the epidermis, **a:** *Clarias* (cat fish); e: epidermis, f: part of a fibroblast x 30 000. **b:** *Branchiostoma*, oblique section x 30 000

Cartilage

In cartilage the specific cells, the chondrocytes, are embedded into an extensive extracellular matrix (Fig. 37). Since cartilage normally does not contain blood vessels and nerves, the colloidal properties of the matrix are important for the nourishment of the chondrocytes which are lodged in small cavities in the matrix. The matrix is composed of chondromucoproteins, the sulphate groups of which are responsible for the basophilia. Immediately around the

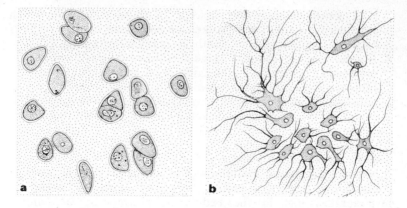

Figure 37.   **a:** Hyaline cartilage from the femoral caput of a frog; **b:** orbital cartilage of the cuttlefish (*Sepia*). After SCHAFFER, 1927

chondrocytes the matrix stains particularly deeply. This area is called capsular or territorial matrix, while the less stainable matrix between the cells is termed interterritorial matrix. In fishes, e.g. sharks, the matrix may contain calcium salts. In the light micro-scope the chondrocytes are elliptical or roundish elements which frequently form small groups (Fig. 37). Each member of the group is derived from a single chondrocyte. In the electron microscope the surface of the chondrocytes is highly irregular. The cytoplasm contains a well developed Golgi apparatus, numerous mitochondria, and an extensive system of rough ER cisternae. Typical inclusions are small lipid droplets and glycogen particles. The periphery contains numerous pinocytotic vesicles. In active cells the rough ER and Golgi apparatus increase in size. The Golgi apparatus produces vacuoles which discharge their contents into the matrix. The chondrocytes synthesize both ground substance and fibrils (Fig. 38).

The tissue surrounding a piece of cartilage is called the perichondrium. It is a transitory zone between cartilage and the dense connective tissue in the neighbourhood.

Three kinds of cartilage can be distinguished in vertebrates on the basis of the amount of matrix and the frequency of fibrils embedded in it.

A. Hyaline cartilage is of particularly wide distribution. In the periphery of a piece of cartilage the chondrocytes are flattened, in the interior roundish or partly angular. In the epiphyseal plates of long bones the chondrocytes form long columns. Hyaline cartilage plays an important role in prenatal life, in adults it is of restricted occurrence, except for those vertebrates which secondarily as adults have a skeleton composed in large parts of cartilage (lampreys, chondrichthyes, many teleosts, etc.).

B. Elastic cartilage contains large quantities of elastic fibres. In mammals it occurs e.g. in the external ear and the epiglottis.

C. Fibrocartilage contains predominantly collagen fibres; ground substance and chondrocytes are relatively rare. It can e.g. be found in the mammalian invertebral disk and at the site of attachment of some tendons to bones.

In fishes and amphibians and during ontogenesis also in higher vertebrates cartilage containing numerous densely packed vesicular chondrocytes occurs. Similar forms of cartilage occur in invertebrates, e.g. in the radula of gastropods. In *Lingula* (brachiopods) a cartilaginous tissue occurs in the lophophore resembling hyaline cartilage with groups of chondrocytes widely separated by matrix (Fig. 38).

Cephalopods have a special type of cartilage. The chondrocytes possess long and branched processes, which, similar to those of the bone cells of vertebrates, are in contact with the processes of neighbouring cells (Fig. 37).

Branchiostoma contains in the pharyngeal bars and in other places an acellular supporting tissue with the mechanical properties of cartilage. In the electron microscope it consists of homogeneous dense masses of fine particulate material and collagen fibrils.

Bone

Bone is a type of connective tissue, which is confined to the vertebrates.

In comparison with cartilage the main differences are: the matrix contains apatite crystals which are responsible for the firmness of bone. The individual bone cells (osteocytes) are in connection with each other by means of long processes, thus the matrix contains countless narrow canaliculi which house these processes; the cell body is lodged in small lacunae. Bone generally is pervaded by blood vessels. No bone cell is further than a fraction of a millimetre away from a capillary.

Because of its hardness its microscopical study requires special techniques: it is either decalcified before the normal embedding and cutting process, or thin-ground sections, which can also be made from fossil material, are investigated.

The organic parts of the matrix consist of typical collagen fibrils and protein-polysaccharides. The fibrils are regularly arranged ensuring a maximal strength of the bone, e.g. in the lamellae of

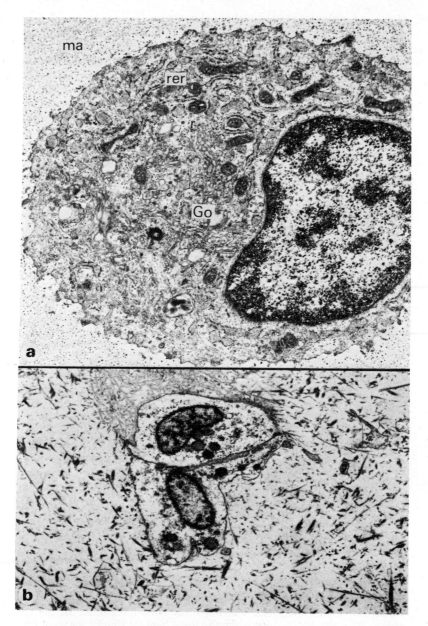

Figure 38. **a:** Cartilage cell from a branchial bar of *Ichthyophis* (Gymnophiona). Note well developed rough ER (rer) and Golgi apparatus (Go), ma: matrix x 12 000; **b:** cartilage-like tissue in the lophophore of *Lingula* (Brachiopoda), two cartilage cells are embedded in collagen fibrils, x 6000

Haversian systems they take a helical course.

The inorganic components are crystals of hydroxyapatite or fluorideapatite, in addition citrate ions, carbonate ions and other ions occur. The calcium ions can be substituted by ingested Pb^{++}, Sr^{++} and Ra^{++}. The incorporation of radioactive Sr^{++} or Ra^{++} ions, as has happened after aerial nuclear bomb tests, is particularly dangerous, since they may destroy the bone tissue including the marrow. The matrix - excluding the fibrils - is also called cement substance.

Two types of bone tissue can be distinguished: mature (= compact = lamellated) bone and immature (= trabecular) bone.

Immature bone occurs in the embryo and growing organisms. It

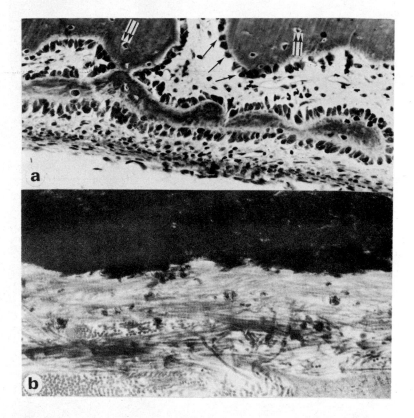

Figure 39. **a:** Bone trabeculae with osteoblasts (arrow) and osteocytes (double arrows) cat x 300; **b:** Calcifying connective tissue from the chordal sheath of *Ichthyophis* (Gymnophiona). Crystals of mineral salts (upper part of the micrograph) are deposited into a matrix rich in collagen fibrils x 18 000

consists of irregularly arranged trabecula of matrix which is relatively rich in collagen fibrils and contains less inorganic material than the mature bone (Fig. 39). In this type of bone the three typical kinds of bone cells can be clearly demonstrated. These three kinds of cells seem to be interconnected by transitory cells and often are regarded only as different functional stages of one cell type. According to another view a stem cell, the osteogenic cell, exists in the surface of bone trabecula which either forms osteoblasts or osteoclasts.

1. Osteoblasts are located at the surface of the trabecula forming epithelium like aggregations (Fig. 39). Their ultrastructure corresponds to that of protein synthesizing cells (a well developed rough ER system and Golgi apparatus, secretion granules). Their granular inclusions presumably contain precursors of the bone matrix. Active osteoblasts contain a large amount of alkaline phosphatase.

2. Osteocytes are resting osteoblasts which are incorporated into the matrix. They possess numerous cytoplasmic processes, lying in canaliculi anastomosing with canaliculi from adjacent cells. In comparison with osteoblasts, they contain reduced amounts of cell organelles. Frequently they store glycogen. They can be activated and transformed to osteoblasts during structural changes and remodelling of the bone.

3. Osteoclasts are those cells which resorb the calcified matrix. The question of their origin is not yet settled. In mammals they either have a separate stem-cell or originate from fusion of osteoblasts and osteocytes; in Amphibia they normally have an own stem-cell but sometimes seem to originate from monocytes. Osteoclasts are large cells containing numerous nuclei. They frequently occupy shallow pits at the surface of the bone trabecula (Howship's lacunae). The plasma membrane facing the surface of the bone matrix extends numerous projections between which apatite crystals and free collagen fibrils can be seen. The cytoplasm contains numerous vacuoles and lysosomes, which may play a role in bone resorption.

The bone is surrounded by the periosteum, which consists of two layers: an outer fibrous layer and an inner osteogenic layer. Cells of the osteogenic layer can transform into bone cells.

Mature bone consists of lamellar structures, into which numerous osteocytes have been incorporated. The collagen fibrils within one lamella are usually of the same orientation, but in adjacent lamellae the direction of their helical course usually is different. In a typical long bone (Fig. 40) the lamellae of the inner (towards the marrow)

Haversian systems

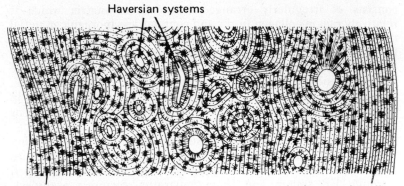

basic inner lamellae   basic outer lamellae

Figure 40.   Cross-section through a metacarpal bone (man). After SCHNEIDER, 1908.

and outer surface completely encircle the bone: inner and outer circumferential (= basic) lamellae. Between these the bone is built up of Haversian systems (= osteons). These consist of a central canal (Haversian canal) containing one or two blood vessels and connective tissue and some osteoblasts and osteogenic cells, and a thick wall of 4-20 concentric lamellae of bone matrix (Fig. 40).

Between the Haversian systems fragments of old osteons are interspersed (interstitial systems). These and the intact osteons are delimited by the cementing lines. Transverse canals interconnecting the longitudinal Haversian canals and leading to the bone surface are called Volkmann's canals. They are not surrounded by concentric lamellae.

Throughout the whole life these various lamellar systems are constantly remodelled.

Also the individual elements of spongy mature bone consist of lamellae, however they normally do not contain blood vessels.

Osteogenesis

Bone either directly originates from primitive connective tissue (intramembraneous ossification) or its formation takes place in pre-existing cartilage models (enchondral ossification). The mode of bone deposition is the same in these two types of ossification; it is first laid down as immature bone, which later is replaced by mature bone.

The ossification of cartilage starts at certain centres of ossification. In a typical long bone at first a collar of bone surrounds the middle region (diaphysis) of the cartilage model (perichondral ossification). The actual replacement of cartilage begins with the invasion of blood vessels into the middle section of the cartilage, the cells of which now hypertrophy, vacuolize, and accummulate glycogen and finally degenerate and die. The cartilage matrix frequently calcifies during this degeneration

Together with the blood vessels cells enter the cartilage model, some of which differentiate into bone marrow cells, others into osteoblasts, which begin to deposit bone matrix. The new bone trabecula fuse with the outer collar and slowly extend to the ends of the piece of skeleton. The terminal sections of the bone, which are called epiphyses, ossify relatively late. The cartilagineous disks (epiphyseal disks) between epiphyses and diaphyses, which appear in later developmental stages mark the zone of active growth, in which various processes occur simultaneously: interstitial growth, maturation, calcification and disintegration of cartilage, and formation, calcification and destruction of bone. The epiphyseal disks disappear when growth stops. The cavities of the diaphyses at first contain the red marrow, i.e. bloodforming tissue; later it is often largely replaced by yellow marrow (mainly fat cells).

Vesicular tissue and notochord

In many invertebrates an assumed supporting function is provided by cells containing voluminous fluid-filled vacuoles. Groups of such cells form the so-called vesicular or chordoid tissue, regardless of their location and origin. Such cells occur in the endoderm of the tentacles of some cnidarians, in turbellarians, enteropneusts and amphioxus in the region of the alimentary canal; the epidermal cells often contain big vacuoles in nudibranchs and tube-dwelling polychaetes.

The structure of the notochord varies in the individual groups of chordates and it does not always consist of vacuolated cells. In the larvae of ascidians the notochord consists of a chord of compact cells containing mainly yolk inclusions and glycogen particles. They closely resemble the cells of the epithelium of the embryonic intestine.

In the notochord of adult appendicularians squamous epithelial cells surround an extracellular space which is filled with an elastic substance.

The notochord of *Branchiostoma* (Fig. 41) consists of flat disk-shaped lamellar muscle cells, the ultrastructure of which resembles that of tonic muscle cells of bivalve molluscs. Even in the light microscope they may be recognized in cross-sections through the animal by the cross-striations with A- and J-zone and a Z-line. The nucleus is small and inconspicuous, cell organelles are - apart from

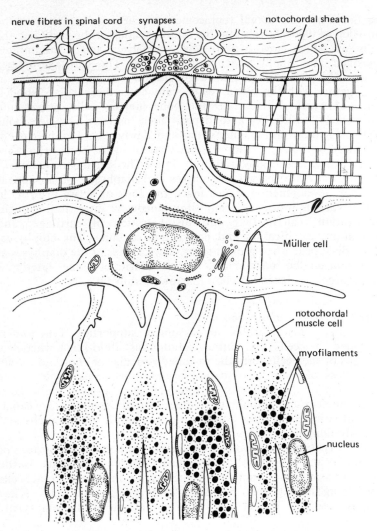

Figure 41.   Schematic representation of the notochord structure in *Branchiostoma*. Longitudinal section through the animal. Extensions of muscle and Müller cells make contact with synaptic endings of the spinal cord. After FLOOD, 1970; WELSCH, 1968

smooth ER cisternae and tubules - rare. Normally two lamellae constitute a cellular unit. They are laterally connected with the chordal sheath and in the dorsal region innervated from the spinal cord (Fig. 41). The significance of the Müller cells, stellate,

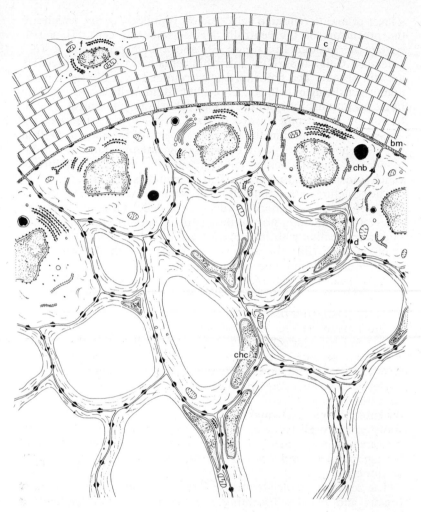

Figure 42. Schematic representation of the lamprey notochord (*Eudontomyzon*). f: fibroblast; C: collagen fibres of the notochordal sheath; bm: basement lamina of the chordoblasts (chb), chc: typical vacuolated notochordal cell, d: desmosomes between notochordal cells

dorsal and ventral elements, is unknown, maybe they are replacement cells.

The notochord of vertebrates is of rather uniform appearance (Fig. 42). It is composed of large vacuolated cells rich in microfilaments and interconnected by desmosomes. In the periphery a layer of undifferentiated cells, the chordoblasts, occur, which are the precursors of the centrally located vacuolar cells. They still contain fair amounts of rough ER and mitochondria and a well-developed Golgi apparatus, microfilaments and glycogen; vacuoles are still absent. The notochord is surrounded by a fibrous sheath, mainly consisting of collagen fibres, but additionally layers of elastic fibres may occur; for example in many sharks the innermost layer of the sheath is a strong *elastica interna*. In some species an *elastica externa* can be found in the peripheral parts of the sheath. Within the notochordal sheath of embryonic gymnophionans and sala-manders a ring of calcified collagen appears, the ultrastructure of which is identical to that of calcified bone matrix (Fig. 39).

The structure of the stomochord of enteropeusts resembles that of the vertebrate notochord. Vacuolized cells form a stratified innervated epithelium surrounding in many species a lumen which is in communication with the anterior gut. In other species the lumen is obliterated, thus the structural similarity with the vertebrate notochord is still more pronounced. The apical cells - if a lumen is present - bear microvilli and cilia.

Reticular connective tissue

This type of connective tissue is characterized by reticular fibres (p. 61) and reticular cells which produce these fibres. Both cells and the fibres provide a loose network into which free cells, e.g. blood cells, can settle down. The reticular cells contain a pale ovoid nucleus and possess long cytoplasmic processes. Often primitive and activated reticular cells are distinguished. The primitive ones resemble the mesenchymal cells of the embryo and are believed to transform into all types of blood and connective tissue cells. The activated cells are macrophages rich in lysosomes and engulfing foreign particles and cellular debris; in the spleen they destroy erythrocytes.

The reticular connective tissue forms a framework in lymphatic organs and blood-cell-forming organs (haemopoietic organs); a similar type of connective tissue forms the *lamina propria* of the intestine in which the reticular cells, however, phagocytize to a markedly lesser extent. Still another type occurs in the thymus, and is scattered in the mucosa of the respiratory and urinary tracts.

Lymphatic tissue (mammals)

Lymphatic tissue consists of a sponge-like framework or stroma and free cells in its meshes. These two components are present in different amounts, in the loose lymphatic tissue the stroma predominates, in the dense lymphatic tissue free cells are the pre-

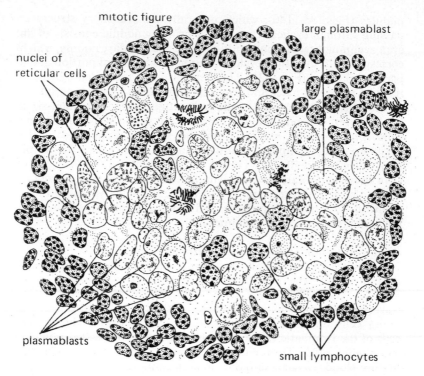

mitotic figure

large plasmablast

nuclei of
reticular cells

plasmablasts

small lymphocytes

Figure 43. Mammalian lymph nodule with a pale germinal centre, which is mainly composed of plasmablasts (precursors of the mature plasmacells). After MAXIMOW, 1927

vailing elements; nodular lymphatic tissue consists of dense aggregations of free cells. In the lymph nodes (see p. 275) the loose lymphatic tissue forms pathways for the lymph, the sinuses, which merely represent particularly loose sections of the tissue with wide intercellular spaces. The reticular cells again have the ability of phagocytosis, occasionally they are concentrated along the sinuses and form the so-called littoral cells.

The typical free cells are the lymphocytes (p. 284), which occur in various sizes and have various functions (p. 275). The small lymphocytes form the vast majority. Other typical free cells are the plasma cells, which develop from the lymphocytes. Other free cells (e.g. monocytes and eosinophils) are rare.

The lymphocytes, which currently are believed to originate in the bone marrow, often form dense accumulations, the lymphatic nodules (Figs. 43, 140), which generally are transitory structures passing through cyclical changes. A primary nodule consists of an even accumulation of small lymphocytes. A secondary nodule, which corresponds to the fully developed form, has a central portion and a peripheral zone (Fig. 43). The central zone (germinal centre = reaction centre) is paler and contains larger cells than the periphery (= corona). The central cells are often called medium-sized lymphocytes, it is now known that they are young stages of plasma cells (plasmoblasts) arising from the small lymphocytes of the periphery. Such lymphatic nodules may arise anywhere. In lymph nodes they are usually found in the cortex (Fig. 139).

In lower vertebrates special lymphatic tissues are rare (birds) or seem to be absent (except for the thymus), although lymphocytes are plentiful. Generally, lymphatic and blood-cell-forming tissues are not as sharply separated as in mammals.

Blood-cell-forming tissues (myeloid tissue)

In adult mammals blood cells are produced exclusively in the red bone marrow. The stroma of this organ is an extremely loose reticular connective tissue with wide intercellular spaces. It is traversed by numerous wide and thin-walled vessels (sinusoids) the lining cells of which are phagocytotic and resemble the littoral cells of the lymphatic tissue (Fig. 44). They are also called reticulo-endothelial cells. Through these extremely thin lining cells the mature blood cells pass into the blood stream.

The connection of the sinusoids with true blood vessels is still unclear.

The free cells constitute an extremely variable assembly of cells. Almost all of them are precursors of blood cells, however also mature types occur frequently.

The following groups of cell types can be distinguished in mammals:

1. Haemocytoblasts, free stem cells for probably all types of blood cells. They are of variable size, basophilic, amoeboid and resemble to some extent lymphocytes. They are possibly derived from reticular cells.
2. Erythroblasts, precursors of erythrocytes. Within about three days they pass through a series of stages: (a) basophilic erythroblasts (rich in ribosomes, well-developed Golgi apparatus, small

Figure 44. Bone marrow, **a:** man, after MAXIMOW, 1927; **b:** activated bone marrow of a chicken, haemocytoblasts (stem cells) may occur intra- and extravascularly. After DANTSCHAKOFF, 1909

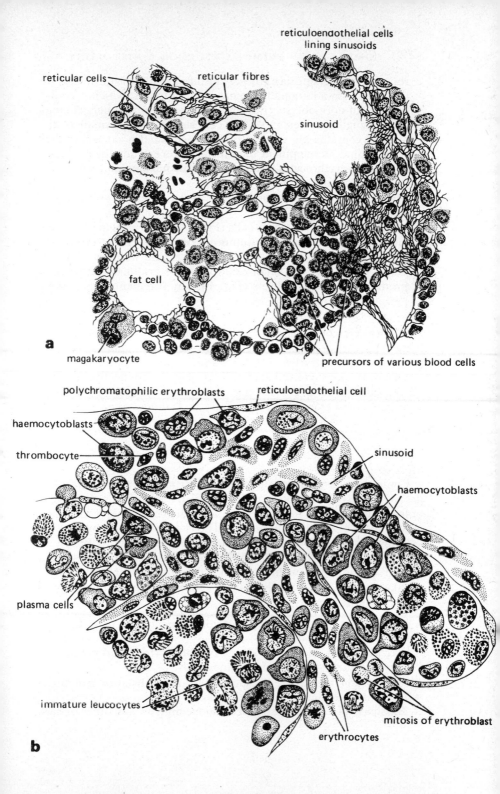

a

reticular cells

reticular fibres

reticuloenaothelial cells
lining sinusoids

sinusoid

fat cell

magakaryocyte

precursors of various blood cells

b

polychromatophilic erythroblasts

reticuloendothelial cell

haemocytoblasts

thrombocyte

sinusoid

haemocytoblasts

plasma cells

immature leucocytes

mitosis of erythroblast

erythrocytes

roundish mitochondria); (b) polychromatophilic erythroblasts (in the cytoplasm additionally haemoglobin appears, which is acidophilic); (c) normoblasts (ribosomes decrease in number, amount of haemoglobin increases, the cell size becomes smaller, the nucleus contains big clumps of heterochromatin, at a terminal stage of their development the normoblasts extrude the nucleus); (d) mature erythrocytes (cells contain only haemoglobin and a few peripheral microtubules).
3. Myelocytes, the precursors of the three types of granulocytes (p. 282).
4. Megakaryocytes, very large cells (Fig. 140) with a highly irregular lobed nucleus containing numerous nucleoli. Their cytoplasm contains many mitochondria, a considerable number of Golgi fields, polysomes and small electron dense granules. These cells produce the blood platelets (Fig. 145) by fragmentation of their peripheral cytoplasm.

In lower vertebrates the haemopoietic tissue is not confined to the bone marrow, e.g. in urodeles and Gymnophiona a cortical peripheral zone of the liver produces three types of blood cells.

One of the most conspicuous cell types in the connective tissue of gastropods and bivalves is the pore cell. These cells have been found to produce and store blood pigments. In *Lymnaea* their cytoplasm contains a well-developed rough ER, which can contain haemocyanin particles.

Mesenchyme

Connective tissue originates from the primitive mesodermal connective tissue of the embryo, which is called mesenchyme. It consists of large stellate cells, the processes of which are in contact with each other, and a few macrophages. The intercellular substance is voluminous and jelly-like and contains thin collagenous fibres. In the umbilical cord it is called Wharton's jelly. In adult animals a similar tissue is present in the cock's comb and in the sex skin of monkeys and in some lower invertebrate groups, e.g. Platyhelminthes and Nemertini.

In summary, the various types of connective tissues of vertebrates contain three groups of cells:
1. reticular cells, having the ability of phagocytosis and possibly being a primitive stem cell of the blood cells.
2. cells producing different types of ground substance and fibres =fibroblasts, chondro - and osteocytes.
3. Bloodcells, free cells arising in the bone marrow and other tissues.

Mesogloea.

The term mesogloea designates an extracellular layer of variable thickness between ecto- and endoderm in Cnidaria and ctenophores. Ordinarily it is composed of a mucopolysaccharide matrix and collagen-like fibres, which usually are non-striated and synthesized by the epidermal epitheliomuscular cells (as demonstrated by auto-radiography). In species with a thick mesogloea (sea anemones, ctenophores) these fibres build up laminated arrangements. In many species also individual cells occur in the mesogloea. In sea anemones they resemble amoebocytes and contain abundant granular inclusions. In the ctenophore mesogloea smooth muscle cells have been described.

Muscle tissue

Muscle cells are highly specialized contractile cells. This property is due to the existence of particular longitudinal filamentous systems in their cytoplasm. The classification into striated and smooth muscle cells is based on the presence or absence of regular cross-striations of the cells.

Smooth muscle cells. In vertebrates this type of muscle cell generally occurs in the viscera, e.g. in the wall of the intestinal tract, of blood vessels, of the genital, urinary and respiratory tracts. It is innervated by the vegetative nervous system.

The individual cells are generally spindle-shaped, occasionally cells with three or more processes occur (Fig. 45). They contain a centrally located elongated nucleus which may become pleated if the cell contracts. It has blunt ends and contains fine granules of heterochromatin and two or more nucleoli. The cell organelles are concentrated near the poles of the nucleus, prominent are mitochondria and in older organisms lipofuscin granules. Glycogen can be abundant and the whole cytoplasm – which in muscle cells is also called sarcoplasm – may contain individual tubules of the smooth ER.

The most important cytoplasmic components are thin myofilaments (diameter about 30 Å), which are longitudinally oriented and generally form bundles of five or more. They can be seen only in the electron microscope. In the course of these filaments electron dense areas occur, where the filaments seem to be embedded into a dense matrix. These areas probably correspond to the Z-lines of cross-striated muscle cells. Similar areas are to be found under the plasma membrane where they are similar to half-desmosomes. Beside the thin filaments individual thicker ones (diameter 60–80 Å) can be demonstrated, which, however, do not stand in a regular geometrical relation to the thinner filaments.

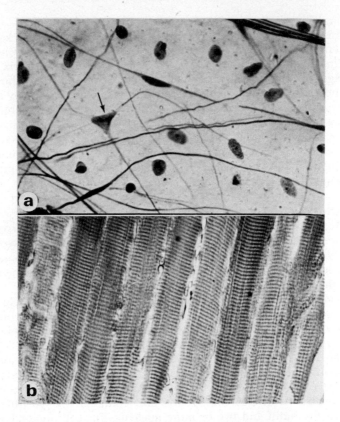

Figure 45.   **a:** Light microscopy of muscle cells. Smooth muscle cells in the wall of the urinary bladder of the frog (*Rana*). Beside elongated spindle shaped cells elements with three extensions occur (arrow), x 250. **b:** cross-striated muscle cells, x 250

Since actin and myosin have been biochemically isolated from smooth muscle cells it is generally assumed that the thin filaments correspond to actin and the thicker ones to myosin. It is believed that the myosin filaments are long and possess lateral spiny projections, to which the actin filaments can become attached. In a contracting cell these filaments presumably pass along each other - a process which principally agrees with the contraction of cross-striated muscle cells.

The plasma membrane under which numerous pinocytotic vesicles occur, is surrounded by a basement lamina. Neighbouring cells either lie individually side by side or are interconnected by tight and gap junctions. The cells may be individually innervated or groups of cells interconnected by junctional complexes are innervated by one nerve fibre.

The belt-shaped or star-shaped basket cells in exocrine glands are typical smooth muscle cells; they lie inside the basement lamina of the gland.

The smooth muscle cells of invertebrates often differ from those of the vertebrates by the conspicuous presence of thin and thick filaments (diameter up to 150 nm. As in the thick filaments of the oblique-striated muscle cells (see below) they contain beside myosin various amounts of paramyosin. Presumably myosin forms a sheath around a central axis of paramyosin. Paramyosin-containing filaments exhibit cross-striations in the electron microscope.

Striated muscle cells. In vertebrates these cells are subdivided into skeletal and cardiac muscle cells. The skeletal muscle cells are responsible for movements and posture and are innervated by spinal and some of the cranial nerves. Cardiac muscle cells are activated by the conducting tissue which can be influenced by the autonomic nervous system.

Skeletal muscle cells because of their extraordinary length are also termed muscle fibres. The individual fibres form bundles; these constitute the whole muscle. Each of these whole muscles, bundles and fibres is surrounded by connective tissue containing collagen fibres. The envelope around the muscle is called epimysium, that around the bundles perimysium and that around the fibre endomysium. In these connective tissue sheaths numerous blood capillaries and nerve fibres occur. Each muscle fibre is surrounded by helically arranged capillaries.

The muscle fibres ordinarily contain several nuclei. Two main explanations exist of how these multinucleated cells arise: (a) by fusion of embryonic muscle cells (myoblasts), in this case the fibre would be a syncytium; (b) the myoblasts grow actively and elongate, but only their nuclei divide during this process, in this case the fibre would be a plasmodium.

The plasma membrane is often also called the sarcolemma. It is surrounded by a basement lamina. In the light microscopic literature plasma membrane, basement lamina and adjacent reticular fibrils together are called sarcolemma. Between basement lamina and plasma membrane individual flattened cells which are poor in organelles occur (satellite cells); their function is unknown.

Light microscopy. The localization of the elongated or oval nuclei varies. In mammals they occupy a peripheral position. Mitochondria form rows in the periphery and between the muscle fibrils. The smooth ER forms a network around the fibrils. The cytoplasm further contains glycogen and often also a few lipid droplets. The colour of the muscle is due to the presence of the protein myoglobin in the fibres. The dominating feature of the cytoplasm are the parallel longitudinal muscle fibrils (myofibrils). Cross-sections through the fibres show that they form groups (Cohnheim's fields). In longitudinal sections of the fibres the individual fibrils exhibit alternating dark and light segments (Fig. 45). In neighbouring fibrils these light and dark zones are usually in

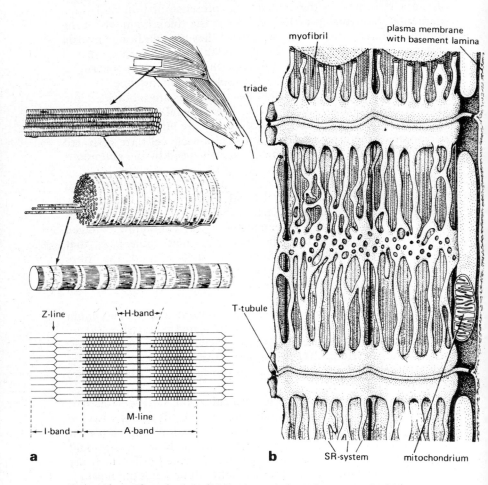

Figure 46.   **a:** Organization of skeletal muscle from the gross to the fine structural level: from top to bottom; muscle, group of muscle cells, muscle cell (=muscle fibre), muscle fibril, muscle filaments; **b:** three dimensional schematic representation of the fine structure of muscle fibrils, the SR- and T-system in a striated muscle cell of the frog. After BLOOM & FAWCETT, 1970

the same position so that the whole fibre assumes a cross-striation. With polarized light the dark bands, as seen in a well-stained preparation, are anisotropic and appear as light stripes; in contrast the light bands of the stained section are isotropic, i.e. dark. The anisotropic bands are termed A-bands, the isotropic ones I-bands. Within the I-band a dark line can be observed, the Z-line. The area between two Z-lines is called a sarcomere. Within the A-band in good preparations a pale H-zone with a dark middle line (M-line) can be distinguished.

Electron microscopic preparations give further information about the structure of the myofibril and the arrangement of the smooth ER. The fibrils consist of a regularly arranged system of coarse myosin and fine actin filaments (Fig. 46). The myosin filaments are located in the A-band and are interconnected in the M-line by dense material. Actin filaments occur in the I-band but also extend deeply into the A-band; they are attached to the Z-line.

Approaching the Z-line one actin filament divides into four Z-filaments which penetrate the Z-line and continue in an actin filament on the other side. That part of the A-band which does not contain actin filaments is the H-zone. In the A-band actin and myosin filaments under certain conditions can be interconnected by cross bridges containing among others ATPase.

The smooth ER (= sarcoplasmic reticulum) forms an inter-connected system of tubes and cisternae (Fig. 46). Individual tubules are also termed sarcotubules. Over the A-band these tubules are longitudinally arranged, over the H-zone they form an anastomosing network. At certain points the longitudinal tubules merge with circular channels, the terminal cisternae. Neighbouring pairs of these cisternae embrace a third tubular element, the T-tubule (transverse tubule), which corresponds to a funnel-like blind ending invagination of the plasma membrane. The three channels together are called triad (if only one terminal cisterna comes into contact with a T-tubule the common structure is called dyad). In amphibians triads only occur at the Z-line (Fig. 46), in mammals at the transition of A- and I-band.

The T-tubules serve the rapid conduction of an electrical impulse into the interior of the fibre. The channels of the sarcoplasmic reticulum (SR-system) contain calcium ions which are essential for contraction and relaxation.

Muscle spindles consist of about six small and modified muscle fibres surrounded by their own sheath of connective tissue. These fibres are called intrafusal fibres in contrast to the ordinary fibres termed extrafusal fibres (Fig. 48). They contain few fibrils, which are concentrated in the terminal parts of the spindle-shaped cells. The nuclei are concentrated in the mid portion of the cell. The intrafusal

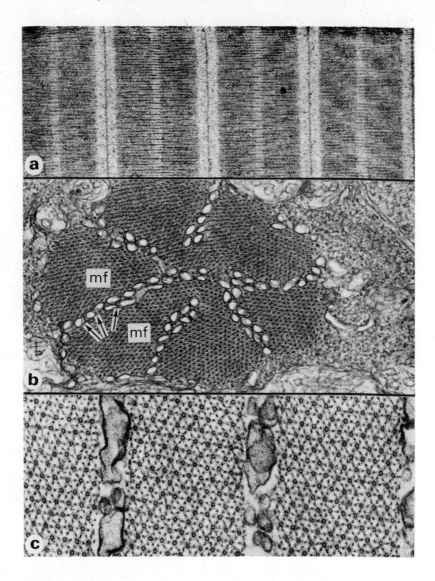

Figure 47. Fine structure of cross-striated muscle cells. **a:** *Oikopleura* (**Appendicularia**) longitudinal section. x 19000, **b:** *Microhyla* (Anura) larva, cross-section, group of muscle fibrils (two of which are labelled (mf)), richly supplied by channels of the SR- and T-system (arrows), x 20 000; **c:** *Sagitta* (arrow worm), cross-section, note regular hexagonal arrangement of myosin and actin filaments; the myosin filament in this animal exhibits a tubular structure. x 50 000

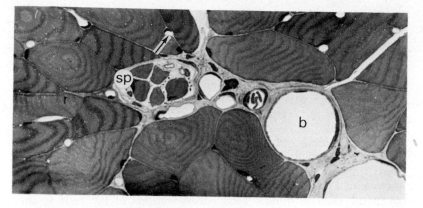

Figure 48. Cross-section through cross-striated muscle cells (rat), note presence of a muscle spindle (sp) with five small intrafusal fibres; b: larger blood vessel, arrow points to blood capillary. x 480

fibres are innervated by sensory and motor nerves. The spindles are loosely distributed in a muscle and represent stretch receptor organs.

Insects only possess striated muscle cells, which are to be found in the walls of heart, intestine and other viscera, of course they are also part of the locomotor apparatus. The contractile elements can be arranged in fibrils of roundish, lamellar or polygonal cross-section. The fine structure of the fibrils resembles that of the vertebrate fibrils, but the relations between actin and myosin filaments vary considerably. In flight muscles of fast flyers a hexagonal pattern occurs: myosin filaments form the angular points of a hexagon in the centre of which an additional myosin filament occurs, which at the same time is an angular point of a neighbouring hexagon. Between two myosin filaments lies one actin filament. In visceral muscles one myosin filament is surrounded by a maximum of twelve actin filaments. In the flight muscles of slow flyers, one myosin filament is surrounded by 7-9 actin filaments. In the flight muscles of fast flyers the I-band is relatively short and the myosin filaments do not terminate at the border of the A- and I-bands, but possess a thin appendage filament reaching the Z-line. Between the fibrils unusually numerous and large mitochondria are intercalated, with very densely arranged cristae which are partly fenestrated. Dyads frequently occur between Z-line and the middle of the sarcomere, but can lie also at the M-band (Heteroptera (Belostomatidae), some Hymenoptera). In the fast asynchronally oscillating flight muscles, e.g. of dipterans, the sarcoplasmic reticulum of the dyads is reduced.

It only forms vesicles along the T-tubule. Triads are relatively rare in insects.

The structure of the arthropod myofibrils shows many more variations; e.g. in some Coleoptera (*Hydrophilus*) and in some Crustacea the sarcomere exhibits further subdivisions; here in the I-band an anisotropic line, the N-band, occurs.

Comparable cross-striated muscle cells occur in many other invertebrates (e.g. chaetognaths (Fig. 47), bryozoans, rotifers, echinoderms).

Cardiac muscle cells of vertebrates. These cells possess several centrally located nuclei; they are branched and at their terminal parts interconnected by particular junctional complexes, the intercalated disks. The myofilaments are arranged in the same way as in the skeletal muscle cells. Cross-sections of the cells in the electron microscope show that they do not constitute fibrils but an anastomosing system filling most parts of the cell. This type of arrangement is termed *Felderstruktur* and can also be found in slowly contracting skeletal muscles, e.g. in amphibians. The fibrillar pattern as seen in most skeletal muscle cells characterizes fast muscles.

Between the contractile elements lie columns of mitochondria between which lipid droplets and glycogen particles are interspersed. The mitochondrial cristae often run in zig-zag and are very numerous. Around the nucleus a zone free of filaments exists containing much glycogen and many lipofuscin granules.

The T-system is particularly well developed, in contrast to the skeletal muscle cells it is lined by a basement lamina. Dyads and triads in mammals are located at the Z-line. The sarcoplasmic reticulum is rather poorly developed and consists of a net of confluent tubules which also occur under the plasma membrane. The intercalated disks are of a complex fine structure and consist of many interdigitating short processes. This area of contact is characterized by extensive *maculae* – and *zonulae adhaerentes* and *zonulae occludentes*. Actin filaments penetrate into the dense material of the desmosomes. At their lateral aspects neighbouring heart muscle cells can form extensive tight junctions (*fasciae occludentes*), serving a rapid spread of electrical impulses. The special conducting tissue consists of cardiac muscle cells poor in filaments and mitochondria and rich in free ground cytoplasm and glycogen (Fig. 49). In the impulse generating and propagating nodes of this system, these cells are very short and form a network into the meshes of which nerve fibres and connective tissue are embedded. In the fibrous part of the system the cells are long and of remarkable diameter. Intercalated disks are rarely to be found.

Obliquely striated muscle cells (= spirally-, = helically-striated

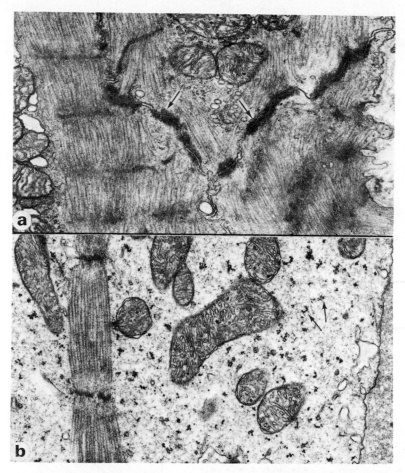

Figure 49. **a:** area of contact (intercalated disk, arrows) between two cardiac muscle cells of *Etmopterus* (shark); **b:** detail of impulse-conducting cell from the heart of *Etmopterus*, note pale ground cytoplasm with glycogen particles (arrows), mitochondria and scarce myofibrils. Both x 18 000

muscle cells). This type of muscle cell is of wide distribution among invertebrates: turbellarians, nematodes, molluscs, annelids etc. The impression of an oblique striation is often due to the fact that the sarcomeres are arranged helically in the cellular periphery. This is particularly obvious in the A-band which runs like a spiral staircase as a dark helix around the cell. These muscle cells will be explained by the description of two examples.

In the nematode *Ascaris* the musculature of the body wall consists of one layer of large longitudinal cells which are subdivided into

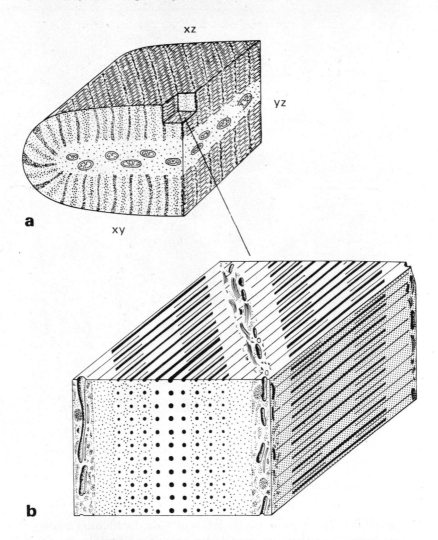

Figure 50. Detail from an obliquely striated muscle cell of *Ascaris* (nematode), in the xz plane the oblique striation is obvious, in the yz plane the myofilaments are arranged in the same fashion as in the cross-striated muscle cell; in the xy plane because of the peculiar arrangement of the myofilaments an additional striation is apparent. After ROSENBLUTH 1965.

three sections. Centrally an inflated glycogen-rich part exists containing the nucleus. A process from this central area extends under the epidermis with the contractile material; a second process either reaches the dorsal or ventral nerve cord. The contractile processes contain in their periphery the myofilaments and in their centre light cytoplasm rich in mitochondria. In cross-sections through the animal the peripheral zone with the myofilaments appears striated (Fig. 50). The regularly oriented stripes run perpendicularly to the cellular surface. In oblique and longitudinal sections variable patterns of striation may be seen, which differ not only in the direction of the striation but also in their width and density.

In *Ascaris* the contractile material is not arranged in fibrils but is evenly distributed in the periphery of the contractile process. The light bands of light microscopy contain cross-sections through myofilaments, in the dark zones accumulations of dense material occur, corresponding to Z-lines and here called Z-bundles. Whereas in cross-sections through myofibrils of vertebrate striated muscle cells only one band or line is met, the cross-sections through the filaments of *Ascaris* show a regular sequence of five bands. Centrally a H-zone occurs, which is characterized by the exclusive presence of cross-sections through coarse filaments. On both sides of it is situated a zone with coarse and fine filaments (A-band) which are each followed by an I-band containing only thin filaments. In *Ascaris*, in cross-sections through the contractile material bands can be seen, which in vertebrates characterize longitudinal sections (Fig. 50). The different images in longitudinal and oblique sections are due to the fact that the filaments of one band do not terminate in common in one plane, running perpendicularly to their long axis. In this animal each filament of one band extends for a short distance the preceding one, so that a line which connects their ends runs obliquely to the long axis of them.

Invaginations of the plasmalemma form together with tubules of the SR system dyads and triads. Neighbouring muscle cells are interconnected by cytoplasmic bridges.

At the area of contact with nerve fibres the processes of the muscle cells closely approach each other so that they are separated only by a space of 1-5 nm (10-50 Å). The synaptic cleft is about 500 Å wide. In the presynaptic region (i.e. in the axon) dense concentrations of synaptic vesicles and big mitochondria occur.

Markedly smaller than the muscle cells of *Ascaris* are those of the body wall of the earthworm *Lumbricus*. The cells constituting the ring musculature are individually embedded in a loose connective tissue. Those cells forming the longitudinal musculature are fixed

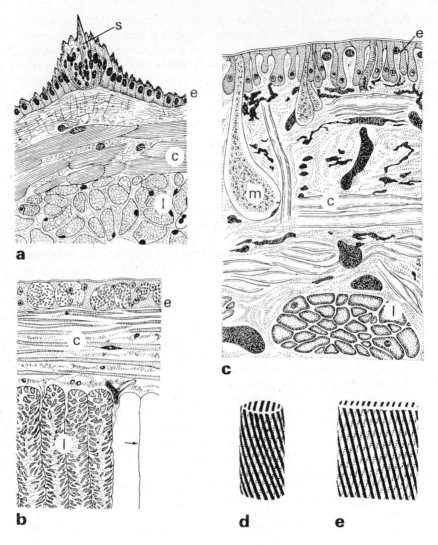

Figure 51. **a:** *Peripatus*, skin, s: group of sensory cells, e: epidermis, c: circularly arranged muscle cells, l: longitudinally arranged muscle cells; **b:** *Lumbricus* (earthworm) skin, e: epidermis with glandular cells, c: circularly arranged muscle cells, l: longitudinally arranged muscle cells; these are of rather small diameter and are attached with one side to connective tissue septa, an isolated one of which is illustrated on the right side (arrow), **c:** *Hirudo* (leech) skin; e: epidermis; m: mucous cell; c: circularly-, l: longitudinally arranged muscle cells, the contractile material is located in the cellular periphery; **d, e:** schematic representation of the contractile material in obliquely striated muscle cells, the A-bands appear as dark lines. After SCHNEIDER, 1908, and BOULIGAND, 1968

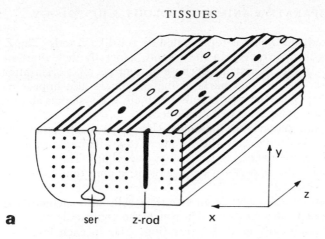

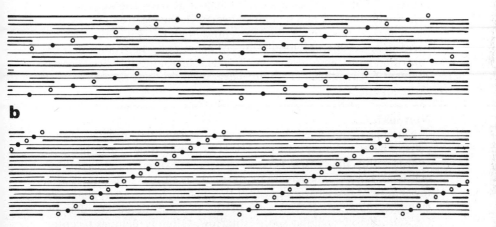

Figure 52. Obliquely striated muscle cells of *Lumbricus,* **a:** three-dimensional schematic representation of the fine structure of a muscle cell. On cross-sections through the cell (xy-plane) beside myofilaments, cisternae of the smooth ER (SR-system ser) and z-rods can be seen; sections in the xz-plane show alternating cross-sections through ER tubules and Z-rods. actin filaments not drawn. **b:** Schematic representation of longitudinal sections in xz-plane of a relaxed (top) and contracted cell. For explanations see text. After HEUMANN & ZEBE, 1967

with an edge of their plasma membrane to long connective tissue septa (Fig. 51). Each muscle cell contains only one nucleus, which together with mitochondria occupies a peripheral part of the cell. As in the vertebrate striated muscle cells A- and I-band and H-zone can be recognized, the Z-line is represented by rod-like Z-rods. The Z-rods are regularly arranged in the I-band, generally they alternate with tubules of the SR system. Because of their peculiar orientation as in *Ascaris* the different parts of the sarcomere also appear on cross-sections. Since the muscle cells are small, a T-system is absent, the SR system, however, is well developed.

During contraction the filaments slide past each other. In addition the line connecting the Z-rods changes its angle with the long axis of the filaments, i.e. it becomes 'raised up'. Therefore this type of muscle cell can perform stronger contractions than the cross-striated one (Fig. 52).

The group of obliquely striated muscle cells also includes the double obliquely striated fibres, in which the contractile elements form two peripherally located layers (Fig. 51). In each layer the sarcomeres are helically arranged but in different directions; the outer ones are wound to the left side, the inner ones to the right side. Outer and inner helices run against each other at an angle of *c.* 50 degrees. Therefore if such a cell is looked at from the outside, one gets the impression of a regular network. In the electron microscope one can see that the Z-line is represented by Z-nodules, which correspond to small accumulations of dense material from which six thin filaments emerge on each side, surrounding each coarse filament hexagonally. These ultrastructural findings refer to several cephalopods.

Nervous tissue

Nervous tissue consists of neurons (nerve cells) and neuroglial cells. The ependymal cells of chordates, which line the fluid-filled spaces within the central nervous system, are often listed as a third cell type; however, observations particularly of lower chordates and lower vertebrates clearly show that they belong to the neuroglial cells (tanycyte glial cells). The cells of the nervous tissue are densely packed; the intercellular space is narrow. Often it includes receptor cells. Only the nervous system of higher forms, e.g. vertebrates and insects, contains blood vessels or air channels supplying this system with oxygen and nutrients. Generally, the nervous tissue is surrounded by particular connective tissue sheaths, the meninges.

Neurons

In light microscopic preparations neurons often stand out by their large size. They contain characteristic processes of various lengths, the number and arrangement of which form the basis for a classification of neurons (Fig. 53). The various parts of one neuron have special names: perikaryon (cell body, soma), axon (neurite),

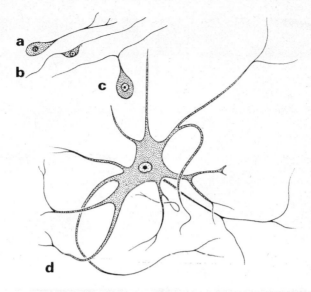

Figure 53. Various types of neurons, **a:** unipolar, **b:** bipolar, **c:** pseudounipolar, **d:** multipolar neuron. After STOEHR, V. MÖLLENDORFF & GOERTTLER, 1963

dendrite, collateral, endings (end-feet, end bulbs, boutons).

The perikaryon is that part of the neuron which contains the nucleus and the majority of cell organelles. In light microscopic preparations it is often the only part of the neuron which can be recognized (Fig. 54). The nucleus generally is large and spherical, it contains mainly euchromatin and a distinct nucleolus (Fig. 54). Because of its light appearance the nucleus often is called 'vesicular'. Its structure and location varies in different types of neurons and can be used for the identification of a certain area of the nervous system. Some nuclei of mammalian neurons have been found to be tetraploid.

The organelles of the perikaryon often are so plentiful or well developed that they may be clearly demonstrated at the light microscopic level (Fig. 2); e.g. the rough ER in many neurons can be clearly recognized as basophilic clumps (Nissl bodies) or the Golgi apparatus forms a distinct network throughout the cytoplasm (Fig. 54). Other components which can be demonstrated clearly with the light microscope are the dense network of microfilaments (neurofilaments) and the usually high number of lysosomes demonstrated by histochemical preparations for acid phosphatase.

In the electron microscope the rough ER often forms numerous

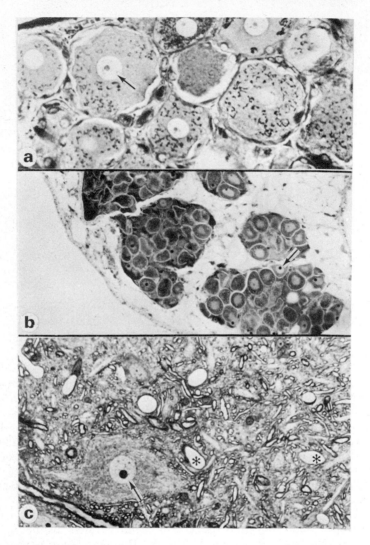

Figure 54. Nervous tissue, light microscopy. **a:** spinal ganglion, cat; a group of perikarya in which the Golgi apparatus has been selectively stained (irregularly arranged dark threadlike structures in the cytoplasm), arrow points to nucleus. x 600; **b:** ganglion of *Echiurus* (Echiurida), arrow points to nucleus with prominent nucleolus in a nerve cell. x 110, **c:** spinal cord of the rat, arrow points to nucleus of a large neuron; the tissue between the perikarya is termed neuropile and contains myelinated (dense outlines) and unmyelinated nerve fibres, glial cells and blood capillaries (asterisks) x 600

stacks of about 5-10 cisternae; smaller individual cisterae also extend into the basal part of the dendrites, but usually are absent from the outermost periphery and the origin of the axon. In addition abundant polysomes occur. The rough ER stacks (corresponding to the Nissl bodies) are largest in large motor neurons, in many sensory neurons, e.g. in the spinal ganglia, they are very small, but still numerous (Fig. 57). The size and number of the rough ER stacks can vary under different physiological conditions.

The cisternae of the extensive Golgi apparatuses are often in connection with smooth tubules frequently thought to be part of the smooth ER. These again are connected with the rough ER. Thus these membranous systems in many neurons appear to be particularly closely related to each other.

The very numerous mitochondria are usually relatively small and almost never contain mitochondrial granules.

The lysosomes may be constant in number and distribution in different types of neurons; e.g. in the brain of newts certain unipolar neurons of the olfactory region generally contain one lysosome per neuron, others of the *primordium hippocampi* contain 2-3, whereas the neurons of the *trigeminus* in the midbrain and of the trigeminal ganglion contain vast numbers throughout their cytoplasm (Fig. 12). Generally neurons contain many lysosomes.

Many neurons are characterized by containing specific pigments, the demonstration of which can show certain neurons particularly clearly. The occurrence of melanin in the neurons of *nucleus niger* in the midbrain and other areas of the human nervous system is well known.

In some animals, e.g. *Branchiostoma*, the perikarya contain large areas of glycogen.

Particularly in invertebrates most neurons contain large numbers of small secretory granules, which are especially abundant in the neurosecretory neurons producing hormones (Fig. 55). But also ordinary neurons contain vesicular and granular inclusions, which, however, normally are concentrated in the terminals of the axons; their contents are transmitter substances.

Axons and dendrites are slender extensions from the perikaryon; both often cannot clearly be distinguished on the structural level; however, they possess different functions. The axon conducts impulses from the perikaryon to the periphery, dendrites conduct impulses from the periphery to the perikaryon. Each neuron possesses only one axon, whereas the number of dendrites varies from none to several. Both types of processes can ramify.

The dendrites often contain small components of the rough ER and occasional mitochondria. Microfilaments and microtubules occur in addition. Usually dendrites have small spiny or roundish projections at their sides, representing areas of contact with other neurons. The axon usually is much thinner than the dendrites. Its place of origin is called axon hillock. It contains a few elongated mitochondria, individual tubules of the ER, microfilaments and microtubules. The branches of axons are called collaterals, the terminal axonal arborization is often termed telodendron.

By various methods it could be shown that a continuous flow of material down the axon exists (axon flow). Labelled protein was observed to migrate at a rate of about 1.5 mm per day. Neurosecretory granules also move down the axon; the mechanism of transport is unknown; microtubules possibly play a part.

The neuronal processes of higher animals are generally ensheathed to various degrees by neuroglial cells (see below). In those animals with a more primitive organization (e.g. echinoderms,

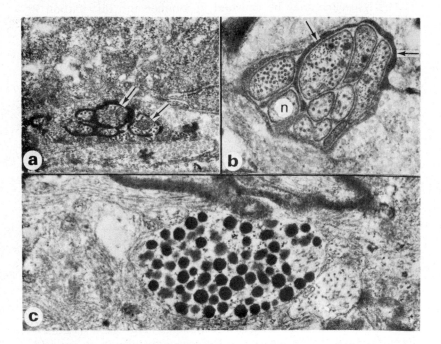

Figure 55.   Fine structure of various types of nerve fibres. **a:** Guinea pig, small bundle of nerve fibres with a positive reaction of acetylcholinesterase on the plasma membrane (arrows), x 18 000; **b:** *Rhacophorus* (tree frog), small group of nerve fibres **(n)** containing microtubules, surrounded by a Schwann cell (arrows), x 24 000; **c:** midbrain of a salamander, neuro-secretory nerve fibre with numerous electron dense granules, x 20 000

enteropneusts, amphioxus, tentaculates, etc.) they generally are naked.

The terminal parts of axons come into contact with other neurons, muscle cells, receptor cells and other cellular elements. The site of contact is called a synapse, it is the region of transmission of nervous impulses from one neuron to another or from neuron to muscle cell. Synapses are not static structures, but can increase and decrease in number. According to their function excitatory and inhibitory synapses are recognized. Synapses may be further classified according to their transmitter: cholinergic, adrenergic, purinergic, peptidergic, etc. According to the localization and structure they may be classified in the following ways:

(a) Synapses between neurons
   (1) Axodendritic synapses connect axonal terminals with the dendrites of another neuron. They are of variable structure, e.g. the dendrites can form dendritic spines which are surrounded by a cup-shaped axonal terminal.
   (2) Axosomatic synapses are areas of contact between axonal terminal and the perikaryon of another neuron.
   (3) Axo-axonal synapses may be found between axon terminals and the axon of another neuron, often at its terminal part.
   Surprisingly high numbers of synapses may be formed by one neuron. It has been calculated that on the surface of one pyramidal cell of the human cerebral cortex 10,000 synapses are to be found; a Purkinje cell of the cerebellar cortex may have several hundred thousand synapses at its dendritic tree. All the above-mentioned synapses are of a bewildering diversity in size and shape. It is striking that some groups of animals generally have bigger synapses (e.g. fishes) than others (e.g. birds).

(b) Synapses between nerve and muscle cells (myoneuronal synapses). The synapses between nerve terminals and smooth muscle cells are of simple structure, those between axon terminal and striated muscle cells (motor end plates) are of a complex structure, in particular in higher vertebrates (Fig. 56).

(c) Synapses between axonal terminals and receptor cells (e.g. in the organ of Corti) are of simple structure.

(d) Synapses between sensory cells and the terminals of sensory neurons. These can be of simple (most taste buds) or of complicated structure (ampullae or Lorenzini); occasionally the nerve terminal forms a big cup surrounding most of the sensory cell (inner ear, Fig. 91).

(e) Synapses between axon terminals and cells of other tissues (endo- and exocrine glandular cells, fat cells, ciliated cells) usually are of simple structure.

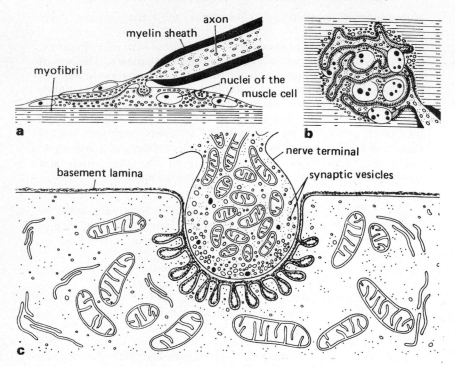

Figure 56. Motor endplate in the light (a,b) and electron microscope (c), **a:** longitudinal section; **b:** surface view; **c:** section through the area of contact between nerve terminal (mitochondria, synaptic vesicles) and muscle cell. After BLOOM & FAWCETT 1970

In the electron microscope one can see that the axonal terminal generally is slightly swollen and free of any ensheathing cells. It contains small vesicles and granules with transmitter substances. In cholinergic synapses predominantly small light vesicles (= synaptic vesicles, diameter 20–60 nm (200–600 Å) occur. Additional bigger electron dense granules may contain a trophic factor. In adrenergic synapses small electron dense granules (diameter: about 800 Å) are characteristic, peptidergic terminals and purinergic ones generally contain bigger dense granules (diameter: more than 1000 Å). Synapses with glycin as transmitter contain elongated light vesicles.

The second regular component of the terminals are accumulations of mitochondria. Microfilaments, microtubules, spined vesicles and glycogen particles are of variable occurrence. The plasma membrane of that area opposing the postsynaptic cell generally is thickened by

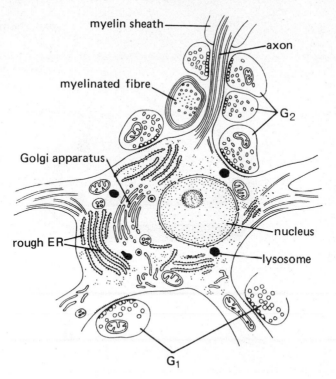

Figure 57. Fine structure of a neuron with synapses. G_1: Gray-1-type-synapse (roundish synaptic vesicles, presumably inhibitory). G_2: Gray-2-type-synapse (oval synaptic vesicles presumably excitatory). After AKERT 1971

apposition of electron dense material to its inner aspect (pre-synaptic membrane), the same phenomenon may often be observed in the opposing cell membrane, with which the area of contact is formed, the postsynaptic membrane. Between these two membranes lies the synaptic cleft. Here the distance between the cells generally is slightly wider (20-30 nm (200-300 Å) in the nervous tissue, about 50 nm (500 Å) in the motor endplate) than in normal areas. The intercellular space can contain electron dense material, which is ascribed to maintain the attachment in the synaptic region. In nerve cells the above-mentioned membrane thickenings are often confined to the points of intersection of a hexagonal network, the meshes of which are just big enough to lodge the synaptic vesicles (Fig. 58). Evidently here the transmitter substance is not liberated by exocytosis, but through narrow 4-4.5 nm (10-45 Å) wide pores

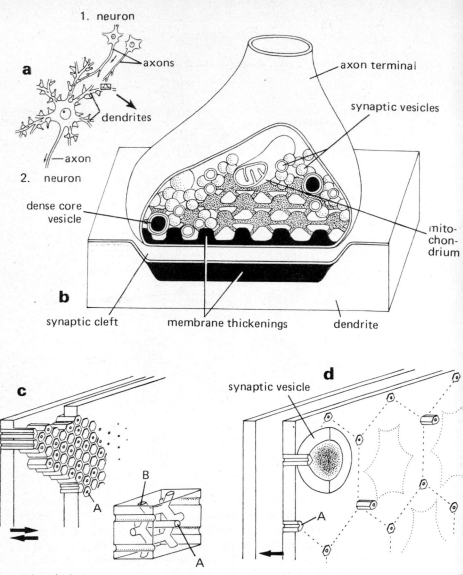

1. neuron

axons

a

dendrites

axon

2. neuron

dense core
vesicle

b

synaptic cleft

axon terminal

synaptic vesicles

mito-
chon-
drium

membrane thickenings   dendrite

c

A

B

A

A

electrical synapse

d

synaptic vesicle

A

chemical synapse

Figure 58. **a:** synaptic contacts between neurons, the small arrows indicate the direction of the flow of excitation. **b:** diagrammatic representation of a typical synapse. **c:** electrical synapse with hexagonal structures interconnecting two opposing membranes, they are perforated by transcellular channels (ionic channels) (A), in detail additional channels of diffusion (B) in the intercellular space are shown. **d:** detail of a chemical synapse. According to this interpretation a hexagonal system for the attachment of the synaptic vesicles exists. Presumably the vesicles empty their contents into channels of diffusion (A), similar in structure to those of the electrical synapse and opening out into intercellular cleft. Electrical synapses conduct into both directions, chemical ones ordinarily only into one. After AKERT, 1971

(synaptopores) in the presynaptic membrane into the synaptic cleft. In other regions of the body the liberation by exocytosis may be an important mechanism of release of transmitter.

Rather often a single neuron seems to fulfil both motor and neurosecretory functions, e.g. in the insect *Rhodnius* the axons which innervate the ventral abdominal intersegmental muscles make typical synaptic contacts with the muscle cells, but are also neurosecretory. In the synaptic area mainly light synaptic vesicles occur, in other parts of the axons groups of neurosecretory granules, which are released by exocytosis around the muscle cells and into the haemolymph.

The synapses mentioned so far are also called chemical synapses, since they transmit the electrical excitation by means of a chemical substance. In the so-called electrical synapses (Fig. 58) the impulse is transmitted without intercalated chemical substance and without temporal retardation, since the membranes of the opposing cells are in touch with each other. At the ultrastructural level small hexagonal structures may be recognized which contain pores representing transcellular channels.

In synapses at glandular and smooth muscle cells the membrane thickenings may be absent. The distance between pre- and post-synaptic membrane may be up to 1000 nm. In invertebrates the membrane thickenings are only rarely to be met with, also the accumulations of mitochondria often are absent or insignificant.

In the central nervous system or in ganglia neurons can form vast accumulations. Thus, in the human brain about 10^{10} neurons occur each with about 10^3-10^4 interconnections. The complete length of the connections between all neurons is about 300,000 km which corresponds to the distance from the moon to the earth. Nerve cells are characterized by an unusually high rate of protein metabolism. In the mammalian brain there is a complete turnover of protein in about fourteen days. About 15,000 protein molecules are synthesized per cell and per second – the cytological expression of these activities is the abundance of polysomes and rough ER cisternae. Some of these proteins are enzymes, another part can be seen in connection of the formation of engrammes. Synthesis of proteins and their transport into the periphery in the cytoplasmic processes can be influenced by the degree of excitation of the neuron. Neurons which are frequently stimulated produce more protein than those which are activated to a lesser extent. In rats fulfilling regularly specific tasks the RNA contents of the neurons increases considerably.

Neuroglial cells

This second component of the nervous system tissue fulfils various tasks, many of which, however, are still imperfectly known. They have a supporting function, play a role in transport between blood or lymph and neurons, they form myelin sheaths and have a protective and scavenger function (phagocytosis of foreign particles and removal of injured or destroyed components of the nervous tissue). Possibly some types of glial cells have a secretory function, e.g. the pituicytes in the neurohypophysis. Neurons and glial cells do not only show structural differences but also biochemical ones, e.g. the mitochondria of glial cells may contain more monoaminooxidase (MAO) and ATPase than those of neurons. The mitochondria of neurons contain particular enzymes associated with protein metabolism.

There is no uniform concept about the number of cell types which are included in the term neuroglial cells. Here we shall include the following cells; in vertebrates the ependymal cells, the glial cells proper (astrocytes, oligodendrocytes, microglia), the satellite (capsular cells, amphicytes) cells; in peripheral nerves the cells of Schwann, and in invertebrates various types of cells ensheathing or surrounding neurons.

Ependymal cells line the ventricles of the brain and the central canal in the spinal cord in chordates. In the lower chordates they are the only type of glial cells present; e.g. in amphioxus they form conspicuous ciliated elements, extending slender and branching processes from their perikarya, lining the central canal, to the periphery of the neural tube, where they terminate with foot-like endings. Their processes provide a coarse framework into which the neuronal processes are embedded. Similar cells occur in the neural cord of enteropneusts and in the epithelial nervous sytem of echinoderms where their origin from specialized supporting cells of the epidermis is particularly evident. Ciliated ependymal cells with long basal processes also occur in lower vertebrates and during ontogenesis of the higher ones. In adult mammals the ependymal cells form an epithelial layer in the choroid plexus and also in the other parts of the CNS they attain an epithelial character: they often bear apical cilia and microvilli and are interconnected by apical junctional complexes; their basal processes freely intermingle with the underlying neurons. In many areas particular organs are formed

Figure 59. Glial cells in mammals. **a, b:** astrocytes with pedicel-like extensions surrounding a blood vessel (**a**), or forming the surface layer of the central nervous system (**b**); **c:** oligodendrocytes in close spacial interrelation with nerve cells; these oligodendrocytes are also termed satellite cells; **d:** microglial cells. After GLEES, 1955

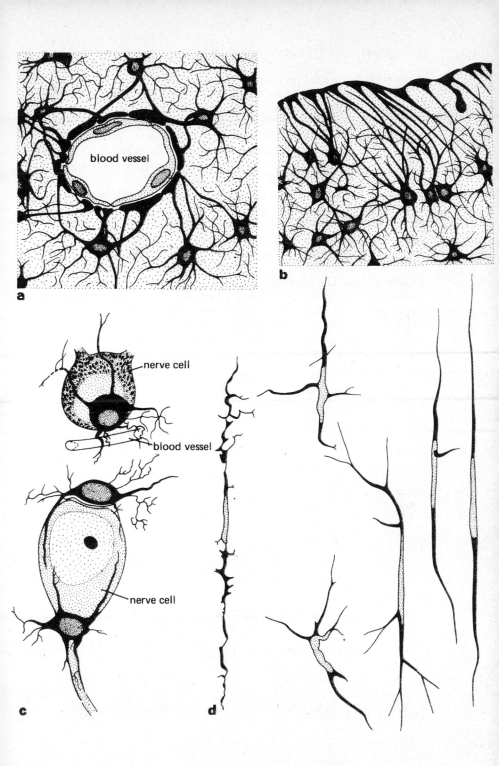

in the ependymal area (periventricular organs).

Astrocytes and oligodendrocytes because of their size are collectively termed macroglia.

Two varieties of astrocytes occur in mammals. Protoplasmic astrocytes with relatively abundant cytoplasm and relatively thick and short processes radiating from the perikaryon. Fibrous astrocytes possess fewer but longer processes containing accumulations of microfilaments. Such glial processes with numerous microfilaments are called neuroglial fibres in light microscopy. Protoplasmic astrocytes predominantly occur in the grey matter, fibrous ones in the white matter of the CNS. Both are interconnected by intermediate types. Their abundant processes fill the spaces between perikarya and processes of neurons and construct a dense three-dimensional network into which the neurons are embedded. The feltwork of neuronal and glial processes is called the neuropile. Particular foot-like processes of the astrocytes reach blood capillaries (Fig. 59) around which they form a continuous sheath, the *membrana limitans gliae perivascularis*. Other astrocytic processes reach the surface of the CNS and here constitute a second boundary layer the *membrana limitans piae* (Fig. 59) which is

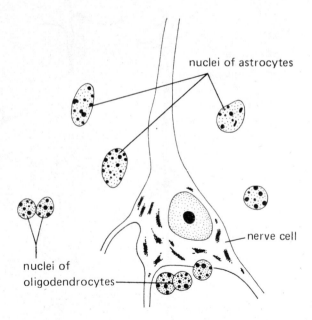

nuclei of astrocytes

nerve cell

nuclei of
oligodendrocytes

Figure 60.   Nuclei of glial cells from the cerebral cortex of man. After HAM, 1965

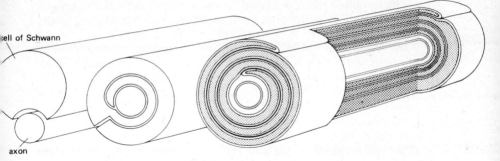

Figure 61. Formation of the sheath of Schwann; on the right the unit membrane is drawn by a double line, left and in the middle by a simple line.

covered by a basal lamina.

The nuclei of astrocytes generally are ovoid and relatively large (Fig. 60), the light ground cytoplasm of their pericarya is relatively poor in organclles, rough ER cisternae are generally absent. They often contain much glycogen.

Injuries of the CNS can induce a marked multiplication of astrocytes which form a scar. Such astrocytes can incorporate foreign material.

Oligodendrocytes are smaller and often are darker than the astrocytes and possess fewer branches. Their nucleus is more or less spherical or ovoid and relatively dark (Fig. 60), their cytoplasm is denser and contains ribosomes and juxtanuclear ER cisternae. Microfilaments are rare or appear to be absent. Transitional forms between astrocytes and oligodendrocytes have been described in particular in young animals. Oligodendrocytes occur in grey and white matter. In the white matter they frequently form rows of cells along nerve fibres. They build up the myelin sheaths (see below) of central nervous neurons and in tissue culture have been seen to exhibit rhythmic pulsatile movements.

The microglial cells are small cells with a dark elongated nucleus and a few processes. The cytoplasm contains among others a few rough ER cisternae, a well-developed Golgi apparatus and lysosomes. These cells act as brain macrophages and increase in size and divide when activated by injuries or invasion of foreign particles.

The Schwann cells surround neuronal processes in the periphery (see p. 112). As the neurons they are of ectodermal origin. Their nuclei generally are flattened and the cytoplasm contains few organelles. Their cytoplasm is drawn out into thin leaflets, in somatic nerves they form the myelin sheaths.

The satellite cells correspond to the Schwann cells in the area of the perikarya of peripheral neurons where occasionally (as in the *ganglion spirale*) they may also form thin myelin sheaths.

In vertebrates peripheral neuronal processes surrounded by Schwann cells are often called nerve fibres. In invertebrates processes of neurons frequently occur without accompanying glial cells and here also they are termed nerve fibres. Often any process of a nerve cell is termed a nerve fibre.

Peripheral nerve fibres of vertebrates. Each neuronal process is enclosed by numerous consecutive Schwann cells forming the sheath of Schwann, which in big and fast conducting neurons in addition can build up the myelin sheath. Small axons, in particular in the autonomic nervous system lack a myelin sheath but are always surrounded by a sheath of Schwann. Thus myelinated and unmyelinated fibres can be distinguished. The myelin sheath can be demonstrated in the light microscope by various methods (osmication, lipid stains and others) as a layer of variable thickness surrounding a usually pale axon or dendrite. Unmyelinated nerves in routine stains usually are difficult to make out.

The sheath of Schwann. In myelinated fibres, in which it is also called the neurilemma, it consists of the outer parts of the Schwann cells containing the flattened nucleus, whereas the inner parts of these cells build up the myelin sheath (Fig. 61). Both sheaths entirely surround one nerve cell process and outwards are surrounded by a basement lamina. Again both sheaths are interrupted at regular intervals by the nodes of Ranvier. These mark the extensions of the individual Schwann cells. The area between two nodes of Ranvier, which is occupied by one Schwann cell, is termed internodal area, it extends from about 200 to more than 1000 μm.

In unmyelinated nerves the sheath of Schwann is of different structure. Here numerous neuronal processes are embedded into deep invaginations of one Schwann cell. They are never entirely surrounded by the cytoplasm of the Schwann cell but in one place are in connection with the surface *via* a narrow cleft (Fig. 55).

The myelin sheath (Fig. 61). The structure of the myelin sheath can be understood by a brief description of its development. The Schwann cells settle down on a nerve cell process at specific distances and surround it by two lateral laminal extensions. One of

Figure 62. Glial cells in polychaetes, **a:** *Nereis* several profiles of microfilament containing glial cells, some of which surround a dendrite (d) of a neuron, arrows point to bundle of microfilaments; **b:** *Arenicola,* central nervous system, glial cell (g) characterized by vesicular and tubular membranous profiles separating perikarya of neurons containing neuro-secretory elementary granules, the vacuolar structures (asterisks) are presumably artefacts. x 18 000. b preparation C. NOWAK

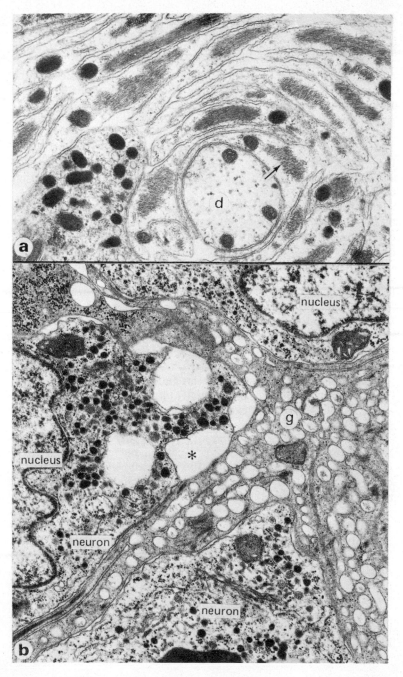

these becomes predominant and spirally surrounds the neuronal process for several times (more than fifty spirals have been found). During this process the cytoplasm is squeezed out of the extension and the final sheath only consists of numerous layers of membranous material. Within the sheath the outer leaflets of the opposing plasma membranes fuse so that it is constructed of alternating lipid and protein layers of different thickness (Fig. 61) As has been mentioned above nucleus and cytoplasm are confined to the outer aspects forming the sheath of Schwann.

Also in invertebrates glial cells are of wide distribution. Often they are characterized by bundles of microfilaments (Fig. 62), occasionally they contain granular inclusions ('granulocytes', Fig. 62).

Sheaths resembling the myelin sheath also occur in various types of invertebrates, especially in arthropods; e.g. in the crustacean *Palaemonetes* such a sheath around individual neurons consists of about twenty spirals, which, however, usually are separated by 20 nm wide intercellular clefts. The thin lamellae usually contain a small amount of cytoplasm and do not correspond to spirals but to individual lamellar processes of a glial cell, the nucleus of which is located in the interior part of the sheath near the neuronal process. Between these lamellar glial cells nodular areas occur, which however are filled by another type of glial cell, extending short finger-shaped projections to the axon and forming tight junctions with it.

Giant fibres. In many invertebrates and occasionally also in vertebrates neuronal processes of unusually large diameter occur (phoronids, annelids, enteropneusts, amphioxus, teleosts (Mauthner's neurons) and others.

Structures formed by the nervous tissue. In higher animals the nervous tissue usually constitutes a central nervous system (CNS) and a peripheral nervous system. In vertebrates the CNS consists of brain and spinal chord, the peripheral nervous system of all the nervous tissue outside the CNS. Those parts of the vertebrate CNS containing the perikarya, the proximal sections of the processes as well as terminals are usually termed grey matter. Specific groups of perikarya in the grey matter we call nuclei. Surrounding the grey matter one finds a zone which contains only neuronal, generally myelinated processes and glial cells called white matter, in which neuronal perikarya are absent. Specific bundles of myelinated processes are called tracts.

Ganglia are smaller concentrations of perikarya. In many invertebrates a large ganglion of central functional importance is located in the anterior region and is also called a brain (arthropods, cephalopods). In vertebrates ganglia are always outside the CNS. Two types can be recognized, sensory and autonomic ones.

Sensory ganglia, e.g. the spinal ganglia and the *ganglion semilunare*, usually contain pseudounipolar neurons with centrally located nucleus and various numbers of multipolar neurons. In the ganglion of the *nervus statoacusticus* bipolar neurons occur. The perikarya are surrounded by satellite cells.

Autonomous ganglia contain multipolar neurons with eccentrically located nucleus. Sympathetic perikarya occasionally contain two nuclei and melanin. An important characteristic of these ganglia is the presence of synapses, transferring impulses from the first to the second neuron. Such synapses are absent in sensory ganglia. The perikarya are generally surrounded by a few satellite cells.

Nerves are branching cord-like structures consisting of bundles of neuronal processes and associated Schwann cells. In invertebrates they generally additionally contain neuronal perikarya and are termed medullary rays.

LITERATURE

AKERT, K. 'Struktur und Ultrastruktur von Nervenzellen und Synapsen.' *Klin. Wschr.* **49**, 509-519 (1971).
ANDREW, W. *Textbook of comparative histology.* Oxford University Press, New York (1959), 652 pp.
—, HICKMAN, C. P. *Histology of the vertebrates.* C. V. Mosby Company, Saint Louis (1974), 439 pp.
BARGMANN, W. *Histologie und mikroskopische Anatomie des Menschen.* 6. Aufl. Thieme Verlag, Stuttgart, (1967) 784 pp.
—'Zur Architektur der Mesogloea.' *Z. Zellsforsch,* **123,** 66-81 (1972).
BLOOM, W., FAWCETT, D. W. *A textbook of histology.* 9th edition. Saunders Co., Philadelphia (1970). 858 pp.
FRANZINI-ARMSTRONG, C. 'The structure of a simple Z-line.' *J. Cell Biol.* **58**, 630-642 (1973).
HALSTEAD, L. B. *Vertebrate hard tissues.* Wykehain Publ., London (1974). 179 pp.
HAM, A. W. *Histology.* Pitman Med. Publishing Co., London. (1975). 7th ed. 902 pp.
HEUMANN, H.-G., ZEBE, E. 'Über Feinbau und Funktionsweise der Fasern aus dem Hautmuskelschlauch des Regenwurms, *Lumbricus terrestris.'* L. Z. Zellforsch. **78,** 131-150 (1967).
HUXLEY, H. E. 'The mechanism of muscular contraction.' *Science.* **164**, 1356-1366 (1969).
KELLY, R. E., RICE, R. V. 'Ultrastructural studies on the contractile mechanism of smooth muscle.' *J. Cell Biol.* **42**, 683-694 (1969).
KOMNICK, H., STOCKEM, W., WOHLFARTH-BOTTERMANN, K. E. 'Ursachen, Begleitphänomene und Steuerung zellulärer Bewegungserscheinungen.' *Fortschritte d. Zool.* **21,** 1, 74 S. 1972.
KRAUSE, R. *Mikroskopische Anatomie der Wirbeltiere in Einzeldarstellungen.* W. de Gruyter, Berlin. (1921), 906 pp.

116   COMPARATIVE ANIMAL CYTOLOGY & HISTOLOGY

LEONHARDT, H. *Histologie, Zytologie Und Mikroanatomie des Menschen.* G. Thieme Verlag, Stuttgart 4th edition (1974). 467 pp.

LUCIANO, L. 'Die Feinstruktur der Tränendrüse der Ratte und ihr Geschlechtsdimorphismus'. *Z. Zellforsch.* **76**, 1-20 (1967).

PANNER, B. J., HONIG, C. R. 'Filament ultrastructure and organization in vertebrate smooth muscle. Contraction hypothesis based on localization of actin and myosin.' *J. Cell Biol.* **35**, 303-321 (1967).

PAH, D. J., PATT, G. R. 'Comparative vertebrate histology.' Harper and Row, New York (1969), 438 pp.

ROSENBLUTH, J. 'Ultrastructural organization of obliquely striated muscle fibers in *Ascaris lumbricoides.' J. Cell Biol.* **25**, 495-515 (1965).

RÜEGG, J. C. 'Contractile mechanisms of smooth muscle.' In *Aspects of cell motility* (P. L. Miller, ed.). XXII, 45-67, University Press, Cambridge (1968).

SCHNEPF, E., WENNEIS, W., SCHILDKNECHT, H. 'Über Arthropoden-Abwehrstoffe XLI. Zur Explosionschemie der Bombardierkäfer (Coleoptera, Carabidae). *Z. Zellforsch.* **96**, 582-599 (1969).

SCHNEIDER, K. C. *Histologisches Praktikum der Tiere für Studenten und Forscher,* G. Fischer Verlag. Jena (1908) 615 pp.

SINGER, I. 'An electron microscopic and autoradiographic study of mesogloeal organization and collagen synthesis in the sea anemone *Aiptasia diaphana.'* Cell Tiss. Res. **149**, 537-554 (1974).

WELSCH, U., STORCH, V. 'Über den Aufbau der Chorda dorsalis niederer Wirbeltiere.' *Zool. Anz., Suppl.* **33**, 601-606 (1970).

Chapter 3
INTEGUMENT

The surface of the animal body is represented by the skin or integument. It consists of two parts of different character and origin: the epithelial ectodermal more superficial epidermis and the deeper mesodermal dermis. Cnidarians and ctenophores only have an epidermis, sponges usually represent a special situation.

The integument has numerous functions: it protects the organism against injuries and in land-living forms against desiccation; it receives stimuli of the surroundings by means of own or associated sensory cells; it can absorb nutrients and excrete waste substances, frequently it has respiratory functions; in higher vertebrates it plays a role in maintaining the water-household and in thermo-regulation. By particular surface structures, colour patterns and associated muscle cells it often is an expressive means of behaviour.

All these functions frequently are due to the properties of the epidermis which in most animals is a simple epithelium, but in vertebrates the epithelium is stratified. The epidermal epithelium may contain specialized cells forming appendages of the body, e.g. setae, feathers or hairs, or producing secretions. Such secretory cells in vertebrates frequently form glands which during ontogeny descend into the dermis.

In numerous, and above all water-dwelling animals the epidermal epithelium is ciliated and bears apical microvilli. In small organisms the ciliary beat serves for locomotion in the water; additionally food particles can be extracted and transported by cilia. Ciliated epidermal epithelia are of wide distribution, e.g. in turbellarians, nemerteans, rotifers, molluscs, annelids, tentaculates, echinoderms, hemichordates. In gnathostomulids the epidermis consists of flagellated cells. In part of the above-mentioned groups, only certain areas of the epidermis bear cilia, e.g. in rotifers.

The surface of sponges is formed by flat epithelial cells (pinakocytes), which easily become detached from each other and form new connections with other cells. Their cytoplasm contains contractile elements. In fresh water sponges the epidermal cells contain contractile vacuoles otherwise known only in protozoans.

The epidermis (ectoderm) of the cnidarians contains specific cell types normally absent in other animals, e.g. desmocytes. cnidoblasts and epitheliomuscular cells (Fig. 64).

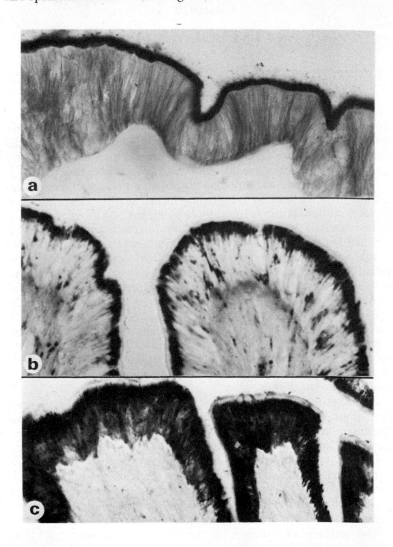

Figure 63. Enzyme histochemical preparations of the integument of the cephalic tentacles of various prosobranch snails. **a:** Cholinesterase, *Aporrhais*, localized predominantly in the brush border. x 380; **b:** Indoxylacetate esterase, (*Neptunea*) predominantly in a zone below the brush border, x 310; **c:** α-naphthyl acetate esterase, *Littorina*, the whole cytoplasm below the brush border gives a positive reaction x 380

epidermis   gastrodermis

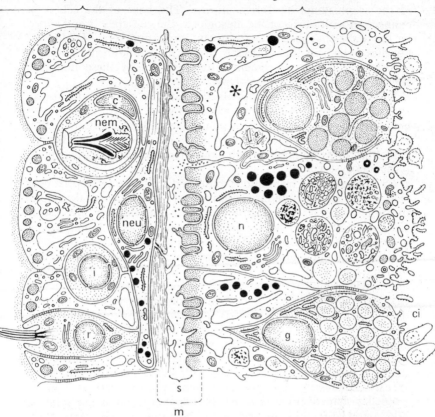

Figure 64. Schematic representation of a longitudinal section through the body wall of *Hydra*, after electron microscopical findings. The epidermis (= ectoderm) is predominantly composed of epitheliomuscular cells (e), which apically contain secretory granules presumably giving rise to a fine filamentous surface coat. In their basal processes they contain longitudinally oriented myofilaments. Between these cells cnidoblasts (c) occur, containing nematocysts (nem) and arising from interstitial cells (i). In addition neurons (neu) and receptor cells (r) are to be found. The latter bear an apical cilium and are basally interconnected with a neuron (secondary receptor cell). Primary receptor cells have also been described. Epi- and gastrodermis are separated by a supporting lamella (s, mesogloea). The gastrodermis (=endoderm) also is composed predominantly of epitheliomuscular cells, here they mainly serve the resorption and digestion of food (nutritive epitheliomuscular cells, n). Their basal myofilaments are arranged in a circular manner. (m indicates the complete contractile apparatus). The nutritive cells contain food vacuoles, lipid and glycogen. As the epidermal cells they often contain large vacuoles (asterisk). In addition glandular cells bear two cilia (ci), difficult to detect in light microscopical preparations. After Lentz 1966

Desmocytes occur in sessile forms, especially e.g. in the foot plate of the scyphistoma of *Aurelia aurita*. The base of the cell is in connection with fibrils of the mesogloea, the cell apex is embedded in the cuticle. These cells produce large numbers of filament bundles (which in the epidermis are termed tonofibrils) and die. Cuticle and mesogloea remain interconnected by these filaments serving as anchorage for the polyps.

Before describing the cnidoblasts – unique cells producing an exploding capsule – a few terms will briefly be defined: cnidoblast = nematoblast = nettle cell. Occasionally the fully differentiated cell is called a cnidocyte or a nematocyte and only those cells are termed cnidoblast or nematoblast which contain a developing nettle capsule (= nematocyst, cnide).

Cnidoblasts arise from undifferentiated cells, the interstitial cells (Fig. 65). These contain large numbers of ribosomes and develop in the following way: Golgi apparatus and granular ER increase in size, the future nematocyst initially appears as a homogeneous matrix in a Golgi vacuole, which constantly increases in size since numerous small Golgi vesicles fuse with it discharging their contents into its lumen. While the nematocyst becomes bigger a striking increase in rough ER can be observed. The immature nematocyst at first develops an apical process also containing matrix and later disappearing again. The matrix differentiates a marginal zone, forming the future capsule and being of low electron density. In the centrally located electron dense matrix stilettes and spines make their appearance which are separated from the matrix by particulate dense material which is in contact with the capsule. In addition a thread develops in the matrix which in cross-sections appears propeller-shaped (Fig. 66). At the apex of the nematocyst an operculum differentiates, evidently being a special part of the capsule. While differentiating the cyst is surrounded by parallel-arranged microtubules converging towards the nearby Golgi apparatus. They are thought to transport material, but this is speculative. When the cyst is fully differentiated the rough ER disintegrates into individual vesicles and free ribosomes. Also the Golgi apparatus decreases in size. This regression is irreversible; if a nematocyst has exploded, the cnidoblast degenerates.

By being stimulated the operculum opens; stilettes, spicules and thread are eversed. The underlying mechanism of this explosion is still unknown.

In the light microscope almost twenty types of nematocysts have been distinguished, of which *Hydra* possesses four. Two main groups can be recognized: astomocnides, the thread of which does not have a terminal opening, and stomocnides with a terminal

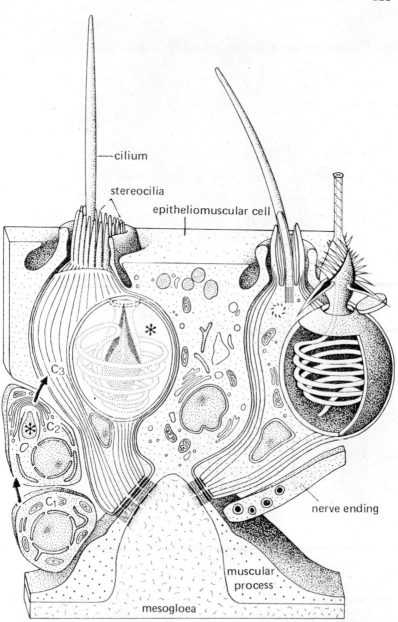

Figure 65. Fine structure of cnidoblasts in the epidermis of *Hydra*, arrows indicate process of maturation of cnidoblast (C_1 to C_3), asterisk: early stage of nematocyst near Golgi apparatus in C_2, mature cyst in C_3 From REMANE, STORCH, WELSCH, 1974 after SLAUTTERBACH, 1961

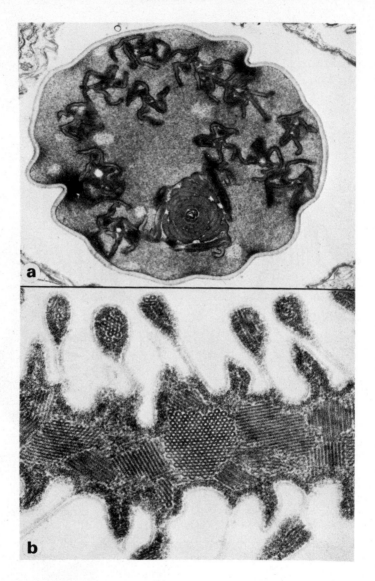

Figure 66. Nematocyt of *Pachycerianthus* (Ceriantharia, Anthozoa). **a:** Nematocyst with profiles of the thread (propeller shaped) and the stylet (below) both of which are embedded into the matrix, x 18 000; **b:** thread, longitudinal section, x 50 000. Photo K. MORITZ

opening through which the contents of the capsule can be injected into the prey. The first group e.g. includes the desmonemes (also termed volvents) with a spirally wound up thread, the second the haplonemes with a simple thread (into this sub-group fall the glutinants) and the heteronemes with a clearly recognizable shaft, which can bear stilettes (penetrants).

Cnidoblasts are at the same time receptor and effector elements. Several cnidoblasts are connected via special zones of contact with an epitheliomuscular cell, containing near the mesogloeal supporting lamella coarse and fine filaments. In the area of contact between the two cell types, both contain microtubules vertically oriented in relation to the surface. Associated with this cellular complex are nerve endings containing partly neurosecretory granules. Possibly the epitheliomuscular cell activates the cnidoblasts connected with it.

The receptor pole of the cnidoblasts exhibits its own differentiations: around a modified cilium stout specialized microvilli ('stereocilia') can be found in regular arrangement. This grouping is also known from the apex of mechanoreceptor cells (Fig. 86). The whole formation is called in cnidarians cnidocil.

The nematocyst of myxosporidians (Protozoa) agrees largely in its structure with that of the cnidarians.

One ctenophore species (*Euchlora rubra*) is also said to have its own cnidoblasts in the epidermis. If found in other invertebrates they have originated from the food of these animals (e.g. nudibranchs) consisting of cnidarians (kleptocnides).

The epitheliomuscular cells form the majority of cells in the ectoderm of cnidarians. Their basal extensions contain myofilaments and together form a closed layer of longitudinal muscular elements. The endodermal epithelium (gastrodermis) forms a corresponding layer of circular muscle elements.

Among the most complicated cell types of the animal kingdom are the colloblasts (Fig. 67), which occur in groups lying closely together on the tentacles of ctenophores. Their sticky secretion is responsible for capturing and glueing planctonic organisms to the surface of the tentacles. They are stalked cells which are anchored in the superficial parts of the mesogloea and which additionally are connected by extracellular fibrils with the smooth muscle cells of the highly contractile tentacles. The apex of the stalk bears the head of the colloblast, in the periphery of which secretory granules occur. These are interconnected by strings of electron-dense material (radii) with the peculiar centrally located star-shaped body, to which also the long nucleus is attached which in the area of contact is without a nuclear envelope. The nucleus extends into the stalk. Also extending from the star-shaped body is a tubule with electron-dense walls

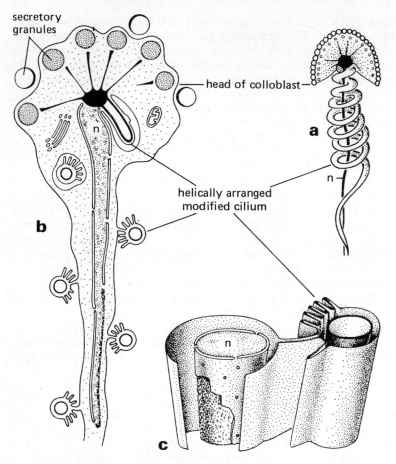

Figure 67.   Schematic representation of the colloblast. **a:** light microscopy (after
Komai 1922); **b, c:** electron microscopy; **b:** longitudinal section; **c:** three-dimensional
reconstruction of the neck-region, n: nucleus, which partly lacks a nuclear envelope.
Basally the cell is attached to the basement membrane by a root-shaped basal process

which winds spirally around the stalk and terminates basally in a
specific root-like structure. Both straight oriented nucleus and
spirally arranged tubule are surrounded by the plasma membrane
which forms only a thin bridge between the two (Fig. 67). Star-
shaped body and tubule are derived from a specialized cilium, as
studies of differentiating colloblasts have shown.

The epidermis of turbellarians is particularly rich in glandular
cells, and some epithelial cells contain a formed secretory product,

the rhabdites. The cells forming the rhabdites are generally sunk deeply into the subepidermal connective tissue and reach the surface only by means of a narrow neck. The rhabdites are slender pointed bodies of various lengths, which in macrostomides may be everted within seconds when the animals are irritated. During this process the rhabdites elongate and their proximal part forms a so-called thread of discharge. The whole ejection of the rhabdite is considered to be a swelling phenomenon in many cases dissolving the structure of the rhabdite and starting at the proximal end. In the light microscopic literature the similarity in structure and mode of discharge with the trichocysts of protozoans (Fig. 18) is stressed. In the electron microscope the mature rhabdites of macrostomides usually consist of a granular central mass surrounded by layers of microfilaments. Two inner layers of helically arranged filaments and an outer circular layer of filaments can be observed to which still loosely arranged longitudinal filaments can be attached. The rhabdites of *Bothrioplana* consist of numerous electron-dense lamellae, concentrically arranged around the long axis of the rhabdite, which are surrounded by a structureless envelope. These rhabdites are of the discharging type, in which the structure after discharge is changed but not dissolved. Rhabdites of the swelling type dissolve after coming in contact with the surrounding water into mucus-like masses which are repellant to enemies. In land-living forms this secretion together with that of mucus cells of the epidermis forms the cysts.

In trematodes and cestodes the body is covered by a submerged epithelium, in which an epithelial cytoplasmic layer lies upon the basement lamina, whereas the nuclei are located in saccular parts of the cytoplasm submerged into the underlying tissues (Fig. 68). Both parts of the epithelium are interconnected by slender strands of cytoplasm between which cells of the outer muscle layer are to be found. The plasma membranes running vertically to the body surface dissolve, so that the epidermis consists of an syncytium with submerged perikarya.

The outer cytoplasmic rim in trematodes frequently contains spines consisting of proteinaceous material, which can even be recognized in the light microscope. In developmental stages with an intestine the apical surface is nearly smooth or forms cupular projections, in stages without an intestine it differentiates numerous branched microvilli.

In cestodes, which in all of their developmental stages are gutless, the surface of the cytoplasmic rim is always increased by long unbranched microvilli. In rare cases the microvilli exhibit apical inflations (*Tylocephalum*), normally they bear pointed electron dense tips, which often are deflected backwards. Size and frequency

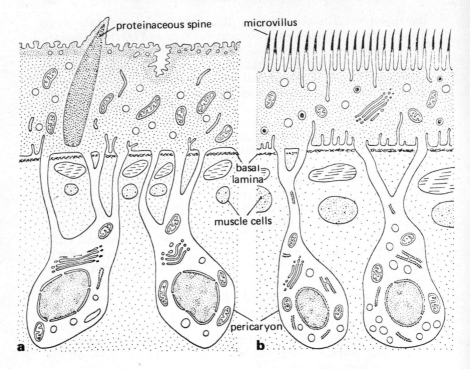

Figure 68. Integument of platy helminths; electron microscopy. **a:** *Fasciola* (liver fluke), **b:** *Abothrium* (cestode), in both cases the perikarya are submerged

of the microvilli differ in the individual stages of development. In *Diphyllobothrium latum* the plerocercoids which live in poikilothermic animals (fishes) have about 4-5 microvilli of 1.5 μm length per μm^2, in the homoiothermic final host (man) the microvilli rapidly increase in size and number; adult animals have about 25-30 microvilli of 4 μm length per μm^2. This apical border has the function of absorbing food and contains numerous enzymes for this purpose. Protein synthesis, however, seems to be confined to the perikaryon. This assumption is supported by electron microscopic observations (lack of rough ER and ribosomes) and autoradiographic studies. Radioactive proline (parenterally absorbed) can first be demonstrated to be incorporated into proteins in the perikaria. It is believed that the proteins are transported from here into the superficial parts of the syncytium.

Mitochondria are rather common in the cestode epidermis; they are small and contain few cristae. They certainly are of little significance for aerobic processes, since adult cestodes live in media

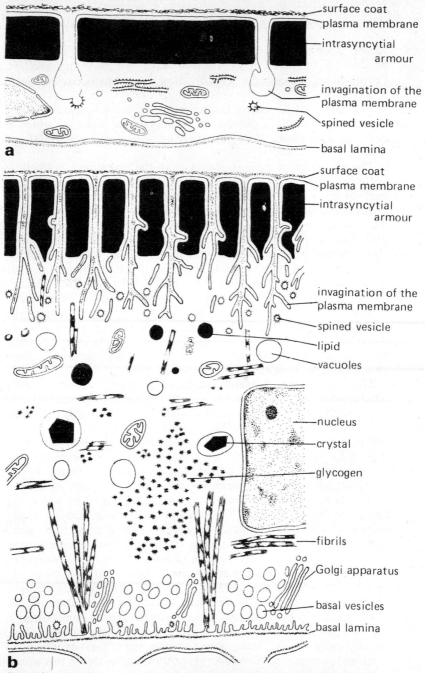

surface coat
plasma membrane
intrasyncytial
armour
invagination of the
plasma membrane
spined vesicle
basal lamina

a

surface coat
plasma membrane
intrasyncytial
armour
invagination of the
plasma membrane
spined vesicle
lipid
vacuoles
nucleus
crystal
glycogen
fibrils
Golgi apparatus
basal vesicles
basal lamina

b

Figure 69. Fine structure of the rotifer (**a**) and acanthocephalan (**b**) integument. In rotifers the body cavity follows below the epidermis, in acanthocephala fibrils and muscle cells lie below the integument. After REMANE, STORCH & WELSCH, 1974

rather poor in oxygen. They play a role in the anoxidative production of ATP in connection with citrulline metabolism. Furthermore, in cestodes CO_2-fixation seems to occur partly in mitochondria.

The epidermis of rotifers and acanthocephalans is also composed of a syncytium. Both possess an intrasyncytial armour, which is perforated by pores, through which an exchange of material can take place.

The ontogeny of rotifers shows that the epidermal epithelium initially is composed of individual cells. Later in the postcoronal parts of the body the vertical plasma membranes are dissolved, only in the epidermal parts of the corona do they remain partly intact; here multi-nuclear cells, in the postcoronal parts a uniform syncytium arises. Next the outer plasma membrane forms minute semispherical invaginations and the intrasyncytial armour develops, which can be of homogeneous structure (*Keratella*), horizontally layered (*Notommata*) or vertically striated (*Mytilina, Brachionus*). Then an active phase of secretory activity begins. Protein and carbohydrate material are combined in the Golgi areas and transported in small vesicles to the apical invaginations, into which the contents are discharged. The material spreads over the whole surface. In the mature animal the hemispherical invaginations change into bottle-shaped structures (Fig. 69).

The integument of acanthocephalan larvae (acanthor) is of a similar structure. In the adult acanthocephalans the number and depth of the invaginations increase markedly thus greatly extending the resorptive surface of this gutless endoparasite. The whole syncytial epidermis is rather thick and can be divided into four zones (Fig. 69). Apically a strong intrasyncytial layer of electron-dense material occurs, which is perforated by numerous finger-shaped invaginations of the plasmalemma (corresponding to the 'armour' of the rotifers). Below it a zone may be distinguished in which the elongated invagination of the plasma membrane and unusually numerous pinocytotic vesicles (generally spined ones) dominate. Next a fibrous layer follows usually containing lipid inclusions and areas of glycogen. The final basal zone is characterized by numerous vacuoles. As in rotifers the syncytium is underlain by a basement lamina. Apically it is covered by a layer of mucopolysaccharides, which are thought to inactivate the digestive enzymes of the host.

The uptake of food through the epidermis has been demonstrated, e.g. in experiments with amino acids, which have shown that female *Moniliformis* in the same time absorb ten times as much L-methionine as males. Also *Macracanthorhynchus* shows this sexual dimorphism; however, to a lesser extent. Protein- and carbohydrate-metabolism of the integument are assumed to take place essentially in the integument of the body region. Lipid metabolism generally is mainly ascribed to the lemniscs. These structures are elongated formations of the syncytium of the neck region, with which they are in direct continuity, and extend into the body cavity. Their cytoplasm contains numerous lipid inclusions and lysosomes, their apical intracellular layer of dense material is thinner than in the body region.

An extracellular layer which is free of cells and covers the whole epidermis, is called a cuticle. A particularly thick cuticle can be called an exoskeleton, the rigidity of which has the consequence that it must be periodically cast off during growth. If a solid layer loosely overlies the epidermis it is called a shell. Finally also the mesoderm can form calcareous exoskeletons which may reach the surface and displace the epidermis.

The epidermis of nematodes may consist either of cells or is a syncytium. The nuclei are concentrated in four longitudinal rows (epidermal cords). Usually the epidermis is covered by a cuticle which in many species consists of three parts: cortex, matrix and fibrous layers (Fig. 73). These three principal layers do not contain chitin and may be further subdivided. *Ascaris* is a genus which has been thoroughly investigated with regard to its cuticle. The outermost layer is the thin lipid-containing surface membrane. Next follows the cortex, which in *Ascaris* is subdivided into an outer homogeneous and an inner fibrous cortex. Below the cortex a loosely structured fibrillar layer can be distinguished which is pervaded by numerous channels connecting cortex and the deeper matrix layer, which in the electron microscope is of homogeneous structure. The matrix consists of proteins, in particular of elastin- and fibroin-like fibrous proteins, and contains enzymes which presumably play a role during growth of the cuticle. Below it three fibrous layers consisting of collagen fibrils occur. Each of these is composed of densely packed fibrils running helically around the body, their direction varies in the three layers. Under these fibrous layers finally a so-called basal lamella can be recognized which also consists of filamentous material. In it and in the fibrous layer channels can be demonstrated originating from the surface of the epidermal cells.

In the free-living marine nematode *Euchromadora vulgaris* only four layers can be distinguished; in many small species the fibrous layers are absent.

In the intestinal parasite *Nippostrongylus brasiliensis*, the matrix layer is replaced by a fluid-filled space containing enzymes and haemoglobin. It also contains electron-dense longitudinal supporting elements, to which correspond the sharp ridges of the

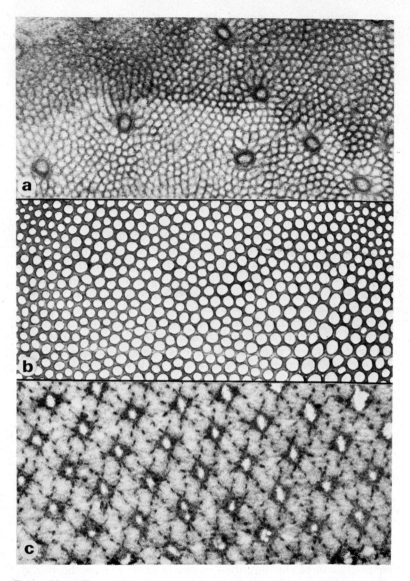

Figure 70. **a:** Tangential section through the relatively loosely constructed intra-syncytial armour of *Brachionus* (Rotatoria), the large circular profiles correspond to the invaginations of the apical plasma membrane. x 45 000; **b:** cross-section through a chaeta of *Echiurus* (Echiurida) x 6000. Photo K. MORITZ; **c:** tangential section through the perforated cuticle of the pharynx of *Trachydemus* (Kinorhyncha). Photo R. STORCH x 45 000

body surface. The fluid-filled space is traversed by collagen fibrils connecting cortex and fibrous layer.

During moulting the material of the old cuticle can be partly reabsorbed, e.g. in plant parasites. In other species the cuticle is completely cast off and no parts of it are reincorporated into the body.

In the epidermal cells the contents of lipid and glycogen is strikingly high. In parasites they may also contain haemoglobin.

The cuticle of the kinorhynchs consists of uniform solid scales which are interconnected by fibrillar areas (Fig. 70). According to electron microscope observations the epidermis consists of individual cells, however, the intercellular space is particularly narrow.

The cuticle of the nematomorphs resembles that of annelids (see below), the epidermis is composed of a syncytium.

Also the epidermis of annelids, sipunculids and pogonophorans is covered by a cuticle, which is composed of collagen fibrils oriented in parallel layers. The direction of the fibres forms right angles in consecutive layers (Fig. 71). Thus a meshwork is formed which in annelids frequently and in Pogonophora always is penetrated by microvilli. In annelids the outermost cuticular layer often is a homogeneous electron dense epicuticle.

The collagen of the annelid cuticle differs from that of vertebrates by its high contents of bound carbohydrates, which can reach 18 per cent (1 per cent in vertebrates). The collagen fibrils do not exhibit any cross-striation.

Rarely a cuticle is absent, e.g. in the polychaete *Chaetopterus variopedatus*. In this species the epidermal cells also secrete collagen fibrils but these, however, become detached from the body surface and form the tube of this sedentary polychaete. The fine structure of the tube corresponds completely to that of the cuticle of other polychaetes.

The same cuticular structure characterizes land-living polychaetes, oligochaetes and leeches, the same is true of sipunculids, the cuticle of which, however, neither in marine nor in land-living (*Physcosoma lurco*) species is penetrated by microvilli.

In the gutless Pogonophora the food is absorbed through the body surface. It is assumed that gases are absorbed through the epidermis of the highly vascularized tentacles, and food particles through the whole epidermis of the body. The exchange of substances may take place at the surface of the microvilli and by pinocytotic vesicles at their bases. The possibility has been discussed that enzymes are secreted by particular epidermal cells into the surrounding water having a function in extracellular digestion. Small molecules can

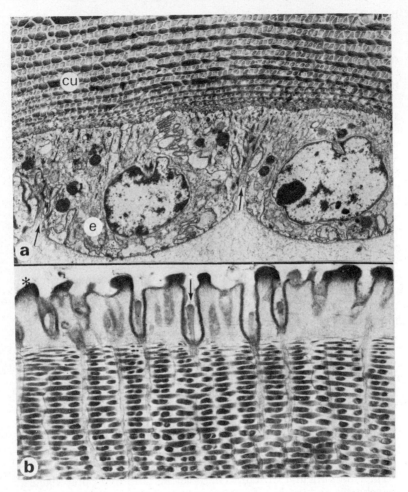

Figure 71.   **a:** *Phascolion* (Sipunculida) epidermis cell (e) covered by a thick cuticle (cu). Arrows point to upfoldings of the subepidermal connective tissue, x 6000; **b:** cuticle of *Ceratonereis* (Polychaeta); note invaginations of the electron dense epicuticle (asterisk) into which microvilli project (arrow) x 14 400

Figure 72.   Three-dimensional reconstruction of a quarter of a chaeta-producing follicle of *Lingula* (Brachiopoda), F: subepidermal fibrils; nf: nucleus of follicular cell; nch: nucleus of chaetoblast, mv: microvilli of chaetoblast; ER: rough ER, Go: Golgi apparatus; mit: mitochondrium; g: glycogen; inspired after BOULIGAND, 1967

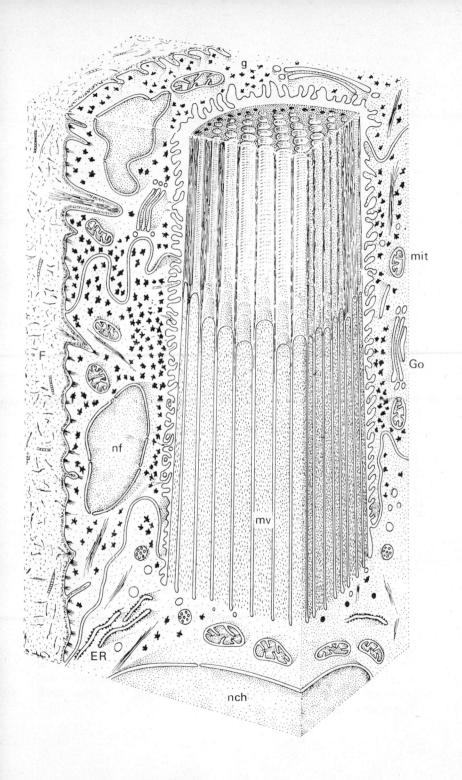

g

mit

Go

F

nf

mv

ER

nch

also be resorbed through the cuticle of polychaetes, which absorb small quantities of glucose, amino acids and other substances through their integument from the seawater.

Not only the structure of the cuticle is almost identical in annelids and Pogonophora, but also mode of formation and structure of the chaetae. Evidently these chaetae are a phylogenetically old structure, for also in primitive brachiopods, e.g. *Lingula*, such setae occur at the edge of the mantle. In late embryonic and juvenile octopods (Cephalopoda) they are also found on the integument (Kölliker's tufts). In all four groups of animals they arise from a single cell, the chaetoblast, which is located at the basis of small follicular invaginations of the epidermis (Fig. 72). The chaetoblast bears a group of long microvilli arising from a circular area of the cellular apex. They secrete fine filamentous material which solidifies in the extracellular space between the microvilli and is pushed into an apical direction into the follicular lumen. It is the construction material for the setae, the space over the microvilli remains free of it. The complete seta thus consists of a system of tight filaments surrounding a number of tubes corresponding to the spaces above the microvilli. The diameter of these tubes continuously decreases from base to tip and from the centre to the periphery. The extreme marginal zone only consists of fibrous material.

The configuration of the apical surface of the chaetoblast changes continuously during secretion. Sequential modulations of the number, size, shape, arrangement and orientation of the microvilli of the chaetoblast seem to be responsible for the modellation of the frequently complicated structure of the annelid setae.

The integument of priapulids (*Priapulus*) consists of cells with euchromatin-rich nuclei, abundant rough ER and basal infoldings. The surface of these cells is covered apically by a thick cuticle, which is composed of apparently randomly oriented fine filamentous material, which does not exhibit any structural peculiarities.

The cuticle of insects forms an exoskeleton consisting of hard and elastic plates which are interconnected by flexible articular membranes. It is secreted by flattened or cuboidal epidermal cells, the height of which varies according to the moulting cycle. Specific epidermal glandular cells liberate their products through cuticular pores to the surface. Derived from the epidermis are the oenocytes which may remain in contact with it or be localized deeper in the body cavity. They are frequently characterized by a dense cytoplasm and crystalloid inclusions. They play a role in the synthesis of cuticulin, a lipid-protein complex, which is found in the endo- and exocuticle and which renders rigidity to it before it is sclerotized. (For other functions, see p. 206.)

The cuticle consists of three layers which can also be seen in the light microscope: an outer thin epicuticle, a usually dark and hard exocuticle and an inner colourless and softer endocuticle. Endo- and exocuticle together are also termed procuticle; they consist of the polysaccharide chitin and various proteins.

The hardness of the exocuticle is due to the presence of chinones the precursors of which are secreted by the epidermal epithelium. In certain areas of the cuticle, e.g. in tendons, wing articulations and ligaments, the protein resilin occurs, rendering these structures extraordinarily elastic.

In the light microscope the endocuticle appears to be lamellated. In the electron microscope it consists of a structureless matrix (protein) into which filaments (chitin) are embedded. The filaments form several layers (laminae) in which they run in parallel to the surface. The laminae appear to be connected by semicircularly arranged filaments giving rise to the so-called parabolic pattern (Fig. 73).

According to an opinion shared by many authors, this appearance is due to the following structural principle: all filaments, also those forming the semicircular structures, run in parallel to the body surface. The filaments of one layer are also oriented in parallel. However, the direction of the filaments in the consecutive layers changes by small angles in a regular pattern. In consecutive laminae the filaments are of antiparallel orientation (Fig. 74).

The lamellation of the endocuticle is not always regular. In Orthoptera the layers are of different structure according to the time in which they are deposited. Layers deposited at night correspond to the above pattern, layers deposited during the day all consist of filaments oriented in one direction.

In the harder exocuticle this structural order is less clearly to be observed. It is supposed that its protein matrix is denser obscuring the chitinous filaments. The epicuticle is free of chitin and again consists of various sublayers. Most important is a sublayer which in the electron-microscopical literature is termed cuticulin layer, which, however, does not contain cuticulin. It is very thin and consists of vertically arranged and polymerized lipid molecules. It is the first layer which is formed and determines the shape of the insect. On top of it a wax and cement layer can be deposited, below a homogeneous layer of dense material (dense layer) can be formed.

Normally the cuticle is pervaded by pore channels originating from the endocuticle and terminating under the epicuticle or at the surface. In the latter case the pore channels branch and penetrate the epicuticle by means of delicate wax-filled canaliculi. Possibly wax is secreted through these canaliculi, since this can be renewed

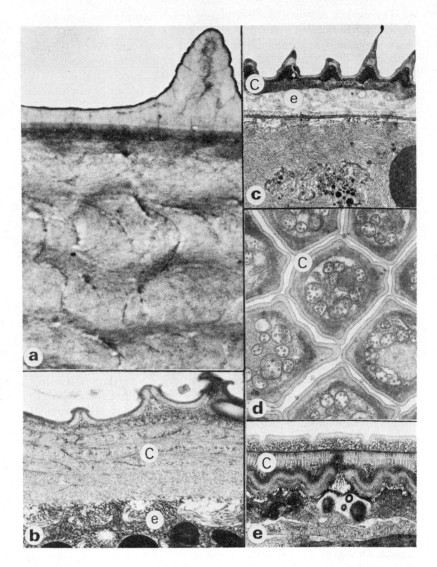

Figure 73. **a:** upper parts of the cuticle of a larva of the Ceratopogonidae, x 30 000; **b:** cuticle (C) of *Podura* (Collembola) e: epidermis, x 18 000 **c:** cuticle (c) with process of *Bdella* (mite), e: epidermis x 5400; **d:** *Porcellio* (Crustacea) projections of an antenna, filled by processes of receptor cells, C: cuticle x 18 000; **e:** *Tobrilus* (Nematoda), C: cuticle x 14 400

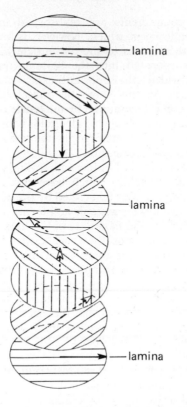

Figure 74. Schematic reconstruction of the insect cuticle. Each disk corresponds to a layer of filaments, the orientation of which is indicated by an arrow. In the consecutive laminae the filaments take an antiparallel course. After NEVILLE 1970

also between two moults. Loss of water might also be due to the presence of these channels.

Moulting may commence by an extension of the epidermal cells and by numerous mitoses. The multiplication of cells leads to a folding of the epidermis. Moulting of the insect exoskeleton is initiated by the separation of the epidermal epithelium from the inner surface of the endocuticle, giving rise to a cleft-like space. A moulting fluid containing inactive proteases and chitinases is secreted into the subcuticular cleft. The first part of the new cuticle, which is formed by the epidermis, is the cuticulin layer. It at first consists of isolated areas which soon fuse to a common layer covering the epidermal cells. After this has happened the enzymes of the moulting fluid are activated and begin to destroy the old endocuticle. Its components are reabsorbed into the epidermis through the cuticulin layer, which, however, is impermeable for the enzymes. While these parts of the old cuticle which now is called exuvia, are reincorporated into the animal, the new procuticle, which is not yet divided into endo- and exocuticle, is formed under the cuticulin layer. At this stage the insect hatches and grows rapidly. Growth soon is terminated by the hardening (sclerotization) of the distal sections of the procuticle which now is called exocuticle. In the articular membranes this exocuticle is absent or very thin and of irregular formation.

Peculiar differentiations of epidermal epithelium and cuticle are the true hairs (macrotrichia) which have flexible joints with the surrounding cuticle. The hair is secreted by the so-called trichogenic cell. A second cell called tormogenic cell forms a membranous ring which is responsible for the flexibility of the hair. If only the cuticle forms thread-like projections these are called false hairs (microtrichia). Finally parts of the integument may grow deep into the body (entapophyses, anterior and posterior gut, tracheae).

The fine structure of the cuticle of spiders and crustaceans corresponds to that of insects. In Crustacea the filaments of the procuticle can form bundles, so that the electron microscope image of them resembles that of the annelid cuticle. Between these bundles vertically oriented filaments occur. In crustaceans salts are frequently deposited in the cuticle.

The cuticle of Tardigrada resembles that of arthropods. It is composed of a chitinous procuticle and a set of non-chitinous layers (wax layer, intracuticle layer, epicuticle (with a surface mucous coat). The procuticle corresponds to the arthropod endocuticle. Parabolic patterns do not occur, but the procuticle is also composed of filamentous material, which however, do not show a definite orientation.

The epidermis of tunicates consists of flat or cuboidal cells which are covered by a thick extracellular layer of various consistencies cartilaginous, fibrous, leathery, etc). This layer can bind iodide and consists of a voluminous matrix containing fine filaments which form a superficial condensation, and in most species contains wandering cells of mesodermal origin (these are absent in appendicularians). In pyrosomes these cells can be contractile and form vascular channels between the individual animals.

The cuboidal or low prismatic epidermal cells of *Branchiostoma* contain a well-developed system of intracellular microfilaments constructing a complicated peripheral framework. The apex is characterized by a few stout microvilli and urn-shaped invaginations (Fig. 75) containing a secretory product. The cytoplasm of many

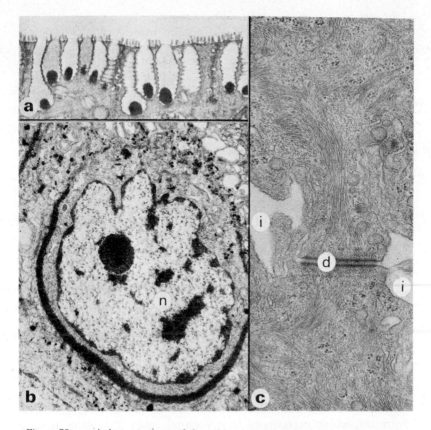

Figure 75.   **a:** Apical cytoplasm of the epidermal cells of *Branchiostoma*, note urn-shaped invaginations x 10 000; **b:** epidermal cell of *Myxine* (hagfish) with cup-shaped layer of microfilaments below the nucleus (n) x 18 000; **c:** desmosome (d) between two epidermal cells of the carp (*Cyprinus*); i: intercellular space, note the abundant microfilaments, which in part converge to the desmosome, x 30 000

cells contains pigment granules and protein crystals. Neighbouring cells are interconnected by numerous cytoplasmic interdigitations. Below the epidermis a layer of collagen is deposited which is of particular regularity (Fig. 36).

In the integument of vertebrates the two components mentioned at the beginning of this chapter are always clearly to be recognized. The outer thin layer is the epithelial epidermis and the inner layer is the dermis (corium), consisting of connective tissue. The dermis is usually very inconspicuous in invertebrates and only consists of a few collagen fibrils and fibroblasts.

In sections the sharp interface between dermis and epidermis of the vertebrate skin normally is of irregular wavy outline (Fig. 79). This is due to the presence of a pattern of projections on the deep surface of the epidermis which fit a complementary pattern of ridges and grooves on the underlying dermis. The projections of the dermis are called dermal papillae, together they form the papillary body which above all serves the attachment of the epidermis to the dermis and is particularly well developed in areas of strain, e.g. on the palms of the hands of primates, or in mammals with an especially thick epidermis, e.g. hippopotami. The free surface of the epidermis on palms and soles of mammals forms the epidermal ridges, which usually are underlain by dermal projections.

Below the dermis the so-called hypodermis (subcutaneous layer) is situated which generally is not considered to be part of the integument. It consists of collagen fibrils and in particular in mammals often houses large accumulations of fat cells.

The glands located in dermis and hypodermis originate from the epidermis.

In fishes the majority of epidermal cells are polygonal elements which build up layers of various thickness. In syngnathids often only two layers of cells exist, in *Gobius*-species the epidermis may consist of more than sixty layers. In teleosts with scales, the epidermis on top of the scales is usually thicker than under them. The basal epithelial cells tend to be prismatic; they divide mitotically and give rise to all the other cells which normally are of uniform polygonal outline, rarely the uppermost cells are flattened and exhibit indications of keratinization (*Periophthalmus*). In individual cases true areas of keratinization occur, e.g. in the pearl organs of cyprinids, which correspond to epidermal cones appearing at the time of spawning. The epidermal cells contain vast numbers of bundles of microfilaments (tonofilaments), which e.g. in *Myxine* (Fig. 75) may form cup-shaped structures below the nucleus. Usually they occur especially at the cellular periphery. Further, the cells contain a well developed rough ER, numerous free ribosomes and often electron dense granules. The cell apex of the outermost layers bears plump microvilli, which are covered by a mucopolysaccharide coat. The cells are interconnected by numerous desmosomes which are located at the end of short cytoplasmic projections (Fig. 75). The intercellular space forms a complex system of channels into which microvilli project. Occasionally the middle layer of cells exhibits particularities: these cells can be unusually large (vesicular cells of gobiids) or extremely flat (mormyrids).

Glandular cells are of wide distribution and may be divided into three groups: mucous slime-producing cells, serous granulated cells and clavate (club-shaped) cells. In Chondrichthyes mucous cells are relatively rare; in lungfish they are abundant and participate in the formation of the cocoon during the dry season, in teleosts they are frequent. The mature cells are in apical location where they extrude their secretory products to the cell surface. The granulated cells, which also in sharks regularly can be found, are usually of roundish shape and contain centrally located granules. The cellular periphery normally contains filaments. They reach the free surface via a long neck-shaped apical process. The clavate cells are particularly rich in filaments and can contain two or more nuclei. They originate in the basal epidermal layer, elongate and assume a club-shaped outline. Later the cellular stalk becomes detached from the base and the cells - under degeneration of their nucleus - become rounder. Their centre contains light material which is believed to be a secretory substance. Clavate cells occur in lampreys and actinopterygians. Occasionally they form glandular complexes (axillary glands of siluroids, to which a toxic secretion is ascribed). Small mixed glands (slime sacks), consisting of mucous and granulated cells, also occur in the myxinoids. Specialized complexes of glandular cells are the variously shaped photophores, which are surrounded by reflecting and dark-pigmented cells. In many cases the photophores consist of granulated cells which are radially oriented around a central lumen which is connected by a small duct with the free surface. The glandular cells produce a light-emitting substance, which partly contains luminescent bacteria. The gland may be covered by a lens, which is of jelly-like consistency if it is derived from the connective tissue. In deep-sea fishes photophores normally are concentrated around the eyes, in *Porichthys* and *Etmopterus* they are distributed all over the body.

The superficial epidermal cells contain numerous secretion granules of different ultrastructure which are the origin of the mucopolysaccharide layer covering the epidermis (the cuticle of light microscopy). This cover can be extremely thick at the suckers of *Blennius* and *Lepadogaster*. The mucous cells presumably do not - or only to small extent - take part in the formation of this coat. The function of the product of these cells is assumed to detach the mucopolysaccharide coat in the panic reaction or to turn the body surface particularly slippery in flight reaction. The epidermis contains free nerve endings which, however, are not in contact with specialized cells as in the mammalian epidermis. In some teleosts, e.g. in *Trigla*, the superficial epidermis of the body contains chemoreceptor cells, resembling taste buds. In the whole epidermis further on excretory chloride cells occur. These elongated elements contain a well developed smooth ER and numerous mitochondria. Finally the fish epidermis may contain free blood cells or chromatophores.

The flat cells in the mormyrid epidermis constitute columns. Their nuclei are in peripheral location, the cytoplasm contains few organelles but abundant tonofilaments. Comparable cells occur in the Gymnotoidei. Both groups of fish possess electroreceptors in the surroundings of which this type of epidermis is situated.

Scales. The structure of the placoid-scales of sharks corresponds to that of teeth (Fig. 124). In sections beside well-developed scales usually others occur which are being resorbed or in early developmental stages. In contrast to the scales of the teleosts they do not have peripheral growth zones. In some species they are rare or absent. Exceptionally also teleosts (South American cat fish) are described to have scales of the placoid type.

The scales of most recent bony fishes are simplified and only consist of dense layers of fibrils, covered by epidermis. Bone cells only occur in *Neoceratodus, Protopterus* and primitive actinopterygians. The scales have a peripheral zone of growth and are surrounded by a fluid-filled space (scale pocket). Quite often they are absent, e.g. in the leather carp, or few in number. In the eel they appear only in animals of several years of age. Modified scales can form integumentary ossifications, which are not enclosed in a scale pocket. In *Aeoliscus* such a dermal armour is fused with underlying ribs. Other modifications are the tubercles of some flat fishes, which can be covered by an enamel like cap or pointed tip and usually contain blood vessels.

During embryogenesis the amphibian epidermis is a simple columnar epithelium, in which briefly before hatching glandular cells arise, the secretory product of which dissolves the capsule of the embryo. The epidermis of the larvae is two-layered and in urodeles and gymnophionans contains large glandular light cells (Leydig cells). In the electron microscope the flat basal cells of the larval epidermis in their basal half exclusively contain tonofilaments, apically free ribosomes occur beside loosely distributed filaments, mainly rough ER cisternae. The cytoplasm of the larger apical cells is lighter and contains fewer filaments. Mitochondria and granular ER are normally concentrated in a zone in the middle of the cell. Directly under the apical plasma membrane which bears a few microvilli secretory granules are located the contents of which is deposited on the free surface. In many species some of the epidermal cells contain pigment granules. The intercellular space is relatively wide in the larval epidermis. After metamorphosis the thickness of

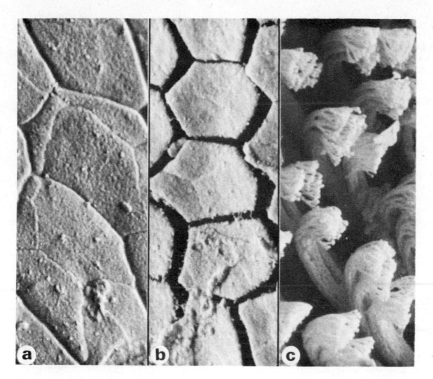

Figure 76. Epidermis as seen in the scanning electron microscope, **a, b:** Tree frog (*Rhacophorus*); **a:** normal epidermis, **b:** epidermis of digital pad, note gaps between the hexagonal epidermal cells; **c:** detail from the adhesive lamellae of a foot of the gecko *Hemidactylus*, the epidermal cells produce tiny hook-like structures, which still are composed of substructures. a, b: x 3600;c: x 20 000

the epidermis increases and one or two apical cells keratinize. The cuboidal to prismatic basal cells contain above all bundles of tonofilaments, ribosomes and rough ER cisternae. The following 4-5 layers of cells are slightly flattened and additionally contain electron-dense granules, the contents of which is delivered partly into the intercellular space. In this zone of cells individual elongated light and mitochondria-rich cells can be demonstrated, the function of which is unknown. In keratinized apical cells densely packed filaments are embedded in a light matrix; the nucleus normally is still recognizable. The intercellular space, which fulfils specific tasks in transport processes, is sealed off near the free surface by tight junctions.

In contrast to fishes, the amphibian skin possesses acinar and tubular glands which maturate briefly before metamorphosis. The acinar glands, which are more frequently to be found, are divided into mucous glands and granulated glands. The mucous cells usually contain light or loosely structured basophilic secretory inclusions (Fig. 77), which frequently in mature cells fuse and form structureless masses. The granulated cells contain electron dense acidophilic secretory granules (Fig. 77). At least in the Urodelomorpha occasionally both cell types seem to occur in one gland. A regular third constituent of these glands are mitochondria-rich cells, with numerous microvilli all over their surface, which seem to be undifferentiated secretory cells. In the periphery of all glands elongated smooth muscle cells occur. In general in one gland the secretory cells are in different phases of their cytoplasmic maturation, therefore the glandular lumen is either wide (most cells are immature) or narrow (some of the cells are fully differentiated). Around the cloaca of urodeles three voluminous glands can be found the lumina of which are particularly wide. Tubular glands are rare (fingers of male anurans, chin of male plethodontids and nasal openings of many species).

The milky secretion of the granulated glands has an irritating effect on mucous membranes of other vertebrates, also the secretion of the mucous glands can be toxic (*Hydromantes*). The glands may be concentrated in certain areas, e.g. the 'parotis' glands in the neck region. Some species, e.g. *Proteus,* only seem to have mucous glands, others, e.g. *Ascaphus*, only granulated glands. Chemical analysis has shown that the secretory product of the granulated glands contains among others tryptamine and adrenaline derivatives. The secretory product of their skin glands are also responsible for the odour of certain species, e.g. smell of onions of some pelobatids, smell of vanilla of some salamanders and toads. The cloacal glands of male urodelans play a role in the formation of the spermatophores.

The dermis frequently contains chromatophores (Fig. 78) and in some gymnophionans bone ossicles. Secondarily bone can appear in the dermis of the head of some anurans (*Brachycephalus*).

The skin of the Sauropsida is characterized by its paucity of glands. Mucous glands are entirely absent. Reptiles have a few holocrine glands: moschus glands at the *angulus mandibulae* of some crocodiles and femoral glands of lizards. Pigeons and galliform birds also possess holocrine glands in the external auditory meatus. An unusual gland, which is found in the majority of birds, is the rump gland, which produces an oily fluid containing vitamin D. In ducks these big glands are composed of individual tubular glands which may be divided into three zones: (a) an outer zone,

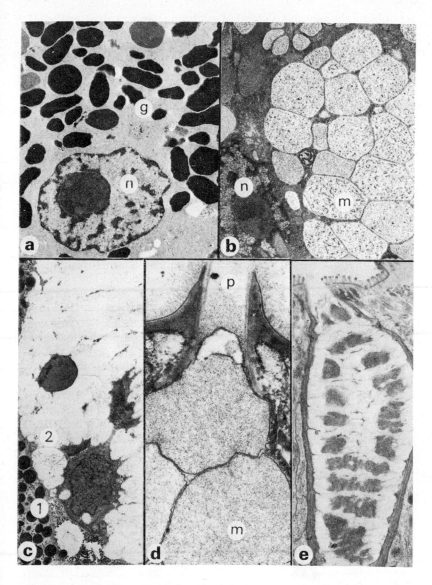

Figure 77. Glandular cells of the skin; **a, b:** *Kaloula* (Anura); **a:** serous granular cell, **b:** mucous cell. n: nucleus; m: mucous droplets; g: secretory granules. a,b x 7500; **c:** *Malacobdella* (Nemertini), two mucous cells, 1: with secretory granules, 2: with an almost unstructured mass of secretory material, x 5400; **d:** *Autolytus* (Polychaeta) apex of glandular cell with mucous droplets (m) and extrusion pore (p) in the cuticle. x 18 000; **e:** *Ceratonereis* (Polychaeta) apex of mucous cell, x 9000

resembling the sebaceous gland of mammals; its stratified epithelial wall contains various lipids; (b) a middle zone with a thinner wall and widened lumen, producing triglycerides; (c) an inner thin-walled zone, which does not synthesize lipids.

The individual layers of the epidermis are comparable to those of the mammals (see below). The filaments of the keratinized cells are of relatively loose arrangement and are embedded in a rather light matrix. Within the epidermal cells regularly lipid inclusions and secretory granules containing mucins are to be found. Fat droplets are particularly frequent in birds. The integument of reptiles can form epidermal (horn) and mesodermal (bone) scales. The thin epidermis of birds gives rise to the feathers which are entirely composed of dead cornified cells.

The epidermis of mammals (Fig. 79) is, as that of reptiles and birds, a stratified keratinized epithelium, the cells of which originate in a basal layer by mitotic divisions. In the rat they migrate within nineteen days (in man in thirty days) from the base to the surface. They undergo a typical process of keratinization which leads to a characteristic stratification of the epidermal cells. The deepest layer, which rests on a basement lamina and the dermis, is formed by the *stratum germinativum* (*stratum basale*). It consists of one row of low prismatic epithelial cells. The next layer is the *stratum spinosum*, its cells are of polygonal outline becoming flattened as they move up from the base of the epithelium to the surface. All of these cells bear short spines that are attached to similar projections from adjacent cells (Fig. 75). The spines of neighbouring cells are separated by a narrow intercellular space and are characterized by their prominent desmosomes and tonofilaments. The *stratum granulosum* is the third layer. It consists of flattened cells, the cytoplasm of which contains basophilic inclusions which in light

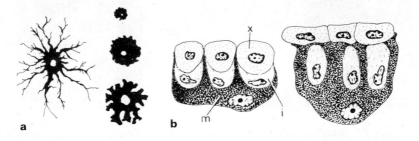

Figure 78. Chromatophores in lower vertebrates; **a:** pigment cells from the skin of the pike (*Esox*) after KRAUSE, 1921; **b:** tree frog (Hyla) functional association of dermal chromatophores (xantho- (x), irido- (i), melanophore (m); left: animal is light green, right: animal is dark green. After SCHMIDT, 1971

microscopy are called keratohyalin granules. In the superficial parts of this layer these granules are very numerous and the nuclei disintegrate. Here the epidermal cells transform into dead elements. Only in the palms and soles the narrow *stratum lucidum* appears in which refractile droplets of a substance called eleidin occur. The terminal layer is the *stratum corneum*. It contains only keratin and rarely also lipid inclusions; all the cell organelles and the nucleus have disappeared. In its uppermost zone the dead horny cells are desquamated in small groups or larger areas.

In the electron microscope the process of keratinization mainly concerns changes of the filamentous components of the cells. In the basal cells individual filaments 5–8 nm in diameter occur.

In the *stratum spinosum* they form very dense small bundles. In the *stratum granulosum* within the filament bundles areas of electron dense material appear (up to 5 µm in diameter). These areas

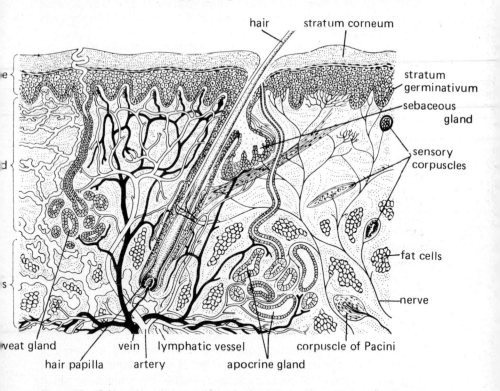

Figure 79. Schematic representation of the mammalian skin. Left: mainly lymphatic vessels; middle: mainly blood vessels, right: mainly nerve endings, **e:** epidermis: **d:** dermis; **s:** subcutaneous layer. After WALDEYER, 1971

contain a protein rich in sulphur and correspond to the keratohyalin granules of light microscopy. In the area of the upper *stratum spinosum* and of the *stratum granulosum* two types of cytoplasmic granules occur: (1) keratinosomes, discharging their contents into the extracellular space. These granules in some species have been found to correspond to lysosomes; possibly their enzymes play a role in the desquamation of the uppermost horny cells; (2) electron-dense granules resembling the mucin-containing granules of lower vertebrates, their contents are also discharged into the intercellular space where it covers the plasma membrane of the epithelial cells (membrane-coating cells). Above the *stratum granulosum* the cells change abruptly. In the *stratum lucidum*, if present, and the *stratum corneum* all cell organelles and the nucleus have disappeared. The cells are completely filled with tightly packed microfilaments embedded in an electron dense matrix, which may have originated from the keratohyalin granules. The transformed desmosomes persist for a long time and dissolve only when the cells are desquamated.

The dermis is composed of a connective tissue in which the amount of fibres (above all collagen) increases from surface to the deeper parts, where they are interconnected with the collagen fibres of the hypodermis. Elastic fibres form a loose network within the dermis, which further contains blood- and lymph vessels, nerves, receptor organs and free cells.

Four groups of skin glands occur in mammals: coiled glands (*glandulae sudoriferae minores,* sweat glands), odoriferous glands (*glandulae sudoriferae maiores*), sebaceous glands, mammary glands.

The coiled glands in higher primates contain secretory cells with the merocrine (= eccrine) type of extrusion; in other mammals they presumably often are apocrine glands, in whales, sea cows and others they are absent. They are usually simple coiled tubular glands. The secretory portions contain basally located smooth muscle cells and two types of epithelial cells, one of which is characterized by numerous apical secretory granules (producing mucopolysaccharides) and abundant ribosomes, whereas the other is poor in organelles and inclusions; since its lateral and basal plasma membranes exhibit complex infoldings and since between these cells small intercellular canaliculi are formed which communicate with the glandular lumen they are believed to secrete a product rich in water. The duct portion of these glands consists of two layers of cuboidal cells, moderately rich in mitochondria, which modify the composition of the secretory product.

The apocrine odoriferous glands (Fig. 26) are characterized by

wide lumina of their secretory portions. In men their secretory
activity starts at puberty and in women shows a cyclical activity
correlated with the menstrual cycle. They also contain a basal layer
of smooth muscle cells and e.g. occur in the axilla.

The holocrine sebaceous glands originate from hair primordia
and usually open into the necks of hair follicles. In some areas they
are not associated with hairs (lips, *labia minora,* corners of the
mouth, etc.). The secretory portions are roundish acini. Normally
several adjacent acini open together into a short duct. At the
periphery of the acinus a layer of flat cells can be distinguished.
Towards the centre of the acinus most of the cells increase in size
and gradually fill with fat droplets. The nuclei shrink in the course
of this process and slowly disappear. The cells finally disintegrate
into fatty detritus. Closely resembling typical sebaceous glands are
parts of or the complete big facial glands of bats (Fig. 26), antelopes
and deer.

A particular group of holocrine glands are the frequently
pigmented and branched perigenital glandular organs of many
mammals, e.g. rodents and bovids. The significance of the pigments
secreted is not entirely clear. Possibly they colour and modify the
urine and have a function in marking a territory. A similar function
is ascribed to the antorbital glands of many artiodactyles the
secretory product of which contains a number of scent substances.
These glands often contain two parts, a pigmented one with
holocrine extrusion and a light one, consisting of coiled glands with
apocrine secretion.

The mammary gland presumably represents a modified and
specialized sweat or odoriferous gland. It is a compound tubulo-
alveolar gland. In monotremes the individual glands open separately
to the free surface of the skin at the basis of hairs, in the other
mammals the individual glands open *via* separate ducts at the nipple
of the breast, which is free of hairs. This gland is subjected to vast
changes during a reproductive cycle. The resting gland consists
principally of the main duct system from which secretory portions
rapidly develop during pregnancy. In the active gland the basophilic
secretory cells surround wide lumina, which are filled with the main
products of the gland: fat and protein. In the cells the fat globules
frequently bulge the apical plasma membrane into the lumen.
During its extrusion it usually is surrounded by bits of cytoplasm
and the plasma membrane. Precursors of the protein (casein)
accumulate in dilated Golgi cisternae (Fig. 9), where they are
concentrated to form larger units (the casein micelles). Within the
glandular epithelium again smooth muscle cells occur, which are
highly branched.

In the epidermis of many mammals branched cells occur, termed Langerhans cells. They can be demonstrated by metal inpregnations and often also by histochemical tests for unspecific esterases. In the electron microscope they are characterized by specific disk-shaped granules. They probably are particular monocytes, which enter the epithelium. Recently they have also been found in the epithelium of the oesophagus and the rumen of bovids.

Hairs (Fig. 79)

Each hair arises in a tubular invagination of the epidermis, the hair follicle. The deepest part of this epithelial down-growth is of bulbous shape and called the germinal matrix, since it gives rise to the hair. A connective tissue papilla containing capillaries invaginates this germinal area from below. Fig. 79 shows some details of the structure of a hair and the hair follicle. The external root sheath is a downward continuation of the epidermis connecting the matrix with the surface, the hair forms by proliferation of the matrix cells, which grow upward within the external root sheath of the follicle. Being pushed up the cells keratinize. The peripheral zone (cuticle and cortex) consists of particularly hard keratin, whereas the medulla, which often is absent, is composed of soft keratin. The proliferating matrix cells form still another structure, a tubular sheath, separating the hair from the external root sheath, and being called internal root sheath. It extends only partway up the follicle and can be subdivided into three sublayers (an inner cuticular layer, Huxley's layer (middle), Henle's layer (outside).

Hair growth is cyclic, which is particularly obvious in mammals of cold climates. In man one hair lives about 2-6 years. Sinus hairs are particularly long and thick hairs the basal parts of which are surrounded by a blood space. They are in contact with numerous nerve endings and represent receptors of touch.

Further keratinized epidermal structures of interest are: nails, hooves, the sheath of horns in the bovids and antilocaprids, the horn(s) of rhinoceroses, claws.

Pigments

The colour of tissues and organs can be either due to exogenous material (exogeneous pigments) taken into the body, like carotenoids, dust particles, mineral salts (silver, lead) and colour crystals artificially driven into the skin (tattoo marks) or to endogenous substances (endogenous pigments) generated inside the body from non-pigmented precursors.

Among the endogenous pigments various groups may be distinguished which usually are confined to a special cell type each, which in general are called chromatophores (= chromocytes). Melanin is the brown pigment in skin, hairs, the eyes, certain nuclei of the brain of mammals. In lower vertebrates it is even of a wider distribution and occurs in the serous lining of the body cavities and in the connective tissue of many other organs. Melanin is produced in the irregularly shaped melanophores (melanocytes), which in vertebrates have their origin in the neural crest. The pigment is concentrated in ellipsoidal electron dense granules, the melanosomes, which arise in the Golgi apparatus. In early stages of its formation the melanosome is limited by a membrane and contains longitudinally oriented lamellae. In the course of maturation melanin is deposited upon these lamellae until it completely obscures the internal structure. In the epidermis of vertebrates melanosomes can be transferred from the melanocytes to epidermal epithelial cells. A particular type of melanin, phaeomelanin, is a yellow, orange or red pigment.

Iridophores (guanophores) function to reflect or scatter light. They contain reflecting platelets which are composed of crystalline deposits of purines (guanine, hypoxanthine). These cells occur in poikilotherms and in the iris of birds. Xanthophores (yellow) and erythrophores (orange, red) are chromatophores which only occur in lower vertebrates. In xanthophores pteridines are the more prevalent pigments; these compounds are synthesized in the pigment cell and are stored in granular inclusions that are composed of concentric lamellae. They occur both in xantho- and erythrophores. Carotenoids are contained in light vesicles and predominantly occur in the erythrophores. However both pigments (pteridines and carotenoids) may often be found in the same xanthophore or erythrophore. Since the carotenoids are soluble in lipid solvents these chromatophores have also been termed lipophores.

In fishes, amphibians and reptiles pigment cells mainly occur in the dermis, in birds and mammals they are particularly frequent in the epidermis, into which, however, they move from the dermis.

The melanocytes frequently invade the epidermis and can inject their pigment granules into epidermal cells. This process can clearly be observed in the development of feathers in birds. Here the melanocytes are voluminous cells extending a long apically directed process, which closely associates with some cells of the feather. Fine branches of this process penetrate into the feather cells and supply them with pigment granules.

The degradation of haemoglobin gives rise to various pigments. Phagocytizing cells in the spleen, the liver and the bone marrow accumulate in their cytoplasm a golden brown iron-containing pigment, termed haemosiderin, which usually is localized in membrane-bound granules, which in the electron microscope can be recognized by the presence of 90 Å dense ferritin particles; pure ferritin crystals are rare.

Lipofuscin is a brownish pigment and considered to be an end stage of lysosomal activity. It usually increases progressively with advancing age (see page 22).

LITERATURE

BAGNARA, J. T., HADLEY, M. E. 'Chromatophores and color change.' Prentice - Hall, Inc., Englewood Cliffs, New Jersey (1973). 201 pp.

BARTH, F. G. 'Die Feinstruktur des Spinneninteguments. I. Die Cuticula der Laufbeine adulter häutungsferner Tiere (*Cupiennius salei* Keys.).' *Z. Zellforsch.* **97**, 137-159 (1969).

BIRD, A. F. *The Structure of Nematodes*. Academic Press, New York, London. 317 pp. 1971.

BRÅTEN, T. 'The fine structure of the tegument of *Diphyllobothrium latum* (L.).' *Z. f. Parasitenkunde*. **30**, 104-112 (1968).

BROCCO, S. L., O'CLAIR, R. M., CLONEY, R. A. 'Cephalopod integument: The ultrastructure of Kölliker's organs and their relationship to setae.' *Cell. Tiss. Res.* **155**, 293-308 (1974).

BRODIE, A. E. 'Development of the cuticle in the Rotifer *Asplanchna brightwelli.' Z. Zellforsch.* **105**, 515-525 (1970).

BRODY, I. 'Variations in the differentiation of the fibrils in the normal human stratum corneum as revealed by electron microscopy.' *J. Ultrastruct Res.* **30**, 601-614 (1970).

BYRAM, J. E., FISHER, F. M. 'The absorptive surface of *Moniliformis dubius* (Acanthocephala). II. Functional aspects.' *Tissue and Cell*. **6**, 21-42 (1974).

CLELAND, J. B., SOUTHCOTT, R. V. 'Injuries to man from marine invertebrates in the Australian region.' *National Health and Medical Research Council Special Report Series No. 12*. Commonwealth of Australia, Canberra (1965) 282 pages.

EAKIN, R. M., BRANDENBURGER, J. L. 'Ultrastructural features of a gordian worm (Nematomorpha).' *J. Ultrastruct. Res.* **46**, 351-374 (1974).

- GUPTA, B. L., LITTLE, C. 'Studies on Pogonophora. 4. Fine structure of the cuticle and epidermis.' *Tissue and Cell*. **2**, 637-696 (1970).

HARDER, W. 'Zur Feinstruktur der Elektrozeptorepidermis der Mormyridae (Teleostei, Pisces).' *Z. Zellforsch.* **114**, 262-270 (1971).

KOEHLER, J. K. 'Some comparative fine structure relationships of the Rotifer integument.' *J. Experim. Zool.* **162**, 231-243 (1966).

LEE, D. L. 'Moulting in nematodes: the formation of the adult cuticle during the final moult of *Nippostrongylus brasiliensis.' Tissue and Cell*. **2**, 139-153 (1970).

LENTZ, T. L. 'The cell biology of *Hydra.'* North-Holland Publishing Company, Amsterdam, 199 S. 1966.

—'Rhabdite formation in *Planaria*. The role of microtubules'. *J. Ultrastruct. Res.* **17**, 114-126 (1967).

LUMSDEN, R. D. 'Cytological studies on the absorptive surfaces of Cestodes II.' *Z.f. Parasitenkunde*. **28**, 1-13 (1966).

—'Ultrastructure of mitochondria in a cestode, *Lacistorhynchus tenuis* (v. Beneden, 1858).' *J. Parasitology*. **53**, 65-77 (1967).

MATOLTSY, A. G., HUSZAR, T. 'Keratinization of the Reptilian epidermis. An ultrastructural study of the turtle skin.' *J. Ultrastruct. Res.* **38**, 87-101 (1972).

MORITZ, K., STORCH, R. 'Zur Feinstruktur des Integumentes von *Trachydemus giganteus* Zelinka (Kinorhyncha).' *Z. Morph. Tiere.* **71**, 189-202 (1972).

NEVILLE, A. C. 'Insect Ultrastructure.' *Symposium of the royal entomological society of London No. 5.* Blackwell Scientific Publ. Oxford, Edinburgh, 1970, 185 S.

O'CLAIR, R. M., CLONEY, R. A. 'Pattern of morphogenesis, mediated by dynamic microvilli: chaetogenesis in *Nereis vexillosa.' Cell Tiss. Res.* **151**, 141-157 (1974).

RIFKIN, E., CHENG, T. C., HOHL, H. R. 'The fine structure of the tegument of *Tylocephalum* metacestodes: with emphasis on a new type of microvilli.' *J. Morph.* **130**, 11-24 (1970).

SMITH, D. S. '*Insect Cells, their structure and function'.* Oliver and Boyd, Edinburgh, 1968. 372 S.

SPEARMAN, R. J. C. *The integument.* Cambridge University Press (1973). 208 pp.

STARCK, D., SCHNEIDER, R. 'Zur Kenntnis insbesondere der Hautdrüsen von *Pelea capreolus* (Foster , 1790) (Artiodactyla, Bovidae, Antilopinae, Peleini).' *Z. Säugetierkunde.* **36**, 321-333 (1972).

STORCH, V., LEHNERT-MORITZ, K. 'Zur Entwicklungsgeschichte der Kolloblasten (Klebzellen) der Ctenophore *Pleurobrachia pileus.' Marine Biol.* **28**, 215-219 (1974).

—, WELSCH, U. 'Ultrastructure and histochemistry of the integument of air-breathing polychaetes from mangrove swamps of Sumatra.' *Marine Biol.* **17**, 137-144 (1972).

TAYLOR, A. E. R., MULLER, R. ed. 'Functional aspects of parasite surfaces.' *Symp. Brit. Soc. Parasitol.* **10**, 1-114 (1972).

WELSCH, U. 'Beobachtungen über die Feinstruktur der Haut und des äußeren Atrialepithels von *Branchiostoma lanceolatum* Pallas.' *Z. Zellforsch.* **88**, 565-575 (1968).

WHITEAR, M. 'Cell specialization and sensory function in fish epidermis.' *J. Zool. Lond.* **163**, 237-264 (1971).

WRIGHT, R. D., LUMSDEN, R. D. 'The acanthor tegument of *Moniliformis dubius.' J. Parasit.* **56**, 727-735 (1970).

Chapter 4

RECEPTOR CELLS (SENSORY CELLS).

Sensory cells usually, but often not in a completely satisfactory way, are classified according to their connection with the nervous system and the position of their receptive process (receptor pole).

1. Primary sensory cells (Fig. 80). They possess a rather long basal process (axon) which contacts with a nerve cell or directly with an effector cell (muscle cell, mucus producing cell etc.) and an apical extension which reaches the free surface of the epithelium. The perikaryon may be situated within an epithelium, or beneath it. Shape and structural organization of these cells may closely resemble that of neurons and especially of sensory neurons so that particularly in primitive forms it may be difficult to separate them. They are of wide distribution in invertebrates, in which they occasionally form groups (Fig. 23); they also occur in vertebrates (olfactory epithelium) and may form chemo-, mechano- and photoreceptors.
2. Secondary sensory cells. They are always located in epithelia and do not possess basal processes. Instead, at their base they are interconnected by synaptic contact with a sensory nerve fibre. They used to be known only in vertebrates, however electron microscopy has revealed their wide distribution also in invertebrates (Cnidaria, (Fig. 64), molluscs, priapulids, annelids, arrow worms, etc.). Typical secondary sensory cells of the vertebrates are the receptor cells of the inner ear (Fig. 91), the taste buds and the lateral line system.
3. Sensory nerve cells. The perikarya are located under an epithelium and extend basal processes (axons), which make contact with other neurons, and distally directed sensory processes (dendrites), which terminate in the area of stimulus perception. The latter type of process may enter an epithelium but does not reach the free surface. They may be enveloped by special adventitial cells, rarely so in invertebrates, frequently so in vertebrates. If such enveloping cells are absent, the terminals

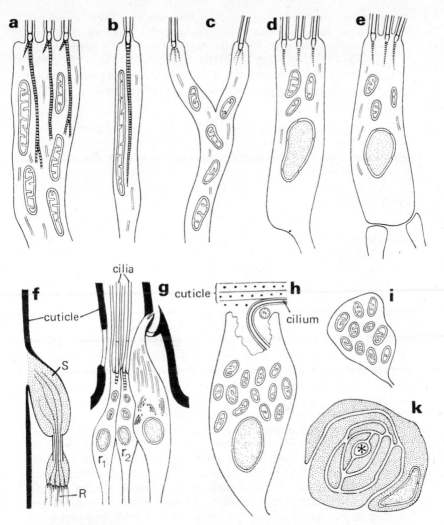

Figure 80. Different types of sensory cells in invertebrates. Schematic drawings after electron micrographs. **a-d:** apices of various receptor neurons. **a:** nemertean; **b:** nemertean; **c:** turbellarian with two dendrites reaching the surface, **d:** mollusc (snail), **e:** secondary sensory cell of a snail with basal nerve endings. Cell types of **a-e** reach the surface of the epidermis and bear cilia; **f:** amphid (lateral organ) of a nematode, a cuticular invagination is filled with slime (s), basally ciliary receptor cells (R) are located. **g:** Kinorhyncha, an apically open spine is invaded by two receptor cells (r_1, r_2) distally bearing cilia, **h:** oligochaete, receptor cell with numerous mitochondria and an apical cilium lying below the cuticle, **i:** inflated nerve ending with numerous mitochondria located in the epidermis of polychaetes and nemerteans. **k:** lamellar body composed of central dendrite (asterisk) and surrounding glial cells. Polychaeta. After STORCH, 1973

are called free nerve endings. In invertebrates these dendrites may form bundles, which invade epithelia pushing aside the basal parts of the epithelial cells. Sensory nerve cells normally are considered to represent specialized neurons. They are often mechano- and thermoreceptors. Sensory nerve cells and primary sensory cells together may be called receptor neurons.

If sensory cells perceive stimuli from the external surroundings they are termed extero(re)ceptors, if they receive stimuli arising within the body they are called intero(re)ceptors. In the following text the sensory cells are grouped according to the types of energy they perceive: chemo-, thermo-, electro-, mechano-, and photoreceptors.

Chemoreceptors

Among chemoreceptors we find interoreceptors, e.g. regulating respiration, the osmotic balance, concentration of various constituents of the blood, etc., and exteroreceptors, e.g. receptors of smell (low stimulatory threshold) and taste (high stimulatory threshold).

Relatively few details are known about the interoreceptors. In vertebrates many specialized neurons in the brain stem act as interoreceptors. Small organs composed of interoreceptors are the carotid and aortic bodies, which are situated on the carotid artery and the aorta. They consist of clusters of epithelium-like cells which are closely applied to the endothelia of small blood-vessels and which are surrounded by enveloping cells. Their cytoplasm contains catecholamines and numerous electron-dense granules, which may contain the amines. The cells are in synaptic contact with nerve endings and presumably register changes in the blood (fall in pH, rise in carbon dioxide, or decrease in oxygen content). In invertebrates with a soft body surface, the exteroreceptors may be formed by primary and secondary sensory cells. They often are located in exposed parts of the body: on tentacles and along the margin of the head in Cnidaria, Turbellaria, Nemertini, annelids and molluscs, along the pallial edge and in siphos of bivalves, in the ambulacral feet of echinoderms, etc. Generally they correspond to cells which apically bear several cilia and often they stand together in small groups. In water-dwelling species the cilia may project above the cuticle (annelids) or above the apical microvilli (nemerteans, molluscs), or they may be embedded in these structures. In the latter case the structure of the cilia frequently is altered: the central tubules may be absent or replaced by an a-b pair

of tubules; then in the periphery only 7-8 a-b pairs occur.
Furthermore they frequently lack rootlets (Fig. 80). Such modified
cilia also regularly occur in land-living molluscs, polychaetes and
oligochaetes.

In gastropods, above all in many archaeogastropods, the cephalic
appendages bear groups of ciliated secondary sensory cells, which
are also thought to represent chemoreceptors. However, ultrastructural criteria allowing in each case a safe distinction between
mechano- and chemoreceptors have not yet been established.

In insects various types of chemoreceptors occur in the antennae,
on the epipharynx, the palps of the maxillae and the tarsi of the
extremities. They contain one or several bipolar receptor cells, which
are connected with a cuticular apparatus, which is produced by a
trichogenous and tormogenous cell, surrounding the receptor cell.

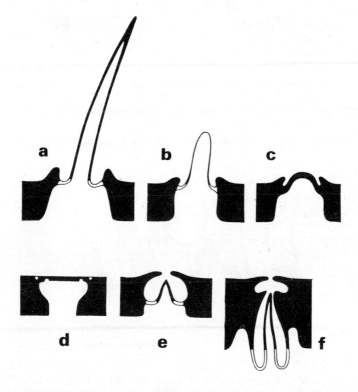

Figure 81. Schematic representation of the cuticular parts of insect sensilla. **a:**
sensillum trichodeum; **b:** *s. basiconicum;* **c:** *s. campaniformium;* **d:** *s. placodeum;* **e:**
s. coeloconicum; **f:** *s. ampullaceum.* After SEIFERT, 1970

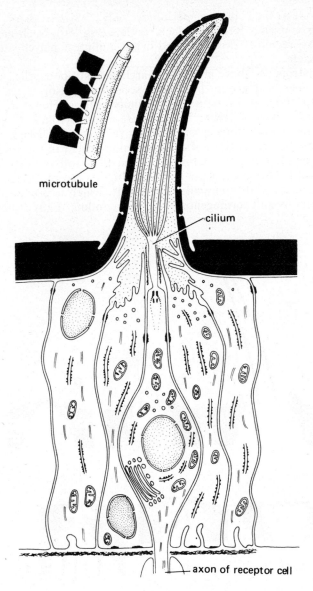

microtubule

cilium

axon of receptor cell

Figure 82.   Schematic representation of an olfactory sensillum on the antenna of *Necrophorus* (cadaver beetle). The bipolar receptor cell bears an apical cilium, which branches into several individual elements each containing a microtubule (enlarged top left). These lie below the cuticle of the sensillum, which is perforated by pores. The branches are surrounded by a fluid-filled extracellular space, which is delimited by the cells at the basis of the cilium. After ERNST, 1969

The whole complex is termed a sensillum.

Various types of sensilla exist (Fig. 81) the structure of which, however, does not indicate their function.

In olfactory sensillae the cuticle forms a hair and is perforated by numerous pores (Fig. 82). In contact chemoreceptors the tip of the cuticular hair is characterized by a rather wide opening. The dendrite of the receptor cells bears a cilium, which distally branches into several slender projections, each of which contains a microtubule (Fig. 82).

Olfactory sensillae occur in the form of a *sensilla trichodea* in Orthoptera, Lepidoptera, Diptera and Coleoptera – and in the form of a *sensilla coeloconica* in Orthoptera and Hymenoptera. *Sensilla coeloconica* and *ampullacea* can react specifically to carbon dioxide and moist air. The same function may be assumed for Tömösvary's organ (postantennal organ) of anamorphic Chilopoda, many Diplopoda and Symphyla. In *Scutigerella* these organs have been studied with the electron microscope. They are located in a cephalic epidermal groove behind the basis of the antennae. More than half of the groove is filled by a meshwork of cuticular rods into which – from the interior of the body – cilia of bipolar receptor cells project. Each dendrite bears two distal cilia, which branch in the meshwork. The cuticle surrounding them only consists of a thin epicuticle which is perforated by tiny pores; exo- and endocuticle are confined to the bottom of the groove. Outside this groove a normal type of cuticle occurs. As in insects the receptor cell is surrounded by an inner and an outer enveloping cell, also termed trichogenous and tormogenous cells. A fluid secretory product of these cells bathes the distal projections of the sensory cell from cellular apex to the cuticular meshwork.

Also the chemoreceptors of arachnids can be constructed according to this scheme. In the tick *Amblyomma americanum*, the sensillar cuticle either is perforated by a system of pores or by a slit-like opening near the tip. Frequently these sensilla contain in addition two mechanoreceptive dendrites, which are fixed to the base of the hair. The cilia of the receptor cells ordinarily exhibit an 11 + 0 pattern. Of similar structure are the scalids of the kinorhynchs (Fig. 80).

The vertebrate olfactory epithelium is either located in the nasal groove or sac (fishes) or forms parts of the epithelial lining of the nasal cavity (tetrapods). In teleosts the olfactory epithelium is a pseudostratified epithelium consisting of extremely tall supportive cells (*c*. 150 μm long), with basally located nuclei, basal cells and sensory cells the nuclear region of which can be found in various heights of the epithelium (Fig. 83). They extend a distal slender process often bearing cilia to the free surface, and a basal axon leaving the epithelium. Some of the distal processes lack cilia. In elasmobranchs the olfactory cells are also located in pseudostratified epithelia, which differ from that of teleosts by the fact that the nuclei are evenly distributed throughout it instead of being concentrated at the epithelial base. Basal cells also occur. The supporting cells are ciliated, the nuclear region is located near the epithelial surface. Below this zone containing the nuclei of the supporting cells several layers of bipolar perikarya of the sensory

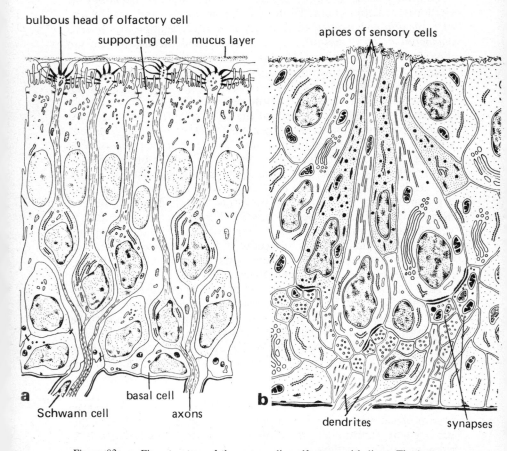

Figure 83. **a:** Fine structure of the mammalian olfactory epithelium. The bulbous heads of the olfactory cells bear up to 50 μm long cilia embedded in a mucous layer. **b:** fine structure of a teleost taste bud; the secondary sensory cells bear apical microvilli and are at their bases synaptically interconnected with sensory nerve terminals. After REMANE, STORCH & WELSCH, 1974

cells are found, the distal process of which never bears cilia (only a few stout microvilli) and reaches the free surface, which is not covered by mucus.

In *Petromyzon* the olfactory epithelium is located within 15–18 pouches of the nasal sac. It is composed of tall ciliated supporting cells (70–80 μm high) with basally located nuclei and bipolar olfactory cells the distal process of which again reaches the free surface and bears cilia. Their perikarya are located in the middle of the epithelium above the nuclei of the supportive cells.

Of basically similar construction is the olfactory epithelium of the tetrapods. In mammals often three cell types can be recognized (Fig. 83): (1) receptor, (2) supporting, (3) basal cells. In all species tight junctions occur apically in the epithelium.

1. The receptor cells again are of bipolar shape, and can be considered as specialized neurons. Their perikarya are located in the middle of the pseudostratified epithelium (about 60–70 μm thick). The distal process bears a bulbous head which projects slightly above the general surface of the epithelium. Radiating from its surface are six to eight cilia originating from basal bodies and assumed to play an important role in chemoreception. They are non-motile and extremely long, in the frog up to 200 μm. The short, relatively thick proximal segment of each cilium is of normal structure, the longer distal part is much narrower and only contains individual microtubules; it courses in parallel to the surface of the epithelium and is embedded in a thick layer of mucus. By its extraordinary length the surface of the olfactory epithelium is considerably enlarged. Infrequently, receptor cells with a slender apical process bearing only a few stout microvilli have been described. The basal processes penetrate the basal lamina and constitute the unmyelinated olfactory nerve.

2. Between the receptor cells numerous supporting cells are to be found, the nuclei of which generally are concentrated distally to the sensory cells. They are characterized by apical microvilli, a well developed system of microfilaments, supporting their basal extensions and constructing a terminal web, fairly abundant smooth ER tubules. Their function seems to be the production of mucosubstances. Most of the mucus layer covering the epithelium, however, originates from the olfactory glands of Bowman, which are serous elements containing numerous secretory granules.

3. In the basal part of the epithelium small basal cells occur, which may be subdivided into light and dark elements. In part they correspond to undifferentiated olfactory cells, from which also in

adult organisms mature olfactory cells can develop. Also the supportive cells arise from these basal cells.

The epithelium of the vomeronasal organ (organ of Jacobson) contains receptor cells apically bearing only microvilli and no cilia. In *Natrix* and *Anguis* centrioles have still been detected, in *Lacerta* even these reminiscences of cilia are absent. The sensory cells are very frequent, outnumbering the supporting cells and often lying closely together.

Taste receptors of vertebrates are formed by groups of individual secondary sensory cells, which are located in the epithelium of the oral cavity (in tetrapods often concentrated on the tongue and in the

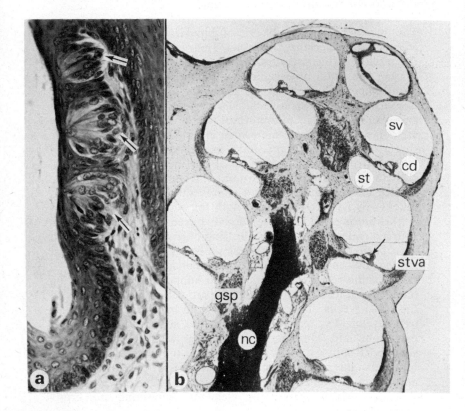

Figure 84.   **a:** Taste buds (arrows) of the tongue of *Galago* (primate) x 500; **b:** cochlea of the guinea pig; sv: *scala vestibuli;* cd: cochlear duct; st: *scala tympani;* gsp: ganglion spirale; nc: *nervus cochlearis;* stva; *stria vascularis,* arrow points to organ of Corti, x 40

dorsal roof of the pharynx) or in teleosts they can be distributed all over the body. Groups of taste receptor cells are termed taste buds (Fig. 84). They are synaptically connected with the facial, glossopharyngeal, and vagal nerves.

In the mammals the taste buds generally are located in various excrescences, the papillae, in the peripheral parts of the tongue. Their ultrastructure seems to be almost the same in all these papillae. The buds are mainly composed of two types of elongated cells which reach the free surface of the epithelium, which often is invaginated in this area (taste pore). The function of these two cell types is not yet definitely known. One type is characterized by a dense cytoplasm and long microvilli extending into the taste pore (taste hairs of light microscopy). Its apical cytoplasm contains electron-dense granules often believed to empty their contents into the taste pore. The second type is rarer than the preceding one. Its cytoplasm is light and contains numerous microtubules and smooth surfaced profiles of the ER. It bears short apical microvilli. Both cell types can be interconnected with nerve terminals. The structure of these synapses varies. Often the sensory cells contain in the presynaptic area vesicles, and the nerve terminals (postsynaptic area) numerous mitochondria. Membrane thickenings can be present or absent. It is a matter for discussion whether both cell types, which apically are connected by tight junctions, are taste cells or whether one of them is a supporting cell. The receptive area is confined to the microvilli. The cells of the taste bud are constantly replaced by basal cells originating from neighbouring epithelial cells.

Thermoreceptors

The structure of thermoreceptors is best known from the pit organs of crotalid snakes (pit vipers). This organ is located in a cavity between the external opening of the nose and the eye. Its floor is formed by a richly innervated membrane, the surface of which is formed by a thin epithelium. The nerve terminals under the epithelium are of peculiar structure, they are branched and exhibit distal bulbous expansions, which are filled with mitochondria (mitochondrial sacs, Fig. 85). These are in close contact with Schwann cells which may nurture them. These terminals, which have a relatively large surface area, are extremely sensitive. Their impulse frequence increases when the temperature rises, it decreases when the temperature falls.

Mitochondrial sacs are of wide distribution in invertebrates and vertebrates (Fig. 80). They may occur in intraepithelial location (nemerteans, polychaetes, vertebrates) or in the connective tissue

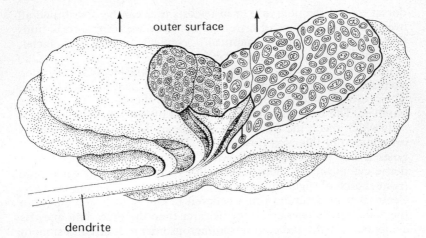

outer surface

dendrite

Figure 85. Thermoreceptor from the pit organ of a crotalid viper; the inflated terminal endings of the sensory neuron are filled with mitochondria. After TERASHIMA, GORIS, KATSUKI, 1970

(reptiles, mammals) or even extend into the ventricular lumen of the central nervous system (vertebrates). Their function is frequently not known, occasionally they may be thermo-, occasionally mechano- or other receptors. In insects thermoreceptors can be located in sensilla covered by a thick cuticle.

Electroreceptors

Electroreceptors occur in the teleost families of gymnotids (South America) and mormyrids (Africa), which use electrical impulses for orientation. Gymnotids produce intermittent electrical discharges, mormyrids produce almost continuous currents.

In the skin of gymnotids two different organs with electro-receptors may be recognized: the ampullar receptor organ, a tonic receptor responding to long-lasting electrical impulses and the tubular receptor organ which adapts rapidly.

The ampullary organs correspond to spherical invaginations of the skin, which open to the free surface by a small duct. The lumina of ampulla and duct are filled by a jelly-like substance. In the ampullary wall supporting and four to eight receptor cells can be distinguished. The latter are particularly large and of roundish shape. At their surface they bear microvilli. The cytoplasm contains abundant cell organelles, among which mitochondria and smooth ER tubules predominate. Into the basal portion of the cells large nerve terminals extend. Ten to fifteen special synaptic areas can be recognized in one nerve ending.

The tubular organs either open to the free surface *via* small ducts (posterior region of the body) or correspond to closed cavities (anterior part of the body). They are surrounded by a basal lamina and are located directly under the epidermis. The wall is composed of elongated cellular processes, resembling those of the basal epidermal cells, and receptor cells, which are relatively tall and can be club-shaped. Their slender bases are underlain by a cushion of supporting cells. Laterally and apically they bear microvilli. In the cytoplasm glycogen particles and mitochondria are particularly prominent. Basally they are in synaptic contact with nerve terminals similar to those of the ampullary receptor cells.

The sensory organs in the epidermis of the mormyrids correspond to jelly filled spaces, at the base of which receptor cells occur. These spaces are interconnected by a narrow duct with a second deeper space, which is filled with mucus and the wall of which also contains sensory cells. Both types of sensory cells resemble those of the gymnotids and are basally interconnected with nerve endings.

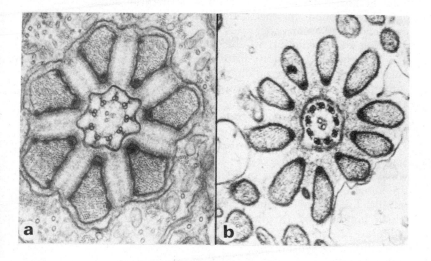

Figure 86.   Cross-sections through the cilia and their surrounding microvilli at the receptor pole of mechanoreceptors. This apparatus is located in a bowl-shaped invagination of the receptor cell. **a:** *Priapulus* (Priapulida), the cilium is surrounded by seven specialized microvilli, x 50 000; **b:** *Rhynchelmis* (Oligochaeta) the cilium is surrounded by ten microvilli, x 36 000

Mechanoreceptors

The simplest type of mechanoreceptors are free nerve endings, which in invertebrates rarely, but in vertebrates frequently, are enveloped by associated cells. In water-dwelling, soft-skinned invertebrates further mechanoreceptors in the form of ciliated primary or secondary sensory cells are of wide distribution. Several cilia often stand closely together and have been described in the light microscope as tactile hairs, e.g. in the Turbellaria, Nemertini, Chaetognatha and others. Often the apex bears only one cilium, which is surrounded by a collar of regularly arranged microvilli containing numerous microfilaments (stereocilia), e.g. in cnidarians (Fig. 65), priapulids (Fig. 86), annelids (Fig. 86), chaetognaths and echinoderms. In annelids the cilia may be surrounded by an epicuticular sheath (Fig. 19).

Similar receptor cells are situated in the wall of the lateral line system of aquatic vertebrates. Here they are secondary sensory cells, the cilia of which are embedded in a jelly-like mass (cupula).

In the statocysts the cilia of the receptor cells can be in connection with concretions (receptors of gravity). The cilia occasionally are characterized by rootlets laterally extending from the basal body in horizontal direction. Similar structural details have not only been found in the statocysts of molluscs, but also in mechanoreceptors of vertebrates. Deflection of the cilium into the direction of the rootlet, in the inner ear of vertebrates, causes depolarization, deflection into the opposite direction hyperpolarization of the receptor cell. The statoreceptor cells can contain voluminous spirally wound lamellar systems, which in part are derived from the rough ER. Also the plasma membrane of the sensory cilia in the static organs of Cnidaria and Ctenophora frequently forms voluminous lamellar systems.

Mechanoreceptors of arthropods may be derived from hair sensilla (Fig. 81). The receptor cells are bipolar and bear a cilium, which is connected with a cuticular sheath (scolops). In the ciliary tip numerous microtubules can frequently be found running in parallel to the longitudinal axis of the cilium (tubular body) and which are believed to play a role in the transformation of the stimulus. Movement of the cuticular sheath of the cilium causes an excitation of the sensory cell.

Hair sensilla, the hairs of which are movable and which act as mechanoreceptors have been described in many arthropods. Trichobothria are specialized hair sensilla, easily movable and arising from a flexible epidermal groove, which react to air currents. They may be found for example on the extremities of spiders, scorpions and pseudoscorpions, on the prosoma of various mites, on the cerci of insects, e.g. cockroaches, furthermore they occur in diplopods, pauropods and symphyla.

They can be deflected in a preferred direction and connected with one sensory cell, e.g. in scorpions. In *Euscorpius* an orientation in space is accomplished by the special arrangement of various groups of trichobothria; these stand in areas of the pedipalpus, which are oriented towards each other at right angles. On the locomotory extremities of the spider *Tegenaria* trichobothria with four sensory cells have been found. In *Scutigerella* which only possesses one pair of trichobothria, sixteen sensory cells are connected with a flexible cuticular membrane, giving rise to a hair, which can be deflected in all directions.

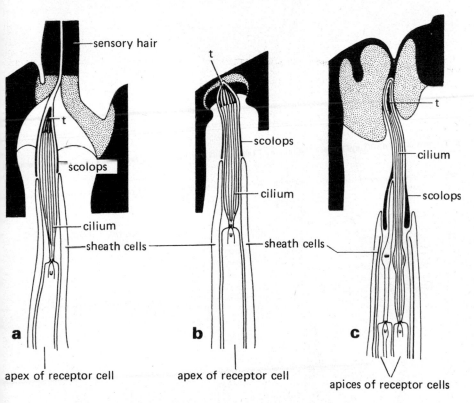

Figure 87. Apices of sensory cells with cilia and cuticular structures in various mechanoreceptors of insects (fine structure); **a:** sensory hair of the honey bee, after THURM, 1964; **b:** campaniform sensillum from the pedicellus of *Chrysopa* (Neuroptera); **c:** Scolopophorous organ from the organ of Johnston of *Chrysopa;* T: tubular body, after SCHMIDT, 1969

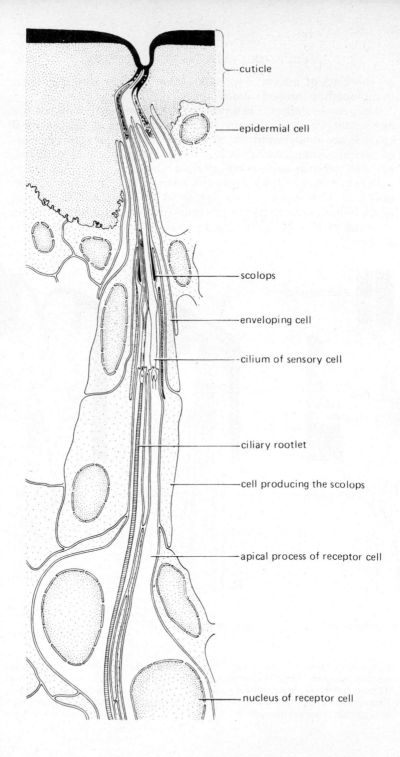

cuticle

epidermial cell

scolops

enveloping cell

cilium of sensory cell

ciliary rootlet

cell producing the scolops

apical process of receptor cell

nucleus of receptor cell

Also derived from the arthropod sensory hairs are the scolopidia (Fig. 88), which are almost exclusively confined to Antennata (but cf. sensory slits). Each scolopidium is composed of two to three sensory cells, the perikarya of which are located deeply under the epidermis. Each sensory cell extends an apical receptive process, which distally bears a cilium. The root of this cilium may be very long and extend down to the perikaryon. Perikaryon and receptive process are surrounded by various cells. The peg cell presumably corresponds to the trichogenous cell of normal insect hairs, the enveloping cell to the tormogenous cell. The cilia project into an extracellular space and are apically connected with a delicate cuticular sheath (cylinder), which originates from the cuticle of the normal epidermis, and probably is formed by the peg cell. This sheath is termed scolops (sensory peg); it can also be seen in the light microscope, and is responsible for the name of the complete organ: scolopidium.

Scolopidia can occur in serial arrangement in the body and in the extremities, such groups are termed chordotonal organs. In the second antennal segment of Thysanura and pterygote insects scolopidia form the wall of a cylindrical structure (Johnston's organ). Their sensory pegs are connected with the soft articular membrane between second antennal segment (pedicellus) and the first segment of the antennal flagellum. Johnston's organ perceives movements of the antennal flagellum.

Scolopophorous organs interconnected with tracheae underlying tightly stretched thin integumentary areas are termed tympanal organs. The specialized part of the integument (ear drum, tympanum) acts as a receiver of sound pressure, the trachea serves the conduction of the stimulus, the complete organ as a phonoreceptor (tympanal organ).

Of basically similar structure as that of the scolopophorous organs, are the cleft sensory organs of spiders. In *Cupiennius salei* more than a thousand of such sensory slits occur. They can be of various sizes and form groups (lyriform organs) or occur singly. In every case the membrane (cuticle) closing the cleft is connected with cilia arising from dendritic processes of bipolar sensory cells. The cilia also contain tubular bodies. These organs perceive various mechanical stimuli: vibrations of the bottom, deflections of the articulations, air sounds.

Figure 88. Longitudinal section through a scolopophorous organ of the organ of Johnston of *Chrysopa*; fine structure. The bipolar sensory cells are deeply located below the epidermis; their apical cilia are interconnected with the cuticle via the scolops. The whole sensory complex is accompanied by different cells (enveloping cell, scolops producing cell and others). After SCHMIDT, 1969

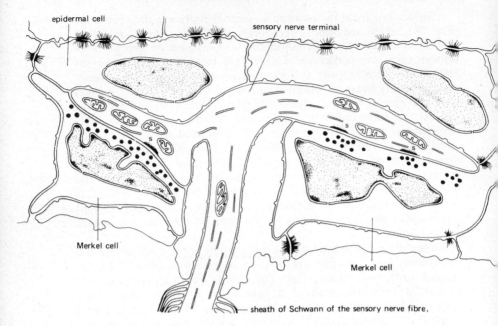

Figure 89. Tactile nerve ending in the mammalian epidermis (Merkel disk). Note synaptic contact (s) between granule containing Merkel cell and nerve terminal, which does not contain synaptic vesicles. After ANDRES, 1966

Various types of mechanoreceptors occur in the epidermis and in the connective tissue of vertebrates. They are best known in mammals. In this group light pressure is perceived by three types of receptor organs: Meissner's corpuscles, Merkel's disks and free nerve endings. The latter e.g. occur in the cornea, in the oral cavity, and in the skin, where they are particularly important tactile organs in hair follicles.

Meissner's corpuscles are located in the dermal papillae of the skin and are particularly prominent in the skin of palms and soles. They are ovoid or elongated structures, which are composed of centrally located irregularly shaped cells between which terminal ramifications of sensory nerve fibres occur. The whole structure is delimited by a thin connective tissue capsule. Merkel's disks occur in the epidermis. They consist of large pale and granule containing epidermal cells (tactile cells), which are in synaptic contact with sensory nerve endings (Fig. 89).

Stronger pressure activates the corpuscles of Pacini, which are found in the deeper layers of the skin, under mucous membranes, in the mesenteries, in the pancreas, along blood vessels and so on. They consist of one or more centrally located nerve endings which are encapsulated by concentric layers of flattened cells (Schwann and connective tissue cells) separated by a fluid containing inter-cellular space. Similar corpuscles also occur in other vertebrates.

In birds they are particularly diversified under the skin of the bills of ducks and geese. In the skin of almost all birds Herbst's corpuscles occur (Fig. 90); here the central nerve terminal is surrounded by an inner layer of cells and peripheral concentric lamellae.

The internal ear (labyrinth) of the vertebrates is derived from the lateral line system. As this system it contains mechanoreceptors, which are activated by fluid currents. In mammals three groups of mechanoreceptive cells are located in the wall of thin walled tubules and sacs constituting the membranous labyrinth, which is suspended in corresponding fluid-filled cavities of the petrous bone (Fig. 84). The canals and cavities in the bone comprise the osseous labyrinth. The fluid of the osseous labyrinth is called perilymph. Also the membranous labyrinth contains fluid: the endolymph.

The sensory cells of the auditory system are located in the organ of Corti, those perceiving rotating movements in the ampullae of the semicircular canals, those of the static sense in utriculus and sacculus. Semicircular canals, utriculus, and sacculus together form the vestibule, the organ of Corti is part of the spirally coiled cochlea.

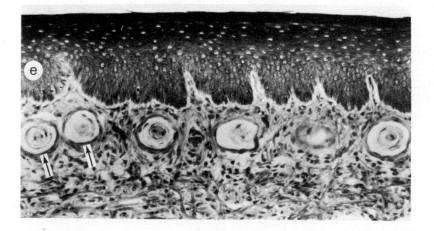

Figure 90.   Encapsulated terminal sensory corpuscles (corpuscles of Herbst, arrows) under the epidermis (e) of the bill of a duck, x 100

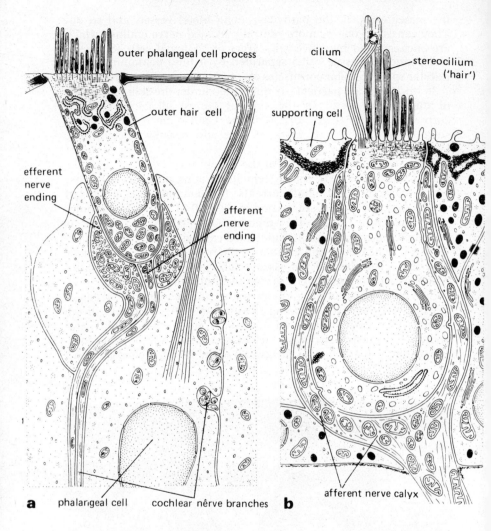

Figure 91.   Schematic representation of the ultrastructure of receptor cells in the mammalian internal ear. **a:** Outer hair cell and its relationship to the outer phalangeal cells, organ of Corti. The sensory cell is innervated by afferent and efferent nerve endings. The cell apex only bears microvilli (stereocilia). **b:** Vestibular type I hair cell in the sensory epithelia of the *crista ampullaris* and the maculae. The cell is surrounded by a cuplike afferent nerve ending (nerve calyx). The apical pole of this receptor cell bears a cilium and stout microvilli (stereocilia). After BLOOM & FAWCETT, 1970

1. Each semicircular canal is characterized by a bulbous dilated portion called an ampulla. These possess a transverse ridge, the *crista ampullaris*, which is covered by sensory and supporting cells. The rest of the semicircular canals is lined by a flat epithelium. The sensory cells bear a single apical cilium and stout microvilli ('hairs', stereocilia), which extend into a gelatinous body above the cristae called the cupula. The sensory cells are activated by deflections of the cupula caused by movements of the endolymph.

2. Utriculus and sacculus contain in their walls fields with a heightened epithelium, which again is composed of sensory and supporting cells: *maculae staticae*. The cilia and microvilli (stereocilia, 'hairs') of the sensory cells extend into a jelly-like mass, which contains countless small crystals ($CaCO_3$ and protein), the otoliths or statoconia, or a bigger statolith. The shifting of these extracellular structures into various directions activates the sensory cells.

   The receptor cells of *crista ampullaris* and *macula statica* are of the same histological structure. Differences seem to concern only their numerical distribution. Two cell types can be distinguished, which mainly differ in respect of the structure of their synapses. Type I is bottle-shaped and has a rounded basal portion, which is enveloped by a large chalice-like nerve ending (Fig. 91). The basally located nucleus is surrounded by many mitochondria, which also are concentrated in the apical cytoplasm. The specializations of the free surface consist of 40–80 stout microvilli (stereocilia) and a kinocilium. The microvilli are arranged upon the cell surface in regular hexagonal array and in successive rows show a progressive increase of length from less than 1 μm on one side to more than 100 μm on the other side of the cell. The longest microvilli occur near the kinocilium. Their basal parts are narrower than their apical portions, centrally they contain longitudinally oriented microfilaments. The kinocilium lacks the central microtubules. Type II is of cylindrical shape and is connected with numerous nerve endings. Otherwise it resembles type I.

3. The receptor cells of the auditory organ are located in the cochlea. Fig. 84 shows a longitudinal section through the complete cochlea of a guinea pig, in which the coils of the cochlea can be seen in cross-section. Fig. 92 illustrates details of the organ of Corti, which lines the floor of the endolymph containing *ductus cochlearis* (*scala media*), which terminates blindly at the apex of the cochlea. The *ductus cochlearis* is accompanied by two perilymphatic ducts, above by the *scala*

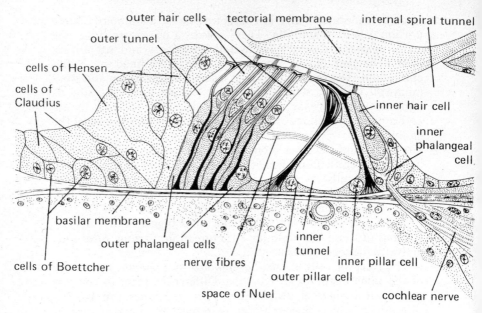

Figure 92.   Schematic representation of the organ of Corti. After HELD, BLOOM & FAWCETT, 1970

vestibuli, below by the *scala tympani*. These two ducts communicate in the helicotrema of the cochlear apex. The organ of Corti is located on the basilar membrane, the basal floor of the *ductus cochlearis,* and it is composed of sensory cells and a complicated system of supporting cells. It is covered by the *membrana tectoria* into which the apical processes of the sensory cells project and which consists of gelatinous material.

The supporting cells are tall slender elements extending from the basilar membrane to the free surface of the organ of Corti. They contain numerous microfilaments. At their bases they can be separated by wide intercellular spaces; apically they are interconnected with other supporting cells and with the sensory cells by junctional complexes. Various types of supporting cells may be recognized: inner and outer pillars (pillar cells), inner and outer phalangeal cells, border cells, cells of Hensen, Claudius, and Boettcher. This complex system of supporting cells encloses several intercellular spaces, which are in communiation with each other. On cross-sections three major spaces can be recognized: inner tunnel, space of Nuel, and outer tunnel (Fig. 92).

In man about 5,600 inner pillars exist and 3,800 outer ones. Three inner ones are connected with two outer ones. The inner phalangeal cells surround the inner haircells (sensory cells), the outer phalangeal cells support the outer haircells and surround their inferior third. The upper parts of the outer haircells are exposed to the fluid-filled space of Nuel and its extensions; apically the sensory cells are again in connection with the outer phalangeal cells (and with the outer pillar).

As in the vestibulum in the organ of Corti two types of receptor-cells occur. The inner haircells are arranged in a row extending through the whole cochlea. In man the outer haircells are arranged in three rows at the basis of the cochlea, in four rows in the second coil, in five rows in the upper coil. The inner haircells resemble the sensory cells in the vestibulum, however in adults they lack a kinocilium although the basal corpuscle remains present. The microvilli (stereocilia) are arranged on the apical surface in form of a U or a W. The microfilaments of the microvilli are anchored in a well developed terminal web. Numerous afferent and efferent nerve endings are attached to their basal surface.

The outer haircells (Fig. 91) are of a slightly different structure. The microvilli on the apex form a W, which is composed of more rows of microvilli than on the inner haircells, and the length of the microvilli varies from long in the periphery to short in the centre. A cilium is absent, a basal body may be present. Below the terminal web lipid inclusions and rough ER cisternae are located. Mitochondria are situated along the plasma membrane and in the cellular bases. Near by the plasma membrane also tubules of smooth ER occur. Each outer haircell is in synaptic contact with afferent and efferent nerve endings. Normally the efferent terminals are larger than the afferent ones, they contain synaptic vesicles. Parallel to the postsynaptic membrane in the receptor cell a flat smooth ER cisterna can be observed, termed subsynaptic cisterna.

The above description of the inner ear refers to mammals. The following paragraph lists a few peculiarities of other vertebrates. In reptiles and birds the organ of Corti (basilar papilla) is located in a sac-like or tubular extension of the sacculus. It is of a much simpler structure resembling the maculae and being composed of a stratified columnar epithelium (without special intercellular spaces) consisting of many (in the pigeon about thirty) rows of rather uniform sensory cells separated by uniform supporting cells. The vestibular membrane, the roof of the *ductus cochlearis*, in mammals consists of two layers of extremely flat epithelial cells. In birds it is relatively thick and contains epithelial ridges with blood capillaries, therefore it is also termed *tegmentum vasculosum*. Its epithelium

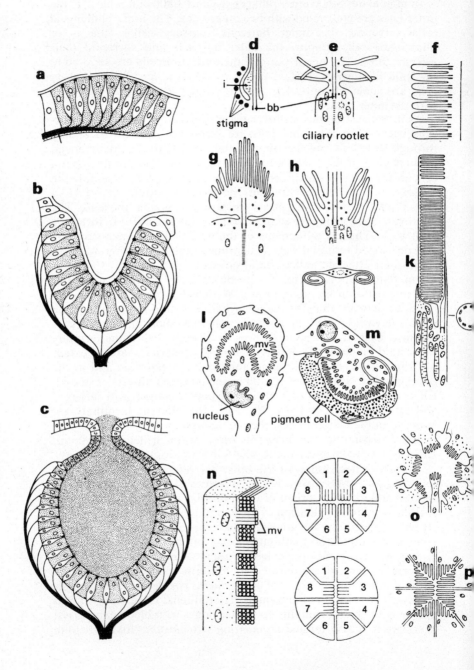

contains prismatic cells with secretory granules. In amphibia the precursor of the cochlea, a pouch of the sacculus, contains sensory cells of the same structure as in the *maculae staticae*. In fishes only the vestibulum occurs. In *Petromyzon* the epithelium of the inner ear is, apart from that of the semicircular canals, ciliated. The sensory organs are similar to those of the higher vertebrates.

Photoreceptors

Two main types of photoreceptors can be distinguished. The first type is characterized by a dense array of microvilli at the receptive surface: rhabdomere type (Fig. 93). Examples can be found mainly among protostomians. The second type represents a modified ciliary cell the cilium of which is transformed in various ways, e.g. its plasma membrane forming lamellar structures: ciliary type (Fig. 93); examples can be found among Cnidaria and deuterostomians. Whether these two types represent two evolutionary lines is not certain. Generally the ciliary type is considered to be primitive, since during embryogenesis also in the rhabdomeric type often cilia can be detected which later become reduced. Generally photoreceptor cells are primary sensory cells.

Usually photoreceptors stand together in formations termed retinae. A primitive retina is a flat epithelial structure. By invagination cup-shaped and vesicular retinae are formed, which respectively form cup ocelli and vesicular ocelli.

Frequently the retina is overlain by a light refractive (dioptric) apparatus (Fig. 94). If the receptive part of the sensory cells is directed towards the light, they are termed everted photoreceptors, if the receptive part points in the opposite direction (away from the light) the photoreceptors are called inverted. The sensory cells are frequently separated by cells containing protective pigment granules, which can screen the photoreceptors (iridial cells, pigment cells). The photoreceptors also may – beside the photopigments –

Figure 93. Light perceptive organs and photoreceptors. **a:** flat retina of the medusa *Aurelia*; **b:** cup-shaped eye of the prosobranch snail *Patella*; **c:** pit-shaped eye of the prosobranch snail *Haliotis*. In **a** to **c** the receptor poles of the sensory cells are painted black. **d-p:** ultrastructure of the receptive pole of photoreceptors; d-k: photoreceptors of the ciliary type. **d:** cilium of *Euglena* (Flagellata), bb: basal body, i: inflation at the basis of the ciliary shaft. **e:** hydromedusa: **f:** sabellid polychaete, **g:** *Ascidia*: **h:** starfish; **i:** ctenophore, **k:** vertebrate, top cone, below rod, right: cross-section through the cilium; **l-p:** rhabdomere type; **l:** leech, mv: microvilli; **m:** opheliid polychaete; **n:** decapode (crustacea), left: longitudinal section through an ommatidium, the microvilli (mv) of two neighbouring sensory cells interdigitate; right: cross-section through an ommatidium at different levels; **o:** fly: open rhabdom, cross-section; **p:** closed rhabdom, cross-section. After EAKIN; from REMANE, STORCH & WELSCH, 1974

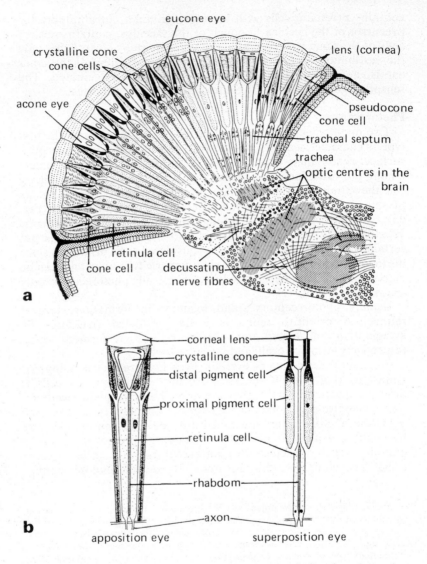

Figure 94. Insect compound eye. **a:** Combined schematic drawing of a section through a compound eye and the associated optic centres in the brain (optic lobe). Below the corneal lens the second part of the dioptric system can be found, the crystalline cone. This structure is formed by the cone cells and can be located outside these cells (pseudocone = exocone, left four and right three ommatidia) and entirely fuse with the lens. The crystalline cone can also be formed inside the cone cells (eucone eye) or the cone cells do not exhibit any structural peculiarities (acone eye). After WEBER, **b:** Schematic drawing of ommatidia of apposition and superposition eyes. After WOLKEN, 1970

contain protective pigment granules.

The space available allows only to describe two photoreceptive organs, the compound eyes and the vertebrate retina. Fig. 93 illustrates further examples of photoreceptor cells.

The compound eyes of insects are composed of single visual units, the ommatidia (Figs. 94, 95), which correspond to narrow, deeply invaginated cup-shaped eyes. In one compound eye a few (some ants) or up to 28,000 (dragonflies) ommatidia may be found. Each ommatidium possesses a dioptric apparatus, which is composed of a transparent lense-shaped area of the cuticle (cornea) and a crystalline cone. Below this structure the photoreceptor cells are situated. Cells containing protective pigments surround crystalline cone and sensory cells (Fig. 94). Differences found in the various species concern number and position of the sensory cells (= retinula cells) in one ommatidium, their distance from the crystalline cone and the position of the pigment cells.

The crystalline cone normally is composed of four crystalline cells (cells of Semper), which themselves can have the function of a lens (acone eyes). In other cases these cells produce an intracellular (eucone eyes) or extracellular (pseudocone eyes) crystalline cone. The nuclei of the crystal cells are located centrally, if no special cone is formed. In eucone eyes the nuclei are located directly under the cornea, in pseudocone eyes they are to be found near the receptor cells.

In the electron microscope the crystalline cone does not exhibit a crystalline fine structure, but consists of randomly oriented fine particular material.

In each ommatidium three to eleven retinula cells may be found, the primitive number in insects seems to be eight. The elongated cells form the wall of a narrow cylinder. They bear a dense array of microvilli, which are directed towards the lumen of the cylinder. Collectively the microvilli of one retinula cell form the rhabdomere (which in the light microscope was considered to be a secretory product of the sensory cells). All the rhabdomeres of one ommatidium together are termed rhabdom. The rhabdomeres of the individual retinula cells can be in close contact in the centre of the ommatidium (closed rhabdom, Figs. 93, 95) or they can be separated by a fluid containing central space (open rhabdom, Fig. 93). The microvilli of the rhabdomeres are oriented at right angles to the longitudinal axis of the ommatidium, microvilli of sensory cells located opposite each other, are often in parallel arrangement (Fig. 95). They presumably contain the photopigment. In pupae of *Bombyx* the first action potentials of the eyes have been recorded at a time when the microvilli became differentiated. The cytoplasm of

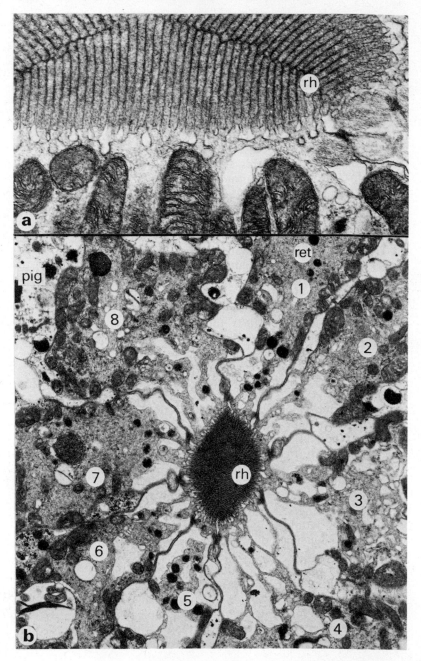

the retinula cells contains abundant mitochondria. If the rhabdom extends to the basis of the crystalline cone, the eye is called an apposition eye. If the rhabdom is only developed at the basis of the ommatidium the eye is termed superposition eye.

Neighbouring ommatidia are separated by various iris or pigment cells. Crystalline cone and cells are mainly surrounded by the distal pigment cells, the sensory cells are surrounded by the basal pigment cells.

In the apposition eye the ommatidia are completely separated by pigment cells, in superposition eyes a middle zone of the ommatidium is free of pigment cells.

In Crustacea compound eyes occur, the rhabdom of which are of a different structure than that of the insect eyes. In longitudinal sections one can see that the rhabdomeres do not consist of a

Figure 95. Ultrastructure of the insect compound eye. **a:** Rhabdom (rh) of *Gomphus* (dragonfly), note the spined vesicles at the bases of the microvilli forming the rhabdomere, x 36 000; **b:** Cross-section through an ommatidium of a bumble bee (*Bombus*). The rhabdom (rh) is composed of four rhabdomeres, which are differentiated by eight retinula cells (ret) (two retinula cells form a common rhabdomere). pig: pigment cell x 12 000

Figure 96. Ultrastructure of the rhabdom of the compound eye of *Neomysis* (Crustacea). Longitudinal section, showing the specific right-angular arrangement of the microvilli, lower right corner: pigment granules in the sensory cell. x 18 000. Photo K. MORITZ

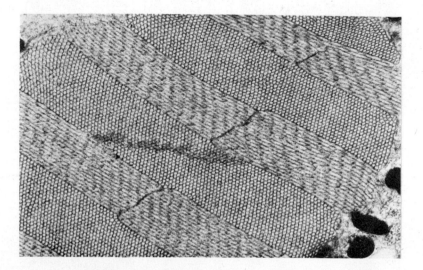

continuous array of microvilli but exhibit gaps (Fig. 93), into which microvilli of other sensory cells project. Thus regularly arranged rhabdoms are formed in which the microvilli not only are oriented at right angles to the longitudinal axis of the ommatidium but also in consecutive layers at right angles towards each other (Figs. 93, 96). The microvilli of one retinula cell always point in the same direction.

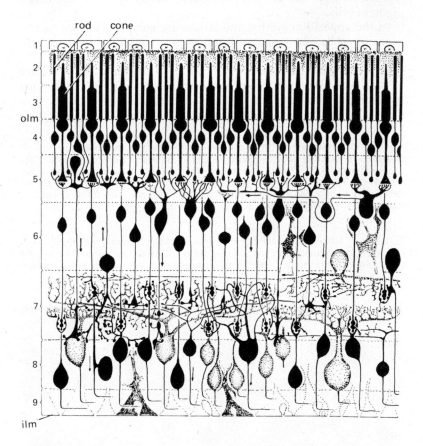

Figure 97. Diagram of the primate retina. 1-9: different layers from outside to inside. 1: pigment epithelium; 2: rod and cone outer segments; 3: rod and cone inner segments; 4: outer nuclear layer; 5: outer plexiform layer; 6: inner nuclear layer; 7: inner plexiform layer; 8: ganglion cell layer; 9: nerve fibre layer. olm: outer limiting membrane (row of desmosomes between sensory cells and extensions of glial cells), ilm: inner limiting membrane (pedicelles of glial cells and basement lamina). 2-4: photoreceptors; 6: mainly bipolar neurons; 8: mainly perikarya of ganglion cells; 5 and 7: zones of synaptic contact. Arrows indicate flow of excitation. After POLYAK, 1950

Compound eyes also occur outside the arthropods, e.g. in polychaetes and molluscs. The individual ommatidia can exhibit an own dioptric apparatus as in arthropods or be covered by a common lens. This situation e.g. can be found in most cephalopods, the everted retina of which groups of receptor cells form rhabdoms. The closed rhabdoms of *Octopus* and *Sepia* are formed by four retinula cells.

The photoreceptors of the lateral eyes of vertebrates are located in a multilayered inverted retina, which is a peripherally located part of the diencephalon and thus mainly consists of nervous tissue. Three principal cell types occur in the retina: sensory cells, the receptive apices of which are directed away from the light, form an outer layer, bipolar neurons form a middle layer, big bi- or multipolar neurons (ganglion cells) form an inner layer.

The arrangement of the nuclei, cytoplasmic extensions and synaptic regions of these cells is responsible for the fact that several sublayers may be recognized in light microscopic preparations of the retina (Fig. 97). The nuclei of layers 4, 6 and 8 belong to the principal cell types of the retina: sensory cells (4), bipolar neurons (6) and the perikarya of big neurons (8), the axons of which build up the optic nerve. The plexiform layers are composed of nerve fibres and synaptic regions.

The arrangement of the cells and the thickness of the retina vary in different regions of the eye and in different species. In certain areas *(foveae centrales)* it is particularly thin and consists almost entirely of sensory cells, in the area surrounding a *fovea centralis* the number of ganglion cells is particularly high and the arrangement of the cells is especially regular. In the peripheral parts of the retina the number of cells decreases and the layered arrangement becomes indistinct.

Two types of sensory cells can be distinguished: rod cells and cone cells. Rod cells are elongated cells (length in mammals 60–40 μm) the cytoplasm of which is differentiated into several regions. The elongated outer segment borders the pigment epithelium and in the light microscope often alone is termed rod. It contains the photopigment and in the electron microscope can be seen to be composed of a large number of parallel lamellae oriented traversely to the axis of the rod (Fig. 98). Each lamella is a closed membrane limited sac flattened into a disk, about 2 μm in diameter and about 14 nm thick. The narrow cavity measures about 8 nm across.

Below the outer an inner segment can be recognized. The two are connected by a slender stalk which corresponds to a modified cilium in which the central two microtubules are absent. The nine outer pairs of double tubules originate from a basal corpuscle which

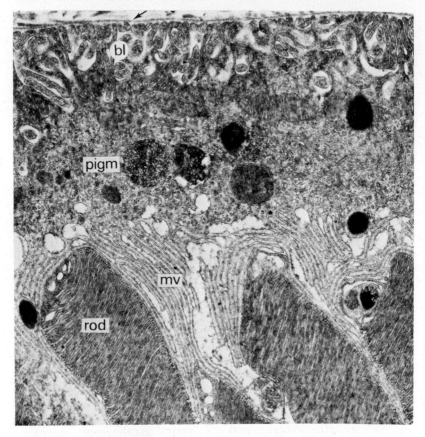

Figure 98. Rat, electron micrograph of the pigment epithelium (pigm) and distal parts of the outer segments of a number of rods (rod). Arrow points to basement lamina of the pigment epithelium; the latter is characterized by a basal labyrinth (b) and microvilli (mv) surrounding the outer segments of the rods. x 20 000

frequently extends rootlets. The inner segment contains abundant elongated mitochondria (collectively called in the light microscope ellipsoid). Next follow the outer rod fibre and the rod body. The outer rod fibre is a slender portion connecting inner segment with the nuclear zone, the rod body.

From the nucleus an axon-like process is extended (inner rod fibre) which makes synaptic contact with the bipolar cells.

The cone cells exhibit a similar ultrastructure as the rod cells. The shape of their outer segment is plumper and resembles a cone. Some of its membranous disks open out into the extracellular space (Fig.

93). The outer cone fibre is usually absent. The cone cell nucleus is paler and larger than that of the rod cells. The inner segments of teleost and amphibian cone cells are contractile.

The material of the outer segments is constantly renewed. In Anuran rod cells every day about thirty new disks are formed. A corresponding number is apically sloughed off and incorporated into the pigment epithelium. In cone cells no new formation of disks can be observed, but autoradiographs show that their molecular components also are regularly renewed.

The receptor cells are surrounded by elongated glial cells (cells of Müller) which are connected with the sensory cells above their nuclear regions by junctional complexes. This row of contact areas appears in the light microscope as a dark line, which is termed outer limiting membrane. Apically of this zone the glial cells extend microvilli into the intercellular space. The cells of Müller contain glycogen particles, which may be important for nutrition of the receptor cells.

The bipolar neurons interconnect receptor cells and ganglion cells. Some of them transmit impulses from sensory cells to ganglion cells, others transmit into the opposite direction. Also located in the inner nuclear layer are the horizontal cells, typical neurons, that interconnect groups of receptor cells. The small oval nuclei of the cells of Müller also occur in this layer.

The inner part of the inner nuclear layer contains a further type of neuron, the large amacrine cells which seem to interconnect groups of ganglion cells. The inner limiting membrane corresponds to pedicle-like terminals of the glial cells, which form a border against the vitreous body.

Within the retina blood capillaries can be observed. Nourishment of the receptor cells is accomplished by vessels of the uvea. The pigment epithelium plays an important role in the exchange of nutrients between these blood vessels and the photoreceptors. It extends long microvilli, which surround the distal parts of the outer segments. The pigment cells further contain pigment granules and stacks of smooth ER, which may have a photoreceptive function regulating the movement of the pigment granules.

The retina forms the innermost coat of the wall of the eyeball and is directly attached to the centrally located vitreous body. The two outer coats are the vascular tunic (uvea) and the sclera, which may contain cartilaginous (Amphibia) and osseous (many birds) tissue.

In the eye of many reptiles and birds a particular structure extends from the wall of the eyeball into the vitreous body. In many birds it is a folded lamellar structure (*pecten oculi*), in others and in reptiles it is a cone-shaped projection. It contains abundant blood capillaries and pigment cells and in the pigeon, e.g. is essential for nutrition of the receptor cells (Fig. 147).

A few further characteristics of the retina of non-mammalian vertebrates may be listed briefly. The inner segment of rod cells in birds, reptiles and amphibia contains oil droplets. In reptiles the layer of ganglion cells is unusually voluminous and the amacrine cells are relatively prominent cells. The rod cells of teleosts are particularly long (about 100 μm). Particularly prominent elements of the teleost inner nuclear layer are the large horizontal cells. In many sharks the pigment epithelium is almost devoid of pigment granules. Also in the retina of *Petromyzon* rod- and cone-cells have been described. The individual layers, however, are less clearly to be recognized.

LITERATURE

ALTNER, H., MÜLLER, W., BRACHNER, I. 'The ultrastructure of the vomeronasal organ in Reptilia.' Z. Zellforsch. 105, 107-122 (1970).

ANDRES, K. H. 'Über die Feinstruktur der Rezeptoren an Sinushaaren.' Z. Zellforsch. 75, 339-365 (1966).

BABEL, J., BISCHOFF, A., SPOENDLIN, H. 'Ultrastructure of the peripheral nervous system and sense organs. G. Thieme Verlag, Stuttgart, 452 pp. (1970).

BARTH, F. G., LIBERA, W. 'Ein Atlas der Spaltsinnesorgane von *Cupiennius salei* Keys. Chelicerata (Araneae).' Z. Morph. Tiere. 68, 343-369 (1970).

BÖCK, P. 'Die Nerven der Papilla filiformis der Zunge vom Meerschweinchen. Arch. histol. jap. 32, 399-411 (1971).

EAKIN, R. M. 'Structure of invertebrate photoreceptors.' In: *Handbook of sensory physiology*, Vol. VII, 1, 625-684, Springer-Verlag, Berlin, Heidelberg, New York (1972).

FOELIX, R. F. AXTELL, R. C. 'Fine structure of tarsal sensilla in the tick *Amblyomma americanum* (L.).' Z. Zellforsch. 114, 22-37 (1971).

GRAZIADEI, P. P. C., METCALF, J. F. 'Autoradiographic and ultrastructural observations of the frog's olfactory mucosa.' Z. Zellforsch. 116, 305-318 (1971).

HAUPT, J. 'Beitrag zur Kenntnis der Sinnesorgane von Symphylen (Myriapoda). II. Feinstruktur des Tömösváryschen Organs von *Scutigerella immaculata* Newport.' Z. Zellforsch. 122, 172-189 (1971).

HAYES, W. F. 'Fine structure of the chemoreceptor sensillum in *Limulus*.' J. Morph. 133, 205-240 (1971).

HERNANDEZ-NICAISE, M. L. 'Ultrastructural evidence for a sensory-motor neuron in Ctenophora.' Tissue and Cell. 6, 43-47 (1974).

HORRIDGE, G. A. 'Statocysts of medusae and evolution of stereocilia.' Tissue and Cell. 1, 341-353 (1969).

SCHMIDT, K. 'Der Feinbau der stiftführenden Sinnesorgane im Pedicellus der Florfliege *Chrysopa* Leach (Chrysopidae, Planipennia).' Z. Zellforsch. 99, 357-388 (1969).

SCHNEIDER, D., STEINBRECHT, R. A. 'Checklist of insect olfactory sensilla.' Symp. zool. Soc. Lond. 23, 279-297 (1968).

SEIFERT, K. 'Die Ultrastruktur des Riechepithels beim Makrosmatiker.' Norm. u. Pathol. Anatomie. Heft 21, 99 S. G. Thieme Verlag, 1970.

SINOIR, Y. 'L'ultrastructure des organes sensoriels des insects.' *Ann. Zool. Ecol. anim.* **1**, 339-356 (1969).

SLIFER, E. H. 'The structure of arthropod chemoreceptors.' *Ann. Rev. Entomol.* **15**, 121-142 (1970).

SMITH, D. S. 'The fine structure of haltere sensilla in the blowfly, *Calliphora erythrocephala* (Meig.) with scanning electron microscopical observations on the haltere surface.' *Tissue and Cell.* **1**, 443-484 (1969).

STEINBRECHT, R. A. 'Comparative morphology of olfactory receptors.' In: *Olfaction and taste* (C. Pfaffmann, ed.). New York: Rockefeller University Press 1969.

STORCH, V. 'Vergleichende elekronenmikroskopische Untersuchungen über Receptoren von Wirbellosen (Nemertinen, Turbellarien, Molluscen, Anneliden, Aschelminthen).' *Verhandl. Deutsch. Zoolog. Ges.* **66**, 61-65 (1973).

SZAMIER, R. B., WACHTEL, A. W. 'Special cutaneous receptor organs in fish. VI. Ampullary and tuberous organs of *Hypopomus*.' *J. Ultrastruct. Res.* **30**, 450-471 (1970).

TERASHIMA, S., GORIS, R. C., KATSUKI, Y. 'Structure of warm fiber terminals in the pit membrane of vipers.' *J. Ultrastruct. Res.* **31**, 494-506 (1970).

THURM, U. 'Untersuchungen zur funktionellen Organisation sensorischer Zellverbände.' *Verh. dtsch. zool. Ges.* 79-88 (1970).

VINNIKOV, Y. A. 'Evolution of the gravity receptor.' *Minerva Otorinolaringologica.* **24**, 1-48 (1974).

WOLKEN, J. *Invertebrate photoreceptors.* Acad. Press, New York, 179 pp., 1971.

WOLSTENHOLME, G. E. W., KNIGHT, J. 'Taste and smell in vertebrates.' *Ciba Found. Symp.* Churchill, London, 402 pp. (1970).

Chapter 5
NERVOUS SYSTEM

Sponges. Electron microscopic and histochemical observations have clearly shown that a primitive type of nervous system exists in sponges. Thus older descriptions of nerve cells in sponges based on metal impregnations and stains with methylene blue have been confirmed; e.g. in *Sycon* cells have been demonstrated with contain 5-hydroxytryptamin (5-HT), adrenaline, noradrenaline, mono-aminoxidase (MAO), acetylcholinesterase and neurosecretory substances, all characters of typical neurons. *Sycon* possesses two types of neurons (Fig. 99): (a) spindle-shaped, bipolar ones which occur in the mesenchyme near pinaco- or choanocytes, in particular in the area of the osculum; (b) multipolar cells. Both types contain neurosecretory products; noradrenaline has been additionally demonstrated in the spindle-shaped neurons, adrenaline and 5-HT additionally in the multipolar ones. In the electron microscope both cell types contain electron-dense granules of the kind which is typical for neurosecretory neurons. In *Tethyia* synapse-like terminals containing neurosecretory granules and typical bouton-like endings in the surface of choanocytes have been described.

Cnidaria. Neurons which occur both in endo- and ectoderm constitute a primitive nervous system, a nerve-net. Secondary sensory cells and receptor neurons cannot clearly be separated from typical neurons. In the light microscope bipolar neurons with short processes and bipolar and multipolar nerve cells with long processes have been distinguished. The first group seems to be concentrated in the foot region of polyps, the other neurons are distributed all over the body. The sensory cells usually are spindle-shaped and bear an apical cilium (Fig. 64). Receptor neurons usually possess large perikarya in the depth of the epithelium and extend a ciliated slender process to the surface. In the nervous system of cnidarians, e.g. acetylcholin, adrenaline, noradrenaline, dopamine, 5-HT, neuro-secretory substances have been demonstrated with histo- and bio-chemical methods.

In the electron microscope the bipolar and probably also the

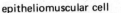
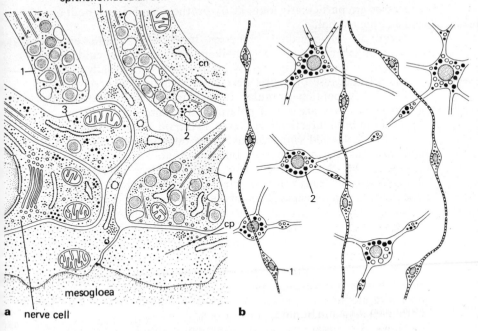

Figure 99.   **a:** different types of nerve endings (1–4) in the epidermis of *Hydra*. The endings contain neurosecretory granules, light vesicles, mitochondria, rough ER, ribosomes, glycogen particles; axon 1 seems to terminate free in the intercellular space, axon 2 near a cnidoblast (cn), axon 3 at a nerve cell, axon 4 at the contractile process (cp) of an epitheliomuscular cell. Apart from the granular and vesicular inclusions the synapses do not show structural specializations. **b:** Catecholamine containing neurons in the sponge *Sycon*. The bipolar cells (1) contain predominantly noradrenaline, the multipolar ones (2) adrenaline. After LENTZ, 1968

multipolar neurons have been shown to contain extensive rough ER cisterns, numerous ribosomes, microtubules and a voluminous Golgi apparatus, surrounded by light vesicles. Many neurons can be termed neurosecretory neurons since they contain numerous dense secretion granules (Fig. 99).

The ultrastructure of the spindle-shaped sensory cells closely resembles that of bipolar neurons, the apical cilium usually is of the 9 + 2 or 9 + 5 pattern.

The processes of the neurons run on top of the myofilament containing basal extensions of the epitheliomuscular cells. Their cytoplasm contains ribosomes, microtubules, glycogen and granular inclusions. Giant fibres with countless neurosecretory granules may frequently be observed at the base of the tentacles. Some of the processes are particularly long, in *Hydra* they can bridge about one-third of the animal.

Terminals of neuronal processes have been found on the contractile extensions of the epitheliomuscular cells, on cnidoblasts and on other neurons (Fig. 99). Synaptic regions are usually difficult to identify because of poorly developed structural characteristics. Usually they contain granular inclusions on both sides of the synapse, i.e. they are not of polarized structure and can transmit impulses in both directions. However, in *Sarsia* and other forms also individual polarized synapses have been demonstrated. Nerve cells can influence the nematocytes, but presumably do not trigger the explosion of the capsule. The neurosecretory substances of cnidarians (and many other invertebrates) are essential for growth, differentiation and regeneration of the animals.

Nerve nets as those found in the Cnidaria are assumed to represent a primitive type of arrangement of the nervous tissue. They also occur e.g. in flatworms, echinoderms and hemichordates. In higher animals they are usually restricted to certain organs, e.g. in the vertebrates to the alimentary canal. The net of the cnidarians consists only of individual processes of neurons, that of the flatworms of medullary rays, i.e. of cords of nervous tissue containing both perikarya and bundles of processes.

Above the cnidarians two developmental trends of the nervous system can be recognized. The first one leads from the nerve net via a concentration in longitudinal cords to the ventrally located nerve cord of the annelids and arthropods (protostomians). The second line also starts with the nerve net and leads to the formation of a dorsal tubular infolding, the neural tube (deuterostomians).

Tentaculates. Generally these animals have a primitive nervous system located within epithelia, and a cerebral ganglion is formed which in bryozoans may contain a lumen. In phoronids giant fibres occur along the whole length of the body.

Flatworms. Some turbellarians, e.g. the acoelans, still maintain the primitive arrangement of a nerve net in the basal parts of the epidermis. Other turbellarians show an advanced condition. Here, within the mesenchymal connective tissue a nervous system can be found which is differentiated into a cerebral ganglion, longitudinal and transverse medullary rays as well as submuscular and sub-epithelial plexus. In contrast to the cnidarians unipolar neurons make their appearance, the bi- and multipolar neurons exhibit a greater degree of branching. The unipolar neurosecretory neurons are located at the posterior aspect of the brain and are assumed to play a role in growth and regeneration. Synapses are of simple structure usually being represented by nerve terminals containing granules. In *Dugesia* synapses with membrane thickenings and typical synaptic vesicles have been found. The cerebral ganglion rarely contains some glial cells. Thus in most turbellarians we can already find all the elements characterizing the nervous system of the bilateral animals. In the following paragraphs only a few characteristics of some selected animal groups shall be described.

Annelids. The central nervous system of annelids consists of a brain (supra-oesophageal ganglion), a sub-oesophageal ganglion and a ventral nerve cord. Usually the majority of neurons are of the neurosecretory type. Glial cells occur regularly. In many annelids giant fibres are located in the ventral nerve cord (Fig. 100).

In the leech *Theromyzon* the brain is surrounded by a layer of connective tissue (perineurium) consisting of collagen fibrils and a few fibroblasts. This capsule of connective tissue extends septa into

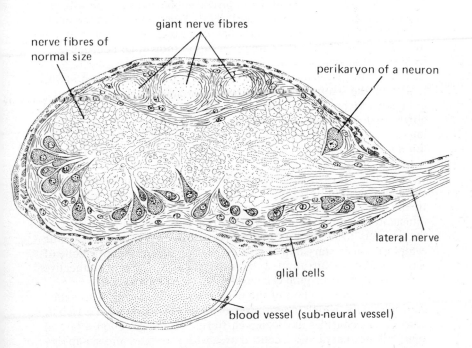

Figure 100. Cross-section through the ganglionic region of the ventral nerve cord of an earthworm (*Eisenia*). The nervous tissue is surrounded by a thin layer of connective tissue and muscle cells which are covered by peritoneal epithelium. The glial cells are mainly located in the periphery and extend pedicelles to the surface. After SCHNEIDER, 1908

the brain, which subdivide the nervous tissue into six symmetrically arranged pairs of compartments. Each compartment contains 1–2 glial cells enveloping several neurons. The neuronal axons penetrate the septa of the connective tissue and merge into a centrally located mass of nerve fibres, the dorsal commissure. Four types of neurons can be recognized. In all of them the perikarya and processes contain numerous granules, which in three of the neuronal types correspond to neurosecretory granules which are released in a neurohaemal organ at the posterior margin of the dorsal commissure. The granules of the fourth neuronal type possibly contain a transmitter substance.

The ventral nerve cord is composed by two chains of ganglia interconnected by commissures and longitudinal connectives. The neurons mainly seen to be of neurosecretory nature e.g. in *Nereis*, in the ganglionic chain mainly neurons with numerous granular inclusions occur (Fig. 62). Only a few perikarya are poor in granules but instead contain abundant glycogen particles. The above-mentioned giant fibres are particularly striking elements of the nerve cord. In *Myxicola* (Polychaeta) they can reach a diameter of 1·5 mm. The giant fibres either are processes of individual neurons (e.g. in *Sigalion*) or arise by fusion of the axons of several neurons (e.g. in *Clymene*). In *Lumbricus* the dorsal giant fibres, which originate by fusion of the axons of 2–3 neurons, are separated by segmental synapses. Here the consecutive fibres lie side by side and differentiate interdigitating pre- and post-synaptic membranes. The lateral dorsal giant fibres possess in each segment two perikarya, the middle one originates from three perikarya, the ventral giant fibres belong to one perikaryon each.

The nerve fibres of *Lumbricus* are frequently surrounded by a thin envelope, resembling a myelin sheath, which is formed by glial cells. In the ventral nerve cord of some leeches the glial cells can be of unusually large dimensions. Within one ganglion the perikarya of the neurons form six groups each of which is embedded into the cytoplasm of six star-shaped glial cells. The central synaptic zone of the ganglion is surrounded by two glial cells. Each connective contains another big glial cell enveloping numerous axons.

Insects. Each ganglion of the insects is surrounded by a so-called neural lamella, which is composed of a fine particular matrix rich in mucopolysaccharides and collagen fibrils. In the ganglion a lateral zone with perikarya and a central area with processes and synapses – together constituting a neuropile – can be distinguished (Fig. 104).

Directly under the neural lamella a layer of glial cells is situated (perineurium) in which the plasma membrane often shows marked foldings. Usually they contain lipid and glycogen and absorb nutrients from the haemolymph. Below these cells a second group of glial cells is located, the processes of which surround the perikarya of neurons, which lie in the deeper parts of the cortical zone. In part these glial cells have been observed to extend processes deep into the neurons. They presumably transfer nutrients and contain a well developed smooth ER. In the cell bodies of the neurons stacks of

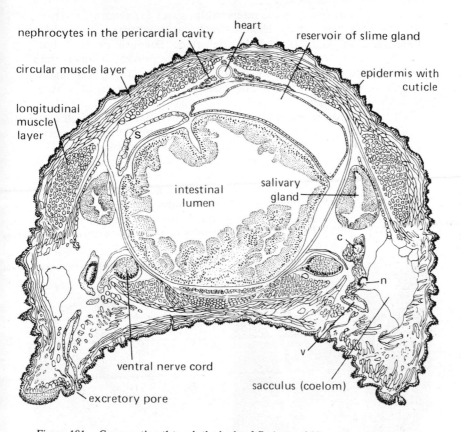

Figure 101. Cross-section through the body of *Peripatus* (skin and muscle cells see Fig. 51). The pericardial cavity is separated from the general body cavity by a horizontal septum. The wall of the heart is only composed of a circular muscle layer, dorsally a nerve is attached to the heart. The epithelial cells of the slime glands (S) contain a polyploid nucleus and produce a proteinaceous sticky slime. The ventral nerve cord is not divided into ganglia and connectives, the perikarya of the neurons are located ventrally, the fibres dorsally. The nephrostome (n) is an open funnel, with a fringe of cilia it leads into a coiled and ciliated tube (c), which contains a vesicular inflation (v), and opens through an excretory pore (nephridiopore). After SCHNEIDER, 1908

rough ER are rare, however, free ribosomes are abundant. The perikarya of neurosecretory neurons, as usual, are filled with electron-dense granules. The perikarya extend one process, the axon, into the neuropil, where it branches extensively. Cross-sections through the neuronal processes in the neuropil which also houses processes of glial cells show that they contain microtubules or neurosecretory granules.

In the area of synapses the intercellular space is extremely narrow (10 nm) and even can be absent (electrical synapses). Only rarely membrane thickenings may be detected. Because of the glial envelopes synapses are not to be found on the perikarya - as is the case in vertebrates - but are confined to the neuropil. The axon terminals may contain synaptic vesicles, the contents of which possibly is glutamate.

The neuronal processes are surrounded by glial cells, which can wind several times around an axon. However, typical myelin sheaths are absent, since each winding still contains some cytoplasm.

A typical ventral nerve cord with segmental ganglia is not present in all articulates, e.g. in onychophores several commissures occur per segment and ganglia and connectives are not clearly separated. In the longitudinal formations, which resemble medullary rays, the perikarya are located in a ventral, the fibres in a dorsal position (Fig. 101).

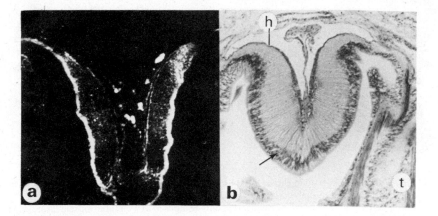

Figure 102.   Nervous system of starfish. **a:** *Astropecten*, fluorescent substances in the apical region of the ectoneural system x 25; **b:** *Asterias*, arrow points to the apical layer of perikarya in the ectoneural system, below which nerve fibres predominate; the basal processes of the supportive cells, which run vertically from the perikaryal layer to the base, are clearly to be seen; h: hyponeural nervous system (a thin layer of perikarya and fibres under the ectoneural system); t: tube foot. x 25

Echinoderms. Primitive, intraepithelial concentrations of nervous tissue in the so-called ecto- and hyponeural and the apical nervous system are present. In the starfish the perikarya of the neurons forming the ectoneural system are interspersed between the epidermal cells at the roof of the ambulacral groove where an apical layer of the perikarya and a basal layer of fibres may be recognized (Fig. 102). The synaptic regions between nerve and muscle cells are peculiar in so far as the muscle cells usually extend a short process towards the nerve fibre. The same phenomenon can be found in nematodes and amphioxus.

Hemichordates. The enteropneust nervous system is primitive, it consists mainly of a nerve fibre layer at the base of the epidermis. It is mainly intraepidermal, some fibres traverse the basement membrane and emerge amongst the muscle cells inserted into the coelomic side of the membrane. No specialized motor end-plates have been observed so far. In the collar region a tubular neurocord exists, which is a submerged strip of epidermis. Here multipolar and bipolar perikarya occur, also mainly in the innermost layers of the epidermal cells. A few giant cells extend one process (axon) each, running posteriorly and anteriorly. The neurons seem to be mainly of neurosecretory nature, since the nerve fibre profiles, varying in diameter between 0.15 to 10 μm, contain numerous vesicles of very varied diameter and contents together with larger granular inclusions, that also occur in the perikarya. The giant fibres also contain vesicles and microfilaments and microtubules. Morphologically recognizable synapses are rare, the majority of fibres are in intimate contact with one another. The central canal of the neurocord, which in primitive species like *Harrimania* and *Ptychodera,* still communicates with the exterior, is lined by typical columnar epidermal cells with cilia and microvilli. Scattered amongst these cells are mucus-secreting cells.

The central nervous system of *Branchiostoma* corresponds to an infolded submerged epithelial nervous system (= neural tube), as has been described in echinoderms. It consists of supporting glial cells and neurons. The anterior end of the neural tube forms a small vesicular structure, which together with the adjacent parts of the tube lying posteriorly to it often is called a brain. The vesicular part contains a fluid-filled space, a ventricle, which is lined by various types of usually ciliated epithelial cells among which two shall be mentioned: an anteriorly located group of cells containing pigment granules and a group of mucus-producing cells in the ventral floor constituting the so-called infundibulum. The mucus substance produced by these cells solidifies in the ventricle and forms the thread of Reissner which extends backwards into the central canal.

Reissner's thread also occurs in numerous vertebrates. In the area immediately behind the anterior vesicle numerous perikarya occur, among which in the dorsal region huge cells (cells of Joseph) are particularly prominent. At the surface of these cells - which presumably represent photoreceptors - a brushborder-like formation of microvilli can be found.

In the same area a supposedly second type of photoreceptor occurs, the plasma membrane of which extends densely packed long lamellar projections into the ventricle. In the ventral region a group of typical neurosecretory perikarya occurs. However, also the other perikarya usually contain beside striking areas of glycogen various vesicles and granules.

Behind the brain area the neural tube is of a more uniform structure. In a cross-section one can recognize a slit-like fluid-filled central canal which extends from the dorsal midline into the centre of the neural cord where it usually is slightly dilated. The central canal is in communication with the ventricle. Around it the peri-karya are located, whereas the fibrous components form a thick peripheral layer. The central canal is lined by usually dark staining ciliated ependymal cells, their basal filament rich processes diverge to the surface of the neural tube. Between the ependymal cells stout and usually ciliated processes of deeper located perikarya reach the

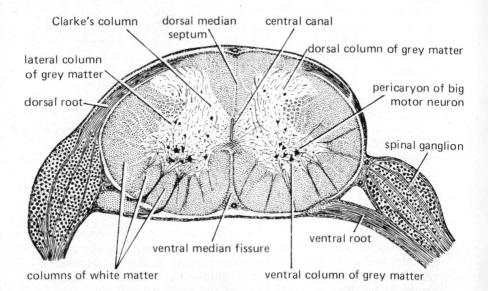

Clarke's column   dorsal median septum   central canal
dorsal column of grey matter
lateral column of grey matter
dorsal root
pericaryon of big motor neuron
spinal ganglion
ventral median fissure
ventral root
columns of white matter
ventral column of grey matter

Figure 103.   Cross-section through the spinal cord of the rabbit. After KRAUSE, 1921

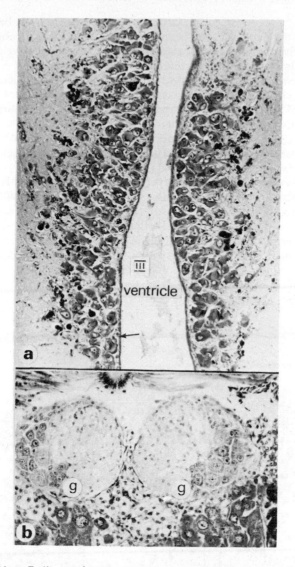

Figure 104. **a:** Perikarya of neurosecretory neurons (*nucleus paraventricularis*) in the dog, stained for neurosecretory material. Left and right *nuclei paraventriculares* are to be seen, separated by the relatively narrow third ventricle. Arrow points to ependymal lining of the ventricle, x 120. **b:** Cross-section through two ganglia (g) in the ventral nerve chord of *Acheta* (Orthopteroidea); perikarya on the lateral aspects of the ganglia; lower margin of the micrograph cells of the fat body. x 100

surface of the central canal. Often neuronal processes can be seen to traverse the central canal from one side of the neural tube to the other. The peripherally located nerve fibres are not enveloped by glial cells and contain numerous types of granular or vesicular components and/or microtubules. Giant fibres occur which mainly contain clear ground cytoplasm. Typical photoreceptors with a border of densely arranged microvilli are covered by semispherical extensions of pigment cells. From the neural tube extend segmentally arranged spinal nerves which have only a dorsal root. The so called ventral root consists of processes of the muscle cells of the body approaching the neural tube.

Vertebrates. The central nervous system of vertebrates is divided into brain and spinal cord. Both contain a fluid filled space, which in the area of the brain constitutes a ventricular system and in the spinal cord the central canal. In the nervous tissue grey and white matter (see p.114) can be distinguished. The distribution of these two components may be demonstrated by various light microscope stains. Staining methods demonstrating the perikarya, e.g. the Nissl or pigment granules, visualize the so-called cytoarchitecture. Procedures staining the white matter, e.g. lipid stains, demonstrate

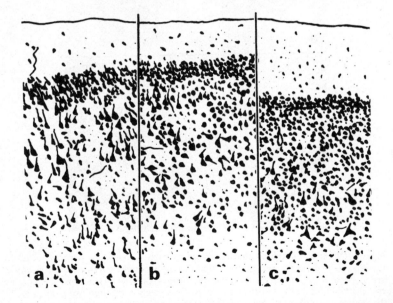

Figure 105.   Cerebral cortex of a dolphin (*Tursiops*), **a:** frontal lobe; **b:** parietal lobe; **c:** occipital lobe. Note the differences in the thickness of the various cortical layers. After TJAN, 1974

the so-called myeloarchitecture. With certain methods both components can be stained in one preparation. For finer distinctions of the grey and white matter histochemical methods demonstrating specific components, e.g. acetylcholinesterase or transmitters like dopamine or 5-HT can be employed.

As in *Branchiostoma* originally the grey matter is concentrated around the fluid-filled spaces. This state of affairs remains typical for the spinal cord of all vertebrates (Fig. 103) and also characterizes the brain of primitive vertebrates, particularly clearly, e.g. that of amphibians. In the course of evolution one can observe that the grey matter in certain parts of the brain, above all in the telencephalon, emigrates from its central location and forms superficial layers which usually are called cortex or cortical areas.

A further characteristic of a primitive type of grey matte. is the apparently irregular arrangement of its frequently rather large perikarya. In a grey matter of a higher type of organization the perikarya often are smaller and form layers, e.g. in the roof of the midbrain of teleosts and anurans and in the cortices of the telencephalon and cerebellum of mammals (Figs. 105, 107).

Fig. 103 shows a typical cross-section through the spinal cord of a mammal. It may be seen that the grey matter forms a centrally located figure with the shape of a butterfly. The dorsal, lateral and ventral projections of it are called dorsal, lateral and ventral horns. In its centre the central canal which is lined by ependymal cells may be recognized. The anterior horn contains large perikarya with coarse clumps of Nissl substance which belong to somatomotoric neurons, and smaller ones in their neighbourhood which belong to the inhibitory Renshaw cells. In the lateral horn the perikarya are smaller; they belong to the autonomic nervous system, the medial ones to the parasympathetic, the lateral ones to the sympathetic system. The perikarya of the dorsal horn usually also are relatively small, they build up interconnections between the various cells of the spinal cord or extend long processes to the brain.

The white matter is composed of various ascending or descending tracts of myelinated fibres, the majority of which cannot be identified on ordinary histological preparations.

In the spinal cord of lampreys and larval amphibians giant fibres occur. In teleosts at the end of the spinal cord a group of neurosecretory neurons is located (see p. 207), forming the urophysis.

At the level of the posterior extremities the avian spinal cord is characterized by an accumulation of glial cells which are almost completely filled with glycogen and which therefore is called the glycogen body.

To give an example of a highly organized cortical area the cortex of the mammalian cerebellum will briefly be described, since it is of a more uniform appearance than the cerebral cortex, the extent and number of layers of which varies considerably in the various mammals, even in one order, and also within various areas of the telencephalon (Figs. 105, 106).

The cerebellar cortex has only three layers: (a) an outer molecular layer, composed of few perikarya and many, in general unmyelinated fibres; (b) an intermediate single layer of large bottle-shaped perikarya belonging to the Purkinje cells, and (c) an inner granular or nuclear layer which is composed of the perikarya of the small granulated cells, which form the vast majority and of a few bigger perikarya belonging to the Golgi and Lugaro cells.

The Purkinje cells are of unusual shape (Fig. 107). The perikaryon gives rise to one or two dendritic stems from which a few main dendrites originate which branch in a fan-like fashion through the molecular layer to the surface. The whole dendritic arborization

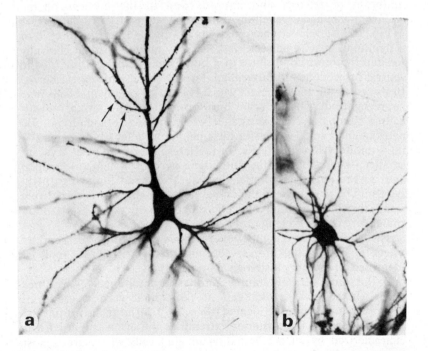

Figure 106. Golgi impregnations of two typical neurons from the human cerebral cortex; **a:** pyramidal cell (note synaptic spines on the dendrites, arrows; **b:** stellate cell (interneuron). x 120. Photo H. BRAAK

is densely covered with tiny spines which indicate synaptic contacts. The axon originates opposite to the dendrites and runs down into the white matter below the cortical area. The cells of the molecular layer which are located roughly at the same level as the perikarya of the Purkinje cells are called basket cells, since the numerous terminal branches of their axons surround the Purkinje cell perikarya.

The vertebrate central nervous system is always surrounded by a basal lamina and a layer of connective tissue (= meninx, plural: meninges), which in fishes is of a loose uniform structure. In amphibia, reptiles and birds a two-layered meninx is described, in which the outer parts are built up of a dense layer of collagen fibrils. In mammals the central nervous system is protected by three coats (Fig. 108): (a) the innermost *pia mater*, a connective tissue layer

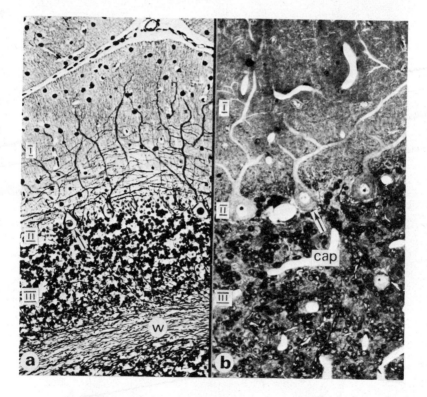

Figure 107. Light microscopical preparations of the cerebellar cortex of the rhesus monkey, I: *stratum moleculare*; II: *stratum ganglionare;* III: *stratum granulosum*. Arrow points to the perikarya of the Purkinje-cells, which constitue the stratum ganglionare. cap: Capillary, w: White matter x 360. Photo W. Lange.

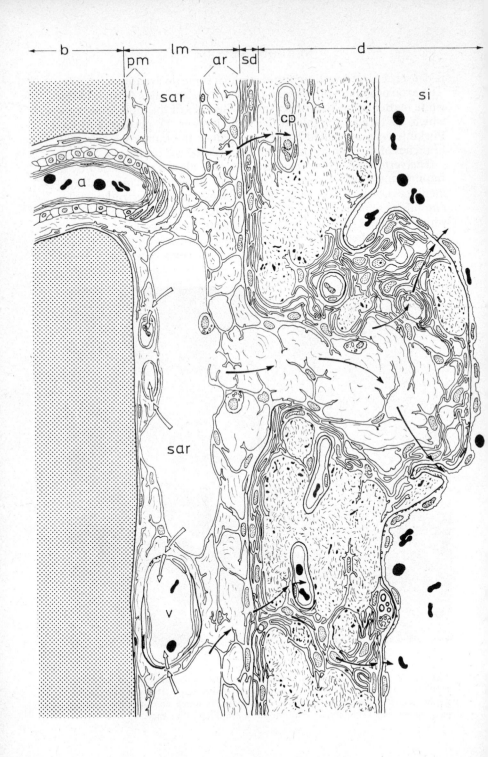

with numerous blood vessels and wide intercellular spaces containing bundles of collagen fibrils; (b) the arachnoid, a middle layer of extremely wide intercellular spaces traversed by collagen fibres, which constitute a cobwebby network of trabeculae. The space between the trabeculae is called subarachnoid space. It is lined by a thin epithelium covering the trabeculae and contains the same fluid as the ventricular system, the cerebrospinal fluid. *Pia mater* and arachnoid together are called leptomeninx; (c) the *dura mater* (= pachymeninx) actually consists of two layers which in the brain fuse: the originally outer, relatively cell-rich layer is the periosteum of the cranial bones. The *dura mater* consists of a system of densely packed collagen fibrils – intermingled with some elastic fibres – and fibroblasts. Within it numerous sensory nerves and venous blood vessels, the sinus, occur, the wall of which is composed only by an endothelium. The inner surface of the dura, which faces the outer relatively dense aspect of the arachnoid, is smooth and consists of a layer of flattened mesothelial cells which constitute the so-called neurothelium. In tissues inadequately fixed within the neurothelium an artificial space, the subdural space, can be observed.

The cerebrospinal fluid is formed by a so-called *tela choroidea,* which occurs in areas where the wall of the brain consists only of a thin non-nervous epithelium (*lamina epithelialis* of the *tela choroidea*). Here the *pia mater* is extremely rich in blood vessels which form extensive plexuses (*plexus choroideus* of the *tela choroidea*). The whole tela is much folded and protrudes into the ventricular space. The simple epithelium consists of cuboidal cells with basal infoldings and club-shaped apical microvilli. The cytoplasm contains numerous mitochondria and lysosomes. The capillaries of the plexus are thin-walled and possess numerous fenestrated pores (Fig. 146). They seem to be unusually permeable. Presumably the capillaries liberate blood plasma which is taken up by the epithelial cells. Here the plasma is modified and secreted as cerebrospinal fluid into the ventricular lumen. This fluid is resorbed by the veins of the meninges.

Figure 108. Schematic representation of the mammalian meninges with an arachnoid villus in the dura mater (d). Black arrows indicate the flow of the cerebrospinal fluid from the subarachnoid space through the arachnoid villus into the venous sinusoid (si) in the dura. White arrows indicate the flow of the cerebrospinal fluid into the veins (v) of the pia mater. b: surface of the brain; a: artery; lm: leptomeninges; pm: pia mater; ar: arachnoid membrane; sar: subarachnoid space; sd: subdural layer of mesothelial and connective tissue cells; cp: capillary. After ANDRES, 1969

204 COMPARATIVE ANIMAL CYTOLOGY & HISTOLOGY

LITERATURE

ANDRES, K. H. 'Feinstruktur der Arachnoidea und Dura mater von Mammalia.' Z. Zellforsch. **79**, 272–295 (1967).

ARIENS CAPPERS, C. U., HUBER, G. C., CROSBY, E. C. *The comparative anatomy of the nervous system of vertebrates, including man.* Bd. 1. 695 S. Bd. 2. 1239 S. Bd. 3. 1845 S. Hafner Publish. Comp. New York, 1960.

BLACKSTADT, T. 'Cortical grey matter', in: *The neuron* (ed. H. Hyden), S. 49–118. Elsevier Publish. Comp. Amsterdam 1967.

BULLOCK, T. H., HORRIDGE, G. A. *Structure and function of the nervous systems of invertebrates.* Vol. I: 798 pp. vol. II: 1719 pp. W. H. Freeman and Company. San Francisco and London. 1965.

CHARLTON, B. T., GRAY, E. G. 'Comparative electron microscopy of synapses in the vertebrates spinal cord.' *J. Cell Sci.* **1**, 67–80 (1966).

DILLY, P. N., WELSCH, U., STORCH, V. 'The structure of the nerve fibre layer and neurochord in the enteropneusts.' *Z. Zellforsch.* **103**, 129–148 (1970).

GOLDING, D. W. 'A survey of neuroendocrine phenomena in non-arthropod invertebrates.' *Biol. Rev.* **49**, 161–224 (1974).

HAGADORN, J. R., BERN, H. A., NISHIOKA, R. S. 'The fine structure of the supraesophageal ganglion of the rhynchobdellid leech *Theromyzon rude*, with special reference to neurosecretion.' *Z. Zellforsch.* **58**, 714–758 (1963).

HAMBERGER, A., BLOMSTRAND, CH., LEHNINGER, A. 'Comparative studies on mitochondria isolated from neuron-enriched and glia-enriched fractions of rabbit and beef brain.' *J. Cell Biol.* **45**, 221–234 (1970).

HERNDORN, R. M. 'The fine structure of the rat cerebellum. II. The stellate neurons, granule cells, and glia.' *J. Cell. Biol.* **23**, 277–293 (1964).

KUHLENBECK, H. 'The central nervous system of vertebrates. Vol. 2. Invertebrates and origin of vertebrates.' S. Karger. Basel, New York. 364 S. 1967.

LENTZ, T. *Primitive nervous systems.* Yale University Press. New Haven. 148 S. 1968.

LEONHARDT, H. 'Ependym.' In: *Zirkumventrikuläre Organe and Liquor,* VEB G. Fischer Verlag, Jena (1969). 286 pp.

MADDRELL, S. H. P., TREHERNE, J. E. 'The ultrastructure of the perineurium in two insect species, *Carausius morosus* and *Periplaneta americana.'* *J. Cell Sci.* **2**, 119–128 (1967).

MEVES, A. 'Elektronenmikroskopische Untersuchungen über die Zytoarchitektur des Cehirns von *Branchiostoma lanceolatum.'* *Z. Zellforsch.* **139**, 511–532 (1973).

PENTREATH, V. W., COBB, J. L. S. 'Neurobiology of Echinodermata.' *Biol. Rev.* **47**, 363–392 (1972).

VAUGHN, J. E. 'An electron microscopic analysis of gliogenesis in rat optic nerves.' *Z. Zellforsch.* **94**, 293–324 (1969).

WESTFALL, J. A. 'Ultrastructure of synapses in a primitive coelenterate.' *J. Ultrastruct. Res.* **32**, 237–246 (1970).

YOUNG, J. Z. 'The anatomy of the nervous system of *Octopus vulgaris.'* Clarendon Press, Oxford. 690 S. 1971.

Chapter 6

ENDOCRINE ORGANS

The endocrine organs are composed of glandular cells of internal secretion; i.e. their secretory products, termed hormones, are secreted into the blood stream or in animals like arthropods into the haemolymph. Typical endocrine glands which are only found in higher animals, usually have a very simple microscopic structure; they consist of cords or small solid or hollow clumps of cells interspersed between capillaries and supported by a delicate connective tissue.

Originally all hormones were produced by neurons, termed neurosecretory neurons. These are of wide distribution among invertebrates and still can be found in the mammalian hypothalamus (Fig. 104). It should be noted, however, that all neurons seem to share the ability to produce secretory substances, in the ordinary neurons these are called transmitters, which in the same way as hormones are extruded into the intercellular space.

A system of neurosecretory neurons and their associated blood spaces, into which the hormone is liberated, is called a neurohaemal system. The structure and function of such systems will be briefly explained in the insects.

The most important hormone-synthesizing and hormone-releasing organs of insects are the brain, the *corpora cardiaca, corpora allata* and the moulting gland (prothoracal gland).

The paired *corpora cardiaca* are situated behind the brain with which they are interconnected by nerve fibres. Only in flies they fuse with the *corpora allata* giving rise to a ring-shaped gland surrounding the heart.

Neurohormones are synthesized in the perikarya of certain neurons of the brain. They are combined with carrier substances and packaged in secretory granules which are transported down the axons of these neurosecretory neurons into the *corpora cardiaca*. Here they are liberated at those parts of the axon terminals which are not surrounded by a glial envelope. After being extruded the hormones pass through a loose basement lamina and a delicate system of collagen fibrils in the *corpora cardiaca* into the haemolymph. In addition the *corpora cardiaca* contain their own neuron-like cells which also produce numerous secretory granules. Their axons differ from those coming from the brain by the presence of small rough ER cisternae and ribosomes. Their secretory products are released in the same way as those of the cerebral neurons. Hormones liberated into the haemolymph from the *corpora cardiaca* play a role in many activities of the body (moulting cycle, growth of the gonads, heart beat, activity of the CNS and others). Further neurosecretory axons pass through the *corpora cardiaca*, coming from the brain and terminating in the *corpora allata*, the intestine, the prothoracal glands, the heart and other organs.

The *corpora allata* are reached by the terminals of neurosecretory neurons in the brain having passed through the *corpora cardiaca*. They are located behind the *corpora cardiaca* and may be closely attached to them. Furthermore they contain non-neuronal glandular cells of variable structure. Frequently they are characterized by fair amounts of smooth ER cisternae *(Schistocerca, Drosophila, Bombyx, Calliphora,* etc.) occasionally rough ER-cisternae are predominant *(Eurygaster, Hyalophora).* In other species smooth and rough ER occur side by side *(Leucophaea, Locusta, Rhodnius,* etc). Generally granules or other definite signs of hormone synthesis are not to be observed. It is assumed that the neurosecretory terminals induce the liberation of substances from the non-neuronal cells. During a long period of the larval life the *corpora allata* produce the juvenile hormone neotenin in the absence of which the development of the imago begins. After the moult leading to the adult animal the *corpora allata* can become reactivated and influence numerous metabolic pathways.

The cells of the moulting gland produce the steroid hormone ecdysone, which initiates the moulting process. The cells possess long interdigitating processes which reach the surface of the organ and which are separated from each other by narrow spaces communicating with the haemolymph. The cytoplasm contains few organelles, there are only individual rough and smooth ER cisternae and relatively small numbers of roundish mitochondria of the crista type.

Oenocytes are polygonal (often polyploid), free cells often forming clusters which among others have been suspected to fulfil endocrine tasks in many insects. Their plasma membrane at least temporarily exhibits deep infoldings. In *Tenebrio* the oenocytes have been shown to synthesize steroid hormones; thus presumably oenocytes and prothorax glands are concerned with the production of the moulting hormone. In many insects also the ultra-structure of the oenocytes corresponds to that of other steroid producing cells. In *Gryllus* e.g. they contain among others abundant smooth ER profiles, which is particularly prominent at times of assumed hormone production (mitochondria are of the crista type). Rough ER also increases in volume at the beginning of secretory activity. Other functions attributed to these cells is detoxification and playing a role in the formation of the cuticle (see p. 134).

The classical neurosecretory neurons of the vertebrates are located in the ventral parts of the diencephalon and produce oligopeptide hormones (Fig. 110). Their axons which usually are unmyelinated – with the exception of the elephant – constitute the hypothalamo-hypophyseal tract which can be demonstrated by specific stains in the light microscope. It passes through the median eminence and the infundibular stalk (together forming the infundibulum) and terminates in the posterior lobe of the pituitary (= neural lobe orlobus nervosus). Median eminence, and infundibular stalk and neural lobe together are called the neurohypophysis. The individual neurosecretory fibres contain abundant electron dense granules 120–200 mµ in diameter. Occasionally they form local accumulations (Herring bodies) in the axons, the terminals of which surround thin-walled blood capillaries with a fenestrated epithelium. The barriers the extruded hormones have to pass are a basal lamina covering the nervous elements, a thin layer of delicate connective tissue, the basal lamina of the blood vessels and their endothelium. The axon terminals also contain synaptic vesicles in addition to the neurosectory granules, which are known to contain the hormone and a protein to which it is bound. On perikarya and axons of the neurosecretory neurons aminergic and cholinergic synapses have been found originating from perikarya of the limbic system and the *formatio reticularis*. The typical glial cells of the neurohypophysis are termed pituicytes.

Other neurosecretory cells of the hypothalamus do not stain with the standard neurosecretory stains, they synthesize the factors influencing the adenohypophysis *via* the hypophyseal portal system.

In fishes the terminal part of the spinal cord contains a group of neurosecretory cells constituting the urophysis (= *neurophysis spinalis caudalis*). Their hormone is among others believed to increase the blood pressure.

In the vertebrates the typical endocrine cells either are located as isolates in other organs, which may represent a primitive condition, or constitute organs of their own. It is striking to realize that many endocrine systems are associated with the alimentary tract including oral cavity and pharynx. The most important exception to this generalization are the steroid-producing cells.

In the electron microscope two basic types of endocrine cells may be distinguished:

(a) Cells found in protein-, glycoprotein- and polypeptide hormone producing organs. They contain numerous electron-dense secretory granules surrounded by a unit membrane. Structure, size and shape of these granules vary and frequently can be taken to characterize individual cell types. These granules do not only store the hormone or hormone precursor but in addition also carrier proteins and biogenic amines (e.g. 5-HT). The latter sometimes are assumed to play a role in the process of hormone liberation. Further characteristics of the cytoplasm are well developed rough ER, especially in activated cells, numerous mitochondria (crista type or type with both cristae and usually triangular tubules as in some amphibians), a well developed Golgi apparatus, microtubules and often bundles of microfilaments. The process of secretion is the same as described for protein-synthesizing cells (p. 56). Of similar structure – especially with regard to the secretory granules – are the adrenal cells producing catecholamines. This brief description shows a fundamental structural similarity between these cells and neurosecretory neurons.

(b) Cells found in steroid hormone-producing organs. They contain a well developed often tubular smooth ER, mitochondria of the tubular or saccular type (in lower vertebrates often also mitochondria with cristae) and lipid inclusions.

A number of ultrastructural and histochemical agreements can be observed in many polypeptide producing cells at various locations in the body: secretory granules, contents of cholinesterase or unspecific esterases, α-glycerophosphate dehydrogenase, and biogenic amines, the ability to take up certain amino acid derivatives (Dopa, 5-HTP) and to decarboxylate them, masked basophilia and others. These cells may be demonstrated in the light microscope by histochemical methods, as with ordinary stains they often are not clearly recognized.

Pituitary gland *(hypophysis cerebri)*

The pituitary gland consists of two major subdivisions, the neurohypophysis, which corresponds to a ventral process of the diencephalon and the adenohypophysis which develops in the embryo as dorsal outpocketing of the roof of the oral cavity. Remnants of this original connection with the mouth are cavities, which may be met with in most vertebrate groups. They are particularly prominent in some primitive actinopterygians, but also in many tetrapods a cleft-like cavity exists between *pars distalis*. and *pars intermedia* which is derived from the original lumen of the outpocketing of the oral cavity, which is also termed Rathke's pouch. In man in the area of this cleft big follicles may occur, which in part may also be derivatives of the lumen of Rathke's pouch, but which in part may also be structures of their own and be an expression of a non-functioning *pars intermedia*. These follicles or cysts should not be confused with the small follicular structures as described below in the *pars distalis,* at least their homology is uncertain. The neurohypophysis has been dealt with in the preceding paragraph.

The adenohypophysis has three subdivisions (Fig. 109): (a) the *pars distalis* (= anterior lobe), (b) the *pars infundibularis* (= *pars tuberalis*) and (c) the *pars intermedia.* The *pars distalis* is the largest part of the adenohypophysis. Its glandular cells are arranged in thick irregular branching cords, which are surrounded by a delicate system of reticular fibres. Between these cords abundant relatively wide capillaries called sinusoids can be found, the endothelium of which is fenestrated and easily permeated by the hormone molecules.

There have been various attempts to classify the endocrine cells according to their stainability with a couple of suitable dyes and to correlate them with the production of specific hormones. With moderately specialized stains three groups of cells can be distinguished in the light microscope: basophilic cells, acidophilic cells (forming together the chromophils) and chromophobic cells. In the pituitary gland the terms basophilic and acidophilic refer exclusively to the stainability of the granular inclusions and not to the typical chromophilic components of the cytoplasm, e.g. the rough ER, as in other cells. The chromophobes do not take up dyes and therefore appear to be devoid of secretory granules. The finer details of these cell types vary considerably in the individual vertebrates. In mammals the acidophils are thought to secrete growth hormone and prolactin. The basophils tend to be larger than the acidophils, their granules are relatively small and stain positively with the PAS method. Their hormones are presumably the glycoproteins thyrotropic hormone, follicle-stimulating hormone and interstitial cell stimulating hormone. The ACTH-producing cell is difficult to establish, possibly it is a basophilic cell. The chromophobes seem to be a group of exhausted or very active cells.

It is assumed that each of the six hormones of the mammalian anterior lobe is synthesized in a separate cell type, with the possible exception of the gonadotropins.

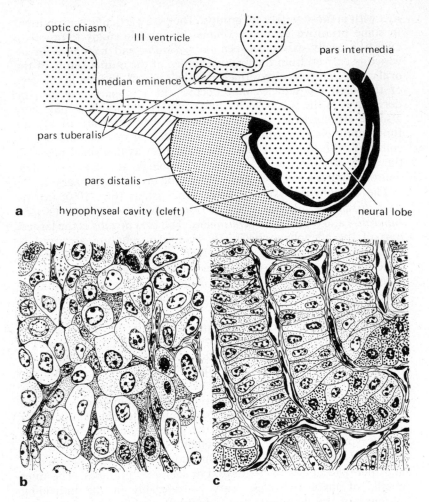

Figure 109. **a:** Schematic representation of the hypophysis of a cat; the third ventricle sends a ventral extension into the neural lobe *(recessus infundibuli);* **b, c:** light microscopical preparations of the adenohypophysis; **a:** intermediate lobe, mouse; **b:** distal lobe, frog *(Rana).* After ROMEIS & KRAUSE, 1921

In the electron microscope the main distinguishing character is the structure of the electron dense granules; e.g. in the rat the granules of the prolactin producing cells have a diameter of 800 nm, those of the ACTH-producing cells are of 100–200 nm in diameter.

An additional component of the mammalian adenohypophysis are star-shaped cells extending their processes between the glandular cells. They are rich in ribosomes and believed either to be a group of embryonic reserve cells or to represent phagocytizing elements. Similar elements may constitute small follicular structures. They are also rich in ribosomes and extend basal processes between the glandular cells. Apically they bear microvilli and occasionally cilia.

The intermedia cells produce the melanocyte stimulating hormone. They are basophilic and contain granules of a size of 200–300 nm. Within the *pars intermedia* different types of nerve endings have been found. In amphibians and some mammals some of these terminals contain neurosecretory granules. A *pars intermedia* is absent in some whales, the manetee and some birds.

The *pars tuberalis* is highly vascularized, its endocrine cells usually form longitudinal rows. In this small part of the adenohypophysis small acido- and basophils as well as chromophobe cells occur. A further component are common cells containing lipid and glycogen inclusions in addition to secretion granules.

In different phases of activity of the endocrine cells of the anterior lobe are correlated with typical structural alterations; e.g. during lactation the prolactin-producing cells are extremely active, which e.g. is indicated by their well developed rough ER and Golgi apparatus. If the secretory activity is experimentally suppressed, e.g by removal of the young ones, the following alterations may be observed. The number of lysosomes increases markedly. They incorporate the secretory granules and digest their contents which is degraded to the level of oligo- or dipeptides. These presumably penetrate the lysosomal membrane and are split into aminoacids in the cytoplasm. The secondary lysosomes receive fresh hydrolytic enzymes *via* small vesicular primary lysosomes originating in the Golgi apparatus. This digestion of hormones in endocrine cells is called krinophagy; it seems to occur in all endocrine cells and differs from autophagy by the exclusive incorporation of secretory granules into the lysosomes.

Stimulation of the gonadotrops leads to particularly striking alterations of these cells. In experimental stimulation, e.g. after castration, rough ER and Golgi apparatus markedly increase in volume. The cisternae of the rough ER become inflated to an unusual extent so that these cells can also be recognized in the light microscope as vacuolated cells (castration cells).

A possible precursor of the vertebrate adenohypophysis is represented by the neural gland (or parts of it) of tunicates and Hatschek's groove (or the whole wheel organ) in the oral cavity of *Branchiostoma*. The electron microscope has not supported this assumption in the tunicates – the epithelial cells of the neural gland do not show any specific indications for endocrine secretory

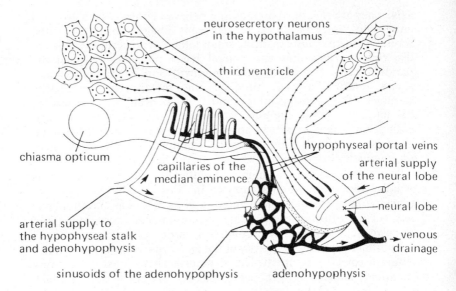

Figure 110. Schematic representation of the blood supply of the mammalian hypophysis and the distribution of the neuro-secretory neurons. Some of the neurosecretory axons terminate at the capillaries of the median eminence, their secretory products are transported *via* the hypophyseal portal veins into the adenohypophysis. Other neurosecretory fibres terminate at vessels of the neural lobe, their products influence peripheral organs. After TURNER & BAGNARA, 1972

activities. In *Branchiostoma,* however, the ultrastructure of some of the epithelial cells favours the idea that the areas of the oral cavity mentioned above might be precursors of the adenohypophysis for they contain numerous secretory granules in their basal parts, which directly come into contact with blood spaces, e.g. in the glomus which has been described as showing rhythmic pulsations.

Endostyle and thyroid gland

The endostyle of tunicates and *Branchiostoma* is the precursor of the vertebrate thyroid gland. In the invertebrate chordates the endostyle forms a narrow band or longitudinal groove of epithelial cells in the floor of the pharynx. These cells usually are columnar and constitute several zones in the endostyle (Figs. 111, 127); e.g. in the endostyle of *Branchiostoma* five zones may be distinguished (Fig. 127). Zones 1 and 3 consist of several layers of slender elongated cells, the apical ones bear one cilium each. It has not yet been decided whether these zones form a stratified or pseudostratified epithelium. Zone 2 consists of tall mucus-producing cells with

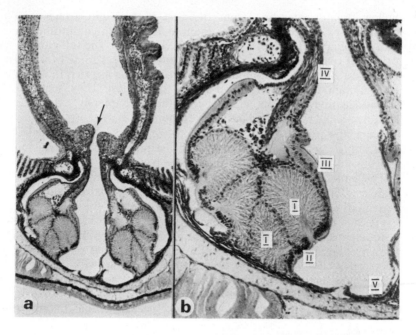

Figure 111. Endostyle of the lamprey larva (ammocoetes), arrow indicates open connection between pharynx (top) and endostyle (below), Roman figures indicate the various zones of the endostyle epithelium, principal sites of iodine binding are zones II, III and parts of zone V. **a:** x 56, **b:** x 140

conspicuous rough ER cisternae and relatively light apical secretory granules. Zone 4 is composed of similar cells, but the rough ER is more abundant and the apical secretory granules are electron-dense. In this area lipid inclusions frequently occur. Zone 5 is composed by one layer of slender columnar cells with one apical cilium. The transitory region between zones 4 and 5 binds iodine, it is therefore occasionaly considered as a separate zone. In all zones ciliated cells occur, those of zones 1, 3 and 5 are extremely long. The different zones may also be characterized by histochemical methods; unspecific esterases e.g. occur in zones 2 and 4. The secretory substances clearly are released at the cellular apex into the pharynx; no indication of an endocrine function has been found so far, although biochemically typical thyroid hormones have been demonstrated. In appendicularians seven zones can be distinguished, in ascidians eight zones. Some of the zones are composed of flattened or cuboidal cells. Ascidians concentrate, appendicularians do not concentrate iodine in their endostyles.

The endostyle of the ammocoetes larva (Agnatha) consists of two hollow organs extending from the first to fifth gill arches and separated by a median septum. Each hollow lumen communicates with the pharynx through a narrow duct (Fig. 111). The tall ciliated epithelial cells can be classified into five or six types some of which concentrate iodine. The main iodine-binding cells are rich in rough ER, contain light vesicles and a few lysosomes. They seem to synthesize thyroglobulin which presumably is apically extruded, hydrolysed and reabsorbed in the intestine.

Thus, the precursors of the thyroid are composed of epithelial cells lining part of the free surface of the pharynx and producing mucous substances for the capture of food particles.

The endocrine cells of the thyroid gland typically form small follicles (Fig. 112). The follicular wall consists of one layer of squamous to columnar epithelial cells. The height of these cells is an expression of their activity. In normal animals inactive follicles have a squamous, active ones a cuboidal or columnar epithelium. The ultrastructure of the epithelial cells differs from that of the other endocrine cells. They are of polarized organization (Fig. 113). A voluminous nucleus with abundant euchromatin and a few nucleoli is centrally located. In the basal and lateral parts of the cytoplasm usually extensive rough ER cisternae occur, which in many

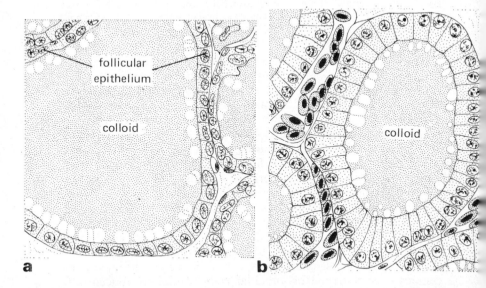

Figure 112.   Thyroid gland of a lizard (*Lacerta*); **a:** follicle with low epithelium, rich in colloid; **b:** follicle with columnar cells of an activated gland. After EGGERT, 1936

vertebrates are dilated, having only slender bands of cytoplasm between them. Relatively numerous mitochondria can be found throughout the cytoplasm, they are often basally concentrated and

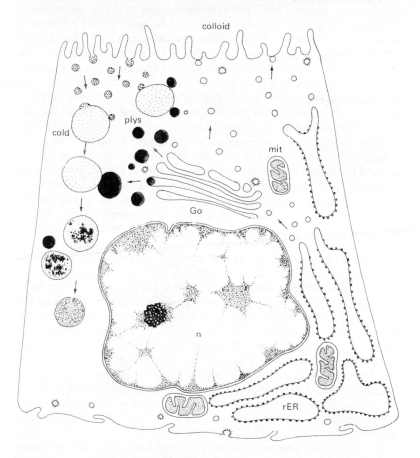

Figure 113.   Ultrastructure of thyroid follicular cell of a mammal. Arrows indicate hypothetical passage of specific products within the cell, into the colloid and from the colloid back into the cell. rER: rough endoplasmic reticulum; nu: nucleus; Go: Golgi apparatus; plys: primary lysosomes; cold: colloid droplets; mit: mitochondrium. Material synthesized in the rough ER is presumably both transported into the Golgi apparatus and directly into the colloid. According to autoradiographs thyroglobulin is transported from the rough ER *via* the Golgi apparatus to the colloid. The resorbed colloid forms colloid droplets (cold), which fuse with primary lysosomes (plys) . It is not yet clear in which way thyroxin and triiodide-thyronin are released from the cell into the blood stream. It is further on an open question, which substances are transported from the apical ER directly into the colloid and how many different populations of apical vesicles exist. After WELSCH (1972)

occupy the space between the rough ER cisternae. In the supranuclear region an extensive Golgi apparatus and various granular and vesicular inclusions may be found. Among these roundish or polymorphic primary lysosomes may be particularly prominent, e.g. in Amphibia. Their role has already been referred to on p. 25. In many species the cells contain vacuoles with resorbed colloid, rarely so in amphibians. Fig. 113 gives a scheme of the possible mode of resorption of colloid and the secretion of material into the follicular lumen. Apically the cells bear microvilli, the number of which is very much dependent on the phase of activity. Resting cells have very few, activated ones abundant microvilli. An apical cilium may frequently be observed.

The follicular lumen contains a substance termed colloid. Its principal constituent is the storage form (= thyroglobulin) of the thyroid hormones (thyroxine, triiodothyronine). Between the deeply stained colloid and the epithelial cells a clear space – often of serrated outline – may frequently be detected, in particular in activated glands in conventional light microscopic preparations. This space corresponds to a zone of liquefied colloid which is going to be resorbed by the epithelium.

Particularly illustrative are the changes in epithelial height and ultrastructure of the follicular cells as well as of the size of the follicles during the development of many Amphibians. In the larva the follicles are relatively small but slowly increase in size, and the epithelium is relatively flat or cuboidal. Briefly before metamorphosis the epithelial height increases rapidly. Rough ER and Golgi apparatus greatly increase in size; the number of primary lysosomes also increases. The follicular lumen may disappear so that the follicles are transformed into irregularly shaped, two layered cords of cells. After the metamorphic climax the epithelial height decreases, the amount of cell organelles becomes reduced, residual bodies appear in greater number than before and the follicles greatly distend.

In most vertebrates the thyroid is a compact organ. In bony fishes its follicles, however, frequently are dispersed along the ventral aorta and may extend caudally into the body. Small accessory groups of follicles may also occur in amphibians and even mammals.

In mammals between the follicular epithelial cells and within the basal lamina of the follicle a second type of endocrine cells is to be found, termed parafollicular or C-cell. These cells ordinarily do not reach the free surface of the epithelium and their hormone is directly delivered into the blood stream. Their ultrastructure differs greatly from that of the normal epithelial cells of the follicle and corresponds to that of typical polypeptide or protein hormone-

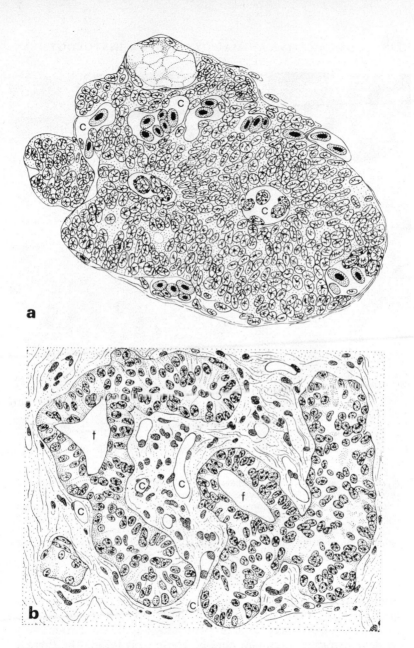

Figure 114. **a:** Parathyroid gland of *Ichthyophis* (Gymnophiona); c: blood capillaries with blood cells. After KLUMP & EGGERT, 1934. **b:** Ultimobranchial gland of *Rana*. In this amphibian species the gland is composed of follicular structures(f), filled with a substance termed colloid (as in the thyroid gland), it is surrounded by numerous blood capillaries (c), after WATZKA, 1932.

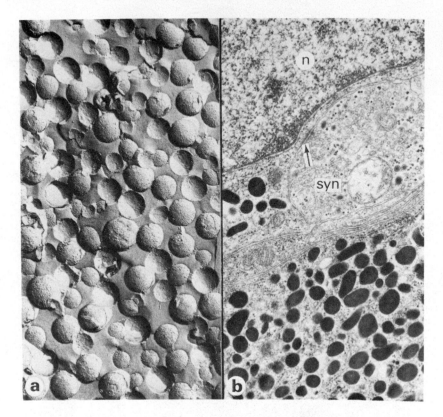

Figure 115.   a: Freeze-etched preparation of part of a C-cell from a mammalian thyroid gland, note the abundance of hormone containing granules, x 18 000. b: Catecholamine (presumably adrenalin) containing cells from the adrenal of a toad (*Bufo*); note synaptic contact between nerve ending (syn) and endocrine cell, typical for the chromaffin tissue of the adrenals. The nerve terminal contains abundant clear synaptic vesicles, arrow points the membrane thickenings of the synapse. n: nucleus x 18 000

producing cells; e.g. they contain abundant electron-dense secretory granules (Fig. 115). By specific methods they often can also be visualized in light microscope preparations, e.g. by silver stains and by demonstration of cholinesterase. These cells invade the thyroid during embryogenesis and are ultimately derived from the neural crest, as has been shown by transplantation experiments in birds. In non-mammals they constitute a separate gland, the ultimobranchial body (see below), but frequently may also be found individually in the thyroid or parathyroid gland or dispersed along the vagus nerve or other structures of the neck.

Ultimobranchial gland

This endocrine gland is derived from the last pouch of the pharyngeal region and contains the C-cells mentioned already. As in mammals their hormone is calcitonin. This gland is of variable appearance and localization. Usually it consists of cell cords and/or follicles (Fig. 114). In birds it has been found to be particularly active in young, growing and in egg-laying animals.

Parathyroid gland

This endocrine gland is only to be found in tetrapod vertebrates. Its secretory product is a polypeptide hormone called parathyroid hormone. The gland is composed of densely arranged cords and clusters of a relatively homogeneous population of rather small epithelial cells, termed principal or chief cells (Fig. 114). Their cytoplasm contains some granulated ER, but in general the cell organelles are relatively few in number. This also applies to the electron-dense secretory granules. In birds it has been speculated that the hormone is not enclosed in typical secretory granules, but in small light vesicles pinching off from the rough ER. Frequently the cells contain rather abundant glycogen particles. So the ultrastructure of these cells differs from that of other polypeptide-producing endocrine cells. This also is true of most light microscope reactions characterizing this group of cells; the high content of leucine amino peptidase in the chief cells is strange. In many mammals chief cells with a darker cytoplasm have been distinguished from chief cells with a lighter cytoplasm. The cytoplasm of some cells seems to contain almost no stainable material, and are occasionally called clear cells. At least part of this light or clear appearance is due to their content of glycogen, although the dark cells also contain glycogen. Presumably a large amount of glycogen indicates a resting condition of the cells.

A second cell type found in the parathyroid glands of some mammals is the oxyphilic cell. It is a rather rare and large element with a small nucleus and a voluminous cytoplasm crammed with mitochondria and intermingled glycogen particles. All the other cell organelles are inconspicuous. The function of these cells is unknown, their number seems to increase with age, possibly they arise from chief cells.

Parathyroid glands of Anuran amphibians undergo cyclical structural changes in response to seasonal fluctuations. In winter the parathyroids of many species of frogs and toads have been reported to degenerate. In general these glands transform into a network of stellate cells, which are vacuolated and occasionally contain disintegrated nuclei. Frogs' parathyroid secretion seems to be interrupted in winter at the level of the Golgi complex: residual bodies occur frequently and part of the Golgi cisternae seem to become degenerate. However rough ER cisternae are numerous and electron-dense secretory granules can be found in the central parts of the cells.

Islets of Langerhans

In tetrapods the endocrine islet cells either are dispersed individually and/or form small groups within the exocrine tissue of the pancreas (Fig. 29). Small aggregations are termed islets of Langerhans. Usually the islet tissue is concentrated in the caudal part of the pancreas, in snakes islet tissue can even be incorporated into the spleen. In teleosts all the islet cells may constitute a large principal islet, which is often attached to the gall bladder. In lampreys this endocrine tissue is attached to the intestinal wall. In tetrapods the individual islet cells frequently lie in the immediate neighbourhood of small exocrine ducts from the epithelium of which they are often believed to be derived.

At least three cell types can be distinguished to each of which the production of a specific hormone is ascribed.

1. The majority of endocrine pancreas cells is formed by the insulin-synthesizing β- (= B-) cells. In the light microscope they can be selectively stained with aldehyde fuchsin, a dye which demonstrates the specific granular components of the cells and thus may be used to demonstrate active and exhausted cells. In the electron microscope the β-cells are characterized by specific secretory granules which in most species contain a crystalline core (Fig. 116); this is due to the regular arrangement of a zinc-insulin complex, in which six insulin molecules surround two Zn ions. Such crystals have not been found in some South American rodents, e.g. the guinea pig, which also seems to lack the zinc component.

2. The product of the second cell type, the argyrophil A-cell is the hormone glucagon. In many mammals these cells are concentrated in the insular periphery, in birds the A and Beta cells can form separate islets. In the electron microscope they contain roundish granules with homogeneous electron-dense contents. Between granular membrane and contents a distinct clear narrow space occurs, the material of which is responsible for the argyrophily of these cells.

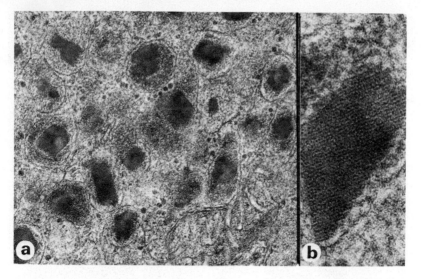

Figure 116.   Details from a Beta cell of the endocrine pancreatic tissue (*Ichthyophis*, Gymnophiona). Note the crystalline contents of the secretory granules. **a:** x 60000; **b:** x 120,000

3. The hormone of the also argyrophilic D-cells is still unknown. In mammals it is often assumed to be gastrin. The D-cells contain secretory granules the contents of which usually is clearly less electron dense than that of the A-cells. Often they also are bigger than the A-cells.

Since both A- and D-cells are argyrophilic, they are also termed α_1- (= D-) and α_2- (= A-) cells.

In many vertebrates, e.g. in teleosts and Amphibia, more – up to five – cell types have been described, whereas in lampreys and hagfish only one or two types are recognized, among these the β-cells are always present. In some species the endocrine islet cells are closely intermingled with nerve cells forming neuroinsular complexes. It seems to be certain that these neurons affect the secretory activity of the endocrine tissue.

In a number of species, e.g. in some Amphibia and mammals, transitory cells between exocrine enzyme-producing and endocrine cells have been observed containing both large exocrine zymogen and the small endocrine secretory granules. The real significance of such cells is unknown, but possibly they represent a primitive

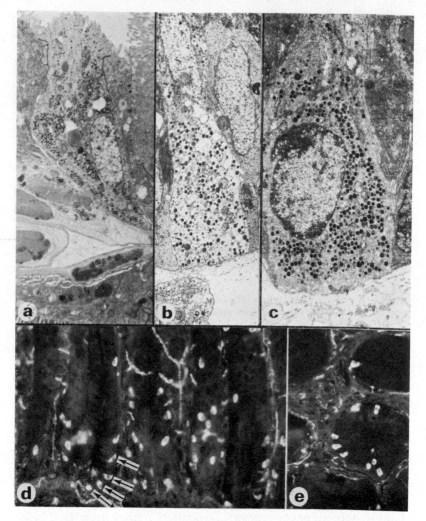

Figure 117. Endocrine cells of the intestine, with secretory granules which are concentrated in the basal cytoplasm. **a-c:** electron micrographs; **d-e:** fluorescence microscopy. In the electron microscope the endocrine cells are characterized by their dense secretory granules. **a:** *Chironomus* (Diptera). *valvula cardiaca*, x 5000; **b:** *Styela* (ascidian), oesophagus x 6000, photo T. TUNAS; **c:** *Erinaceus* (hedgehog) pyloric region of the stomach, x 6000, photo B. WEISE; **d,e:** hedgehog, midgut, endocrine cells (arrows) fluoresce, after Dopa injection, x 100, Photo B. WEISE

condition of a stem cell not yet differentiated into exclusively exo- or endocrine cells.

Gastro-intestinal tract

In the surface epithelium of the stomach and intestine by means of special histological procedures (immunohistochemistry, fluorescence microscopy (Fig. 117), enzyme histochemistry, silver stains, electron microscopy, etc.) individual endocrine cells, usually producing polypeptides, may be demonstrated. These cells usually are denoted by the first letter of their hormone (if known); e.g. the G-cells secrete gastrin, the S-cells secretin. These cells may be abundant and constitute numerous cell types. In the stomach of mammals alone, five different cell types have been described, the hormones of which, however, are not yet always identified. The gastrin-producing cells are concentrated in the pyloric region, the secretin-forming cells in the upper intestine. A special group of these cells—the enterochromaffin (argentaffin) cells - are located in the crypts of Lieberkühn of the whole intestine but have been found also in the stomach. Their products are 5-HT (= serotonin) which reacts with chrome salts, and possibly also a polypeptide.

In the electron microscope all of these cells are typical polypeptide-producing cells, i.e. they can readily be recognized by their numerous electron-dense secretory granules in the lower half of the cells (Fig. 117), the different shapes of which - as in the adenohypophysis - may be used for their identification. Another characteristic feature of these cells is that they often extend a slender process to the free surface of the epithelium, bearing a few stout microvilli, to which is ascribed a receptor function. Similar endocrine cells have been described in the gut of amphioxus, ascidians and rarely also of insects (Fig. 117).

In some respects the endocrine cells of the intestinal tract appear to be primitive, e.g. in respect of their loose distribution and because of the presence of a possibly receptive process reaching the free surface of the intestinal epithelium. Beginning with such cells a developmental series may be constructed which leads over (1) endocrine cells still within the epitheluim but without apical process (e.g. the enterochromaffin cells) and (2) individual cells or groups of endocrine cells below the epithelium (e.g. some endocrine cells below the ducts in the amphibian pancreas which is derived from the intestine) and (3) groups of endocrine cells in the more deeply situated connective tissue (e.g. the islet tissue in lampreys in the intestinal wall or the islets of Langerhans in general).

Adrenals, interrenal and suprarenal bodies; chromaffin tissue

The adrenal gland of mammals consists of two parts of entirely different origin, function and structure: adrenal cortex and adrenal medulla. The cells of the medulla assume a dark brown colour after fixation with solutions containing potassium bichromate and therefore are also termed chromaffin cells. The reaction is believed to be due to the presence of large amounts of catecholamines in this tissue. These cells are derived from the neural crest and correspond to transformed sympathetic neurons. They are always innervated (Fig. 115). Two types may be distinguished secreting noradrenalin and adrenalin respectively. The microscopic appearance of the medulla is very much dependent on the quality of fixation. The elongated cells are closely attached to blood vessels along which they form cell cords resembling columnar epithelia. The cell pole which is in contact with a venule contains the secretory granules, that which is in contact with a capillary contains the nucleus. In the electron microscope these cells are characterized by the presence of polymorphic granules which in the noradrenaline cells are more electron-dense than those in the adrenaline cells (Fig. 115). Also in the light microscope these two cell types can be distinguished, e.g. in azan preparations the noradrenalin storing cells are pale, and further they give a negative reaction for acid phosphatase. The adrenalin-storing cells stain deeply in azan preparations and give a positive reaction for acid phosphatase. Between the medullary cells individual nerve cells occur as well as venules with local muscular thickenings of their walls, which are thought to have the function of sphincters controlling the blood drainage from the gland.

The adrenal cortex is composed of steroid-producing endocrine cells (cf. p. 208) derived from the mesoderm which are arranged into three zones interconnected by transitory cell groups (Fig. 118): (1) an outer *zona glomerulosa* or *zona arcuata* under the tissue capsule, in which the elongated cells form densely packed groups or arcades; (2) a thick middle layer, the *zona fasciculata;* the cells form long cords separated by thin-walled capillaries (sinusoids) disposed radially with respect to the medulla; (3) the inner *zona reticularis* bordering the medulla and being composed of a network of cell cords. The cells are relatively small, usually stain deeply and contain accumulations of lipofuscin pigment.

The cells are typical steroid-producing cells, i.e. they contain smooth ER, lipid inclusions and tubular or saccular mitochondria, but polysomes and rough ER are also present. In the light microscope a typical feature is the vacuolated appearance of their cytoplasm, which is due to the dissolved lipid droplets and which is particularly prominent in the *zona fasciculata.*

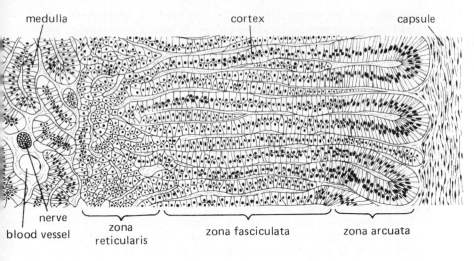

medulla   cortex   capsule

nerve

blood vessel   zona   zona fasciculata   zona arcuata
               reticularis

Figure 118. Adrenal gland with cortex and medulla of the horse. The *zona arcuata* corresponds to the *zona glomerulosa* of other mammals. After KRÖLLING & GRAU, 1960

The meaning of the zonation has been interpreted in two ways (a) the *zona glomerulosa* is a zone of formation of new cells, the *zona fasciculata* is the zone containing active mature cells and the *zona reticularis* is the zone of degenerating cells; (b) each of the zones is relatively independent and produces its own steroid hormones. Much recent evidence favours this second interpretation although some other evidence supports the first interpretation. According to some results the *zona glomerulosa* synthesizes the mineralocorticoids, and the *zona fasciculata* and *reticularis* produce glucocorticoids and sex hormones.

In the other vertebrates the two components of the mammalian adrenal gland are present, too, however usually do not form such a regularly constructed organ.

The chromaffin cells of cyclostomes are concentrated along the walls of the posterior cardinal veins and near the heart. In sharks they mainly constitute small suprarenal bodies along the medial aspect of the kidney tissue. In bony fishes they occur along the posterior cardinal veins but also within lymphatic tissue of the kidney. In amphibians chromaffin cells and interrenal cells (corresponding to the mammalian cortex, see below) are closely intermingled, they constitute in common the adrenal body (= adrenal gland) at the ventral aspect of the kidney. A comparable situation is to be observed in reptiles and birds in which both cell types form a common organ at the kidney, in which however they are of highly variable and intermingled distribution.

The tissue corresponding to the mammalian adrenal cortex, in other vertebrates is usually termed interrenal tissue. In cyclostomes it is loosely distributed along the caudal veins. In sharks it forms one or several interrenal bodies situated between the adrenal bodies, in teleosts it forms groups of cells near the pronephros. In tetrapods it is closely associated with the chromaffin tissue.

Isolated catecholamine-containing chromaffin cells have also been found in invertebrates, e.g. in the purple gland of the snail *Nucella* and in the ganglia of the ventral nerve chord of annelids.

Corpuscles of Stannius

These structures are confined to teleosts and consist of richly vascularized cords of endocrine cells which are attached to the mesonephros. In a number of species two cell types – both containing secretory granules – may be distinguished, differing in the location of the nucleus. Their function is unknown. According to their ultrastructure (abundant rough ER, secretory granules) they may be assumed to produce proteins, which might affect the calcium levels of the blood or physiologically resemble the hormones of the mammalian *zona glomerulosa* (adrenal cortex).

Gonads

The male sex hormones are produced by the Leydig cells (interstitial cells, Fig. 170) of the testes, lying in groups in the connective tissue between the seminiferous tubules. The cells are relatively large and frequently contain two nuclei, their acidophilic cytoplasm contains abundant amounts of smooth ER tubules and variable amounts of lipid inclusions. Resting cells, which occur in most vertebrates during long periods of the year, are inconspicuous elongated cells with few organelles and lipid inclusions.

In the ovary the production of hormones is closely correlated with the maturation of the follicles. In mammals hormone synthesizing tissue can be found in the connective tissue stroma (interstitial tissue) and in the follicular wall. In both cases the cells elaborate steroid hormones and at the ultrastructural level active cells possess as usual abundant smooth ER, tubular mitochondria and lipid inclusions. In the interstitial stroma the endocrine cells produce oestrogens and either form irregularly distributed groups of cells together forming the interstitial gland or a layer of cells around the follicles constituting the *theca interna*. If particularly active (normally during ovulation) these cells accumulate numerous lipid droplets and are termed the theca-lutein cells.

The second group of ovarian hormones – the progestogens – is derived from the follicular wall. These follicular cells increase in number during the maturation stages of the follicle and start to deliberate their hormone when the follicle is transformed into the *corpus luteum*. In the flourishing *corpus luteum* the large endocrine cells constituting its wall contain numerous lipid inclusions and are then termed granulosa lutein cells because of their yellow colour (Fig. 170). In the electron microscope these active cells contain in addition glycogen and abundant smooth ER tubules. If the egg released from the follicle is not fertilized the *corpus luteum* disintegrates.

Placenta

The numerous placental hormones are synthesized in the syncytio-trophoblast, areas with smooth ER are probably responsible for the production of steroid hormones.

Pineal organ

The pineal organ of the vertebrates consists of one or two sacular evaginations (bearing various names) of the roof of the diencephalon which have undergone remarkable alterations in the course of evolution. The characteristic cells of this organ are termed pinealocytes. In the pineal organ of fishes, in the pineal complex of anurans (frontal organ and pineal body) and in the parietal eye of lizards and *Sphenodon* their ultrastructure corresponds to that of the photoreceptor cells of the lateral eyes (Fig. 98). In snakes and lizards the photoreceptor process (the outer segment) becomes degenerated, but can still be recognized as such in the electron microscope. In these two groups the pinealocytes assume clearly characteristics of secretory cells, e.g. in form of electron dense secretory granules in their basal cytoplasmic extensions. Similar granules, however, already occur individually in the typical photoreceptors of the lower vertebrates. In mammals the pinealocytes appear to have entirely transformed into endocrine cells which constitute the bulk of the well vascularized, solid pineal organ (= epiphysis) forming clusters, cords and follicles. Their nuclei frequently are of particularly irregular outline, the cytoplasm containing abundant free ribosomes, some rough ER cisternae and a well developed smooth ER consisting of vesicles and tubules. Further striking features are the abundance of microtubules which form bundles in the partly elongated cytoplasmic processes.

A second type, the interstitial cells, are often regarded as modified glial cells. These cells possess long cytoplasmic processes and contain bundles of microfilaments. In man, extracellular concretions composed of calcium phosphates and carbonates ('brain sand') occur in the pineal organ. It is strange to realize that the pineal organ of numerous mammalian species contains cross-striated muscle cells.

The pinealocytes of birds and mammals are innervated by sympathetic nerve fibres. In the pineal organ of lower vertebrates sensory neurons have been found, which correspond to the ganglion cells of the retina of the lateral eyes.

The hormonal product of the pinealocytes is called melatonin, it exerts an influence on pigmentation and possibly also suppresses the functions of the gonads.

LITERATURE

ARIENS-KAPPERS, J. 'Innervation of the pineal organ: Phylogenetic aspects and comparison of the neural control of the mammalian pineal with that of other neuroendocrine systems.' *Mem. soc. endocrin.* **19**, 27-48 (1971).

BARGMANN, W. 'Die funktionelle Morphologie des endokrinen Regulationssystems.' *Handb. d. allg. Pathologie VIII.* **1**, 1-106 (1971).

BROLIN, S. W., HELLMAN, B., KNUTSON, H. *The structure and metabolism of the pancreatic islets.* Oxford, Pergamon Press, 528 pp. (1964).

CREUTZFELD, W., ed. *Origin, chemistry, physiology and pathophysiology of the gastrointestinal hormones.* G. Thieme Verlag, Stuttgart (1970).

FARQUHAR, M. G. 'Processing of secretory products by cells of the anterior pituitary gland.' *Mem. soc. endocrinol.* **19**, 79-122 (1971).

FUJITA, H., HONMA, Y. 'Some observations on the fine structure of the endostyle of larval lampreys, Ammocoetes of *Lampetra japonica.*' *Gen. Comp. Endocrin.* **11**, 111-131 (1968).

FUJITA, T. 'D cell, the third endocrine element of the pancreatic islet.' *Arch. histol. jap.* **29**, 1-40 (1968).

KRISHNAMURTHY, V. G., BERN, H. A. 'Correlative histological study of the corpuscles of Stannius and the juxtaglomerular cells of teleost fishes.' *Gen. comp. endocrin.* **13**, 313-335 (1969).

OKSCHE, A., UECK, M., RÜDEBERG, C. 'Comparative ultrastructural studies of sensory and secretory elements in pineal organs.' *Mem. soc. endocrin.* **19**, 7-24 (1971).

PEARSE, A. G. E. 'The cytochemistry and ultrastructure of polypeptide hormone-producing cells of the apud series and the embryonic, physiologic and pathologic implications of the concept.' *J. Histochem. Cytochem.* **17**, 303-313 (1969).

ROMEIS, B. 'Hypophyse'. In: *Handbuch der mikroskopischen Anatomie des Menschen.* Ed. by W. v. Möllendorff. Berlin (1940), 513 pp.

SANO, Y. 'Zur vergleichenden Anatomie von hypothalamischen und spinalen neurosekretorischen Systemen.' In: *Gunma Symp. Endocrin.* **1**, 3-8 (1964).

SMITH, D. S. *Insect cells. Their structure and functions.* Oliver and Boyd, Edinburgh (1968), 372 pp.

TOMBES, A. S. *Introduction to invertebrate endocrinology.* New York, Academic Press (1970), 217 pp.

TURNER, C. D., BAGNARA, J. T. *General endocrinology.* 5th ed. Saunders Comp. Philadelphia (1971), 659 pp.

WELSCH, U. 'Die Entwicklung der C-Zellen und des Follikelepithels der Säugerschilddrüse. Elektronenmikroskopische und histochemische Untersuchungen.' *Ergebu. Anat. Entwicklungsgesch.* **46,** 51 pp (1972).

Chapter 7
DIGESTIVE TRACT

The digestive tract is usually a hollow tube traversing the body in longitudinal direction. In its lining we may expect above all various cells specialized for absorbing and digesting food particles. Further we frequently encounter cells the chief function of which is (a) the propulsion of the ingested food (muscle cells, ciliated cells), (b) to provide a slippery and protective surface (mucous cells), (c) to secrete hard substances constituting teeth, etc., which break up and crush the ingested food, and (d) to co-ordinate the activities of the digesting tract (neurons, endocrine cells).

Invertebrates

Sponges

The lining of the absorptive surfaces of sponges is frequently called the gastrodermis (Fig. 119). It is composed of choanocytes (Fig. 120), a cell type which is of relatively wide distribution in the animal kingdom. The sponges, however, are the only group in which these cells form extensive epithelial linings. They are columnar cells which bear a long apical cilium, which is surrounded by a cytoplasmic collar. In the electron microscope it may be seen that this collar is composed of numerous long microvilli interconnected by extracellular mucopolysaccharide material. The plasma membrane of the cilium can form broad lateral wing-like lamellae. The cytoplasm may contain contractile vacuoles. In contrast with the intestinal epithelial cells of higher metazoa, the choanocytes can leave the epithelium and transform - under reduction of cilium and collar - into motile amoebocytes. In addition they may constitute nutritive cells for the developing larvae: they extend processes into the larva, and may even enter it completely and become dissolved. Food particles are taken into the cells by phagocytosis. The tall (up to 20 μm) choanocytes of calcareous sponges digest the nutrients within their cytoplasm (intracellular digestion). The smaller choanocytes of the other sponges transfer the food particles to underlying amoebocytes, which digest them. Sperms transported to the gastrodermis by a water current are also incorporated into the choanocytes and transferred to the egg cells. The versatility of these cells is unique among intestinal epithelial cells. In all other animals we find cells specialized for individual functions being organized into an epithelium.

In Cnidaria, ctenophores and flatworms the digestive tract has only one opening, transport of food particles is mainly achieved by cilia, and phagocytosis plays an important role in food resorption.

Cnidaria

The majority of the intestinal (gastrodermal) cells of the Cnidaria are absorptive epitheliomuscular cells. Their basal myofilament-containing processes are of circular orientation. The cells bear apical cilia, difficult to make out on sections, and pseudopodia engulfing undigested food particles (Fig. 64). These cells also absorb digested nutrients thus extra- and intracellular digestion occur side by side; intracellular digestion is accomplished in food vacuoles,

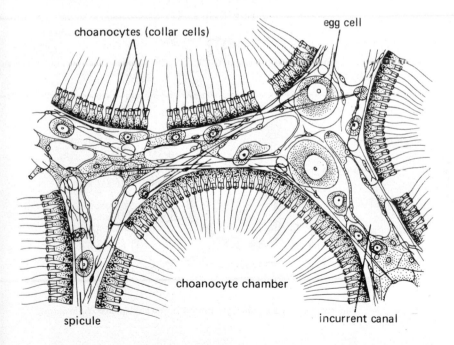

Figure 119. Sycon (sponge), section through the body with parts of four choanocyte chambers, the gaps in the choanocyte epithelium correspond to pores through which the incurrent canals open into the chambers. After SCHULZE from SCHNEIDER, 1908

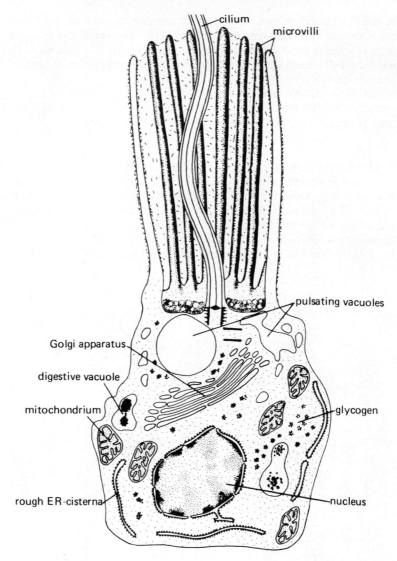

Figure 120. Fine structure of a choanocyte from a freshwater sponge (*Ephydatia*). After BRILL, 1973

which at first are of acid and later of alkaline pH. Two types of glandular cells produce digestive enzymes and mucous substances.

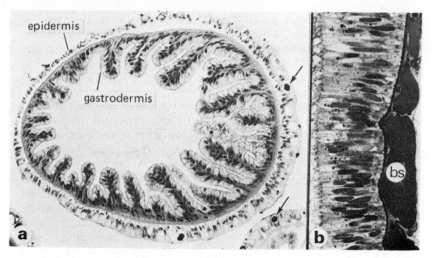

Figure 121. **a:** *Physalia* (Hydrozoa), cross-section through a gastrozooid, the gastrodermis is thrown into longitudinal folds, arrows point to nematocysts, x 90, **b:** ciliated intestinal epithelium of *Branchiostoma*, on the left: intestinal lumen, below the epithelium blood spaces (bs), x 430

The mucous cells are predominantly to be found in the oral region. Furthermore, individual cnidoblasts and sensory cells can be found in the intestinal epithelium. In larger species the food transport is achieved by strands of ciliated cells. In many species the gastrodermis is thrown into folds (Fig. 121).

Flatworms

The intestinal tract of these animals is lined by columnar absorptive and glandular cells. The absorptive cells are ciliated and appear to ingest the food particles mainly by phagocytosis, the glandular cells producing digestive enzymes. A discrete layer of muscle cells and connective tissue is absent in the intestine of flatworms. A peculiar situation is to be found in the famous acoel turbellarians. As an example of this group *Convoluta* is described below.

The whole animal is composed of cells; contrary to older assumptions it does not contain syncytia or plasmodia. The gastro-vascular tube is replaced by a central mass of cells, which are specialized for food uptake and digestion (food vacuoles, lipid droplets, enzyme contents). Zooxanthellae are situated in the extracellular space. This central cell mass is not clearly separated from the peripheral parenchyma. Through the mouth cellular processes protrude into the outer medium. Also in other turbellarians which were believed to possess a syncytial gastrodermis, it was found with the electron microscope, that it is composed of individual cells.

In all other groups of animals the digestive tract (gastro-intestinal tract) usually has two openings: mouth and anus and the anterior and posterior portions are lined by ectodermal epithelium (stomoproctodaeum). Food transport is achieved (a) by ciliary beat: most protostomian groups - except for arthropods and nematodes the intestinal epithelium of which is free of cilia - and deuterostomians, except for the vertebrates, or (b) by muscular activity: above all arthropods and vertebrates. The muscular activity is co-ordinated by nerve cells, however also the ciliated cells can be influenced by nerve endings. In the anterior part the food often is broken up by jaws, teeth, radulae, etc. In the middle part we find extracellular digestion and absorption, the posterior part has numerous functions among which frequently the absorption of water plays an important role. The continuous intestinal tract with two openings is further elaborated by the following structures: increase of the inner surface by folds, villi, etc., branchings, and formation of particular appendages, e.g. salivary and digestive glands, which produce mucus and enzymes.

Selected examples of invertebrate intestinal glands and other specialized structures
In brachiopods midgut diverticula occur, the main function of which is the digestion of food particles. The epithelium of these glandular structures is mainly composed of two cell types: (1) phagocytizing cells incorporate mainly algae by phagocytosis into apical protrusions, basally they store lipid droplets and glycogen. (2) a second cell type extrudes a proteinaceous secretory product into the glandular lumen. Rarely a third cell type with electron dense inclusions occurs (Fig. 122). The intestinal tube, the wall of which is formed by a strikingly tall pseudostratified flagellate epithelium, chiefly seems to serve the transport of food particles.

Many crustacea possess midgut diverticula (hepatopancreas), which have been studied above all in malacostracans. Generally these glands are composed of four cell types: embryonic (E-cells), absorbing (R-cells), fibrillar (F-cells), and vacuolated (B-cells) cells (Fig. 122). The R-cells absorb from the glandular lumen nutrients and store lipid and glycogen. The F-cells are particularly rich in granulated ER cisternae and produce digestive enzymes which are

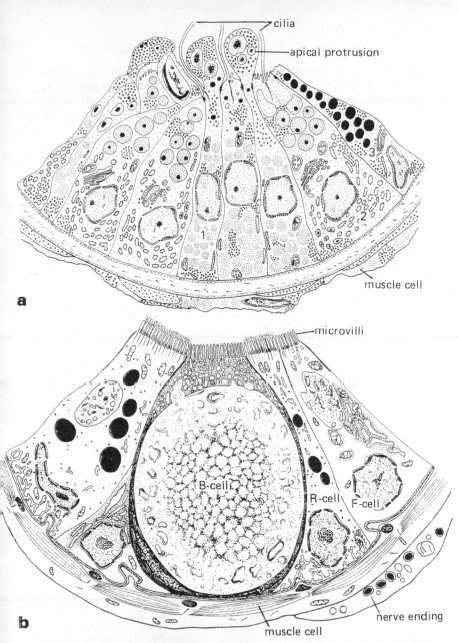

Figure 122. Fine structure of the intestinal diverticula **a:** *Lingula* (Brachiopoda) (1) cell type storing lipid and glycogen with apical phagocytosis, (2) secretory cell, with abundant rough ER and secretory granules, (3) presumably secretory cell, rarely to be found; **b:** *Procambarus* (Decapoda). The epithelia are underlain by muscle cells which are innervated. After LOIZZI, 1971; STORCH, WELSCH, 1975

stored in a supranuclear vacuole. This increases in size by the uptake of nutrients which have been incorporated into the cell by pinocytotic vesicles, until it almost completely fills the cell. At this stage the cell is termed B-cell. Finally the vacuolated cells burst and extrude their contents into the glandular lumen.

The functions of the malacostracan midgut diverticula (e.g. absorption, lipid- and glycogen storage, production of secretory products) can be pronounced in different degrees in the individual species: e.g. in the mysidacean genus *Neomysis* – at least in summer – the gland hardly stores lipid, whereas the land-living hermit crab *Coenobita* possesses a hepatopancreas most cells of which contain numerous lipid droplets. The hepatopancreas of some decapodes contains substantial amounts of calcium, magnesium and inorganic phosphorus. The mitochondria have an enormous capacity for accumulation of Ca.

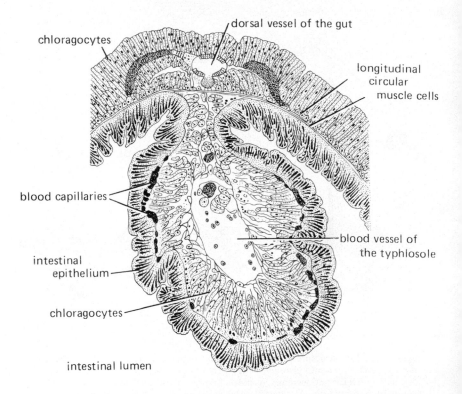

Figure 123. Cross-section through the typhlosole in the gut of the earthworm (*Lumbricus*). After SCHNEIDER, 1908

Ventrally in the epidermis of nematodes a group of glandular cells constitutes the ventral gland. Their cytoplasm contains rough ER cisternae and secretory granules. In intestinal parasites their secretory product, which is rich in enzymes, can attack the mucosa of the host. In other species it may play a role in digestion. In general these cells resemble those of the dorsal oesophageal glands. Evidently they do not take part in excretory processes as has frequently been believed.

In numerous groups of animals the midgut contains peritrophic membranes, which envelope food particles or masses of digested food. Such membranes are continuously produced and extruded with the faeces.

They occur e.g. in all arthropod groups, annelids, molluscs, tentaculates, echinoderms, hemichordates and chordates, but not however, in all species. They e.g. are absent in flat- and roundworms and in chordates are of rare occurrence. Frequently such a membrane is formed by a delamination process by the entire midgut epithelium. It is a secretory product, which often is composed of fibrillar and protein-containing matrix components. In insects the fibrils are composed of chitin and may form various patterns, e.g. hexagonal, rhombic or irregular ones, which are species specific. Its minute pores, which can be seen in the electron microscope, allow the passage of digestive enzymes and digested food. Its function is unclear.

In oligochaetes a characteristic dorsal fold of the midgut is the typhlosole. Its epithelial cells are usually rich in lysosomal enzymes, the tissue below the epithelium is composed of elongated cells called chloragog cells or chloragocytes. These cells contain abundant yellowish-green granules, the chloragosomes. They store lipid and glycogen and are also believed to have an excretory function, storing nitrogen-containing wastes. In the earthworm *Lumbricus* three types of inclusion bodies have been observed in the electron microscope (1) protein vacuoles, containing haemoglobin and often also iron, (2) siderosomes, containing exclusively iron (ferritin), (3) chloragosomes, which are of very heterogenous appearance and which seem to be free of iron. Indications for the storage of metabolic waste products have not been detected in this species, however, a separate cell-type, characterized by crystalline inclusions, possibly urate crystals, has also been described in *Lumbricus*.

Molluscs
The intestine of molluscs is characterized by radula and jaws, diverse associated glands, and a ciliated and innervated epithelium.

Radula and jaws are usually absent in microphagous species (e.g. the bivalves). The radula is composed of numerous, frequently thousands of small teeth, together forming a belt that passes over a supporting rod, the odontophore, which consists of firm cartilagineous tissue. The radula teeth are a secretory product of epithelial cells (odontoblasts) lining the wall of a pouch in the oral cavity·(radula sac). The odontoblasts accumulate apical secretory granules, which participate in the formation of the teeth. Special cells each seem to produce a matrix, mineral salts, and pigments. Salivary glands may be found in the anterior region of the gut of most species. In cephalopods they consist of two pairs. The secretory product of the posterior pair in octopuses contains various compounds, e.g. toxic proteins, which help to kill the prey, and biogenic amines. In the epithelium of the glands different types of cells may be recognized. They either are protein-synthesizing secretory cells (rough ER, secretory granules) or cells, which appear to transport ions and fluids (infoldings of the plasma membrane, numerous mitochondria).

The glands associated with the midgut may frequently be divided into a compact 'liver' region and a loosely constructed 'pancreatic' region. Both synthesize enzymes, among which lysosomal ones and esterases are particularly prominent in histochemical preparations. The pancreatic part in addition seems to fulfil an excretory function.

Considerable differences – in classes as well as in genera – in the structure of the midgut diverticula of molluscs have led to a confusing terminology and the description of various numbers (1-7) of cell types. In cephalopods the hepatopancreas is composed of two parts, 'liver' and 'pancreas'. Coarse food particles do not seem to enter its lumen. In the other molluscs it is of a more uniform structure; its lumen contains food particles which are phagocytized or incorporated into the epithelial cells in other ways. Beside this intracellular also extracellular digestion occurs, since digestive enzymes are secreted into the lumen. In bivalves two cell types correspond to these two functions. The transport of food particles within the gland is achieved by the cilia of these cells or by the particularly long flagella of a third cell type. In pulmonates further cell types occur: elements storing excretory products and calcium cells which contain concretions of calcium phosphate for the formation of the shell.

Also along the terminal parts of the intestine glands may frequently be observed. They are particularly voluminous in cephalopods in which they form the ink sac. The wall of this structure is composed of an inner cuboidal epithelium, a middle layer of circular and longitudinal muscle cells and an outer

connective tissue layer. The gland consists of two chambers, a
reservoir and a chamber in which the ink, which contains melanin,
is produced. The silvery colour of the ink sac is due to iridiocytes in
its wall.

The stomachs of many bivalves contain the crystalline style. It is a
secretory product, which arises from a tubular invagination. It
rotates in its invagination – the cilia of its epithelium provide the
driving force – and contains enzymes, e.g. amylase.

Insects

The anterior part of the insect intestine is lined by a cuticle (Fig.
125). It can form a narrow tube; frequently, however, it is
subdivided into a number of different regions and may even be
provided with lateral diverticula. Because of its cuticular lining it

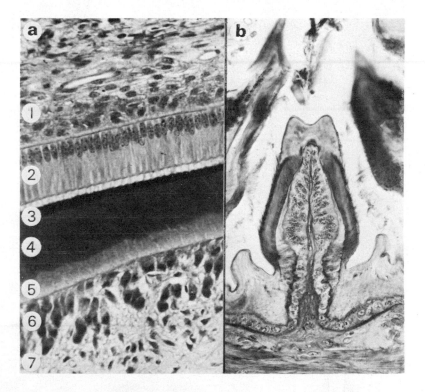

Figure 124. **a:** Section through a developing tooth of a cat: (1) enamel pulp; (2)
ameloblasts; (3) enamel (dense narrow layer) (4) dentin; (5) predentin; (6)
odontoblasts, (7) dental pulp. **b:** tooth from the gizzard of *Acheta.* (Orthoptera) x 300

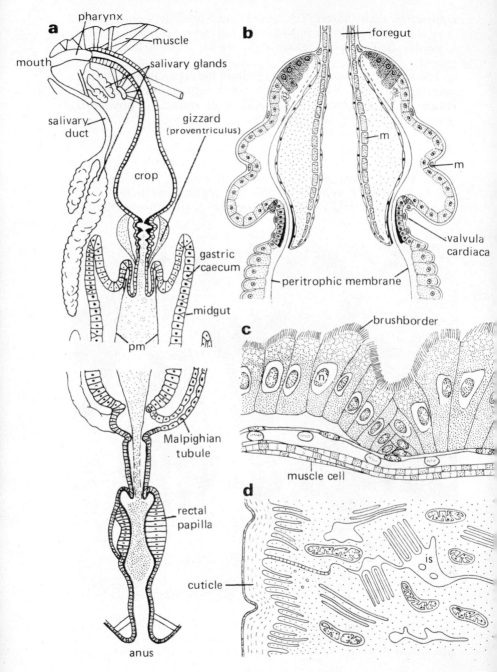

seems to be excluded from absorptive processes, which are confined to midgut (nutrients) and posterior intestine (water, ions).

In the anterior region the following subdivisions can usually be recognized: a pharynx, which may be constricted and dilated by special groups of muscle cells, an oesophagus, with less musculature in its wall, a crop (*ingluvies*), which serves as an extensible chamber of food storage and a chewing stomach (*proventriculus*) the cuticle of which frequently differentiates small teeth (Fig. 124). By means of a circular fold (the *valvula cardiaca*) the anterior gut is pushed into the midgut (Fig. 125). Except for their different shapes the individual segments of the anterior gut may be recognized by the different arrangement of the muscle cells in this region. All the muscle cells are cross-striated, but are, however, characterized by a slow and long lasting type of contraction, as in the smooth muscle cells of vertebrates. Longitudinally arranged muscle cells may be found in the pharynx, at least in its dorsal aspect; they are absent in the oesophagus and are strongly developed in the proventriculus. Circular musculature is well developed in pharynx and proventriculus, in the oesophagus it forms only a thin layer. In the crop both types of musculature form a loose network. Digestion may be initiated in the crop by enzymes secreted by salivary glands or midgut epithelium. The main site of digestion is the midgut (= mesenteron). The epithelial cells of the anterior gut (overlain by a cuticle) often are relatively flat and contain large numbers of microtubules.

The salivary glands are of extremely variable function and structure. If they produce proteins their epithelial cells usually are rich in stacks of rough ER. If their products contain a fluid component, the cells are rich in mitochondria, apical microvilli and basal infoldings. In dipterans the nuclei of the salivary gland cells often contain giant chromosomes (Fig. 7).

In contrast with the anterior and posterior gut, the midgut epithelium is not covered by a cuticle. Except for paired or circularly arranged blind appendages (coeca, chylus glands) in its anterior section, it usually is free of associated glands or other structures. Its wall is composed of a columnar epithelium and a thin muscular layer. The latter consists of an inner circular and an outer longitudinal component. Both are cross-striated and embedded in a

Figure 125. Details from the insect intestine. **a,** Schematic representation of the insect intestine, pm: peritrophic membrane; **b:** *Chironomus* (Diptera), formation of the peritrophic membrane in the *valvula cardiaca,* m: muscle layer; **c:** epithelium of the midgut, n: nucleus; **d:** fine structure of the epithelium of the rectal papilla, note complicated folds of plasma membrane, *Calliphora* (Diptera), is: intercellular space. After WEBER 1954, BERRIDGE 1970, PLATZER-SCHULTZ, WELSCH 1969

thick extracellular matrix containing collagen fibrils. Here also nerve fibres with neurosecretory granules occur. They innervate the muscle cells and possibly also influence the epithelial cells.

The epithelial cells usually are of uniform appearance and their function is absorption of food and production of enzymes. Their basal plasma membrane is characterized by numerous deep infoldings, to which mitochondria are attached. Apically they bear densely arranged microvilli, which are covered by a thin layer of mucopolysaccharides. The cytoplasm is rich in rough ER cisternae, a well developed Golgi apparatus and numerous mitochondria, which are not only confined to the basal parts of the cells. Secretory products often are extruded in the merocrine way, however also the apocrine and holocrine types of extrusion have been described.

Beside resorption and secretion of enzymes these cells fulfil further tasks, e.g. storage and synthesis of specific proteins including those which are incorporated into the yolk of developing egg cells.

Absorption is accomplished by permeation of molecules through the plasma membrane and by pinocytotic vesicles. Phagocytosis does not occur in the insect intestine. Worn out epithelial cells are replaced by groups of embryonic cells, which are located in the base of the epithelium. Occasionally these cells form small crypts protruding into the abdominal cavity (regeneration crypts). As in other undifferentiated cells their cytoplasm contains few lamellar organelles but is rich in mitochondria.

Mucus-producing cells are absent. Those cells termed goblet cells in the midgut of some insects (Ephemerida, Lepidoptera) are elements which are invaginated at the apex, this invagination bears microvilli containing mitochondria. It may be that they are specialized elements for the transport of ions.

The midgut of many larval dipterans exhibits additional functional and structural peculiarities. In *Drosophila* it may be divided into three regions of which the middle one is particularly differentiated. It is characterized by a low pH (about 3) and the occurrence of four cell types. At the beginning of this zone side by side light prismatic so-called interstitial cells and dark cuprophil cells occur. The apex of the latter is marked by cup-shaped microvilli bearing invaginations; these cells specifically accumulate copper. The next region can be recognized by its large flat cells, it is followed by a zone of smaller cuboidal cells which accumulate iron. Usually all these cells bear apical microvilli or lamellar upfoldings and possess a basal labyrinth. In the interstitial cells, which presumably are responsible for the low pH in this region of the gut, the microvilli are short and the basal infoldings deep. In the cuprophil cells the microvilli are extremely tall, the basal infoldings are short. Their cytoplasm contains lysosomes, the number of which increases with a diet rich in copper. In the cuprophil cells of *Lucilia* the apical invagination is absent and the interstitial cells are rich in lipid droplets (= lipochrome cells).

The epithelium of the midgut of many insects also has excretory functions. It can accumulate calcium salts, which e.g. in pupae of *Bombyx mori* completely fill the cytoplasm. Normally such accumulations are extruded into the intestinal lumen. In *Rhodnius* pigments originating from the metabolism of the absorbed haemoglobin, are excreted *via* the intestinal epithelium.

The peritrophic membrane is frequently a secretory product of the entire midgut epithelium. In this case several peritrophic membranes, which are rhythmically produced can be observed, those with a smaller diameter being enclosed by wider ones. In dipterans the peritrophic membrane is produced in different ways (e.g. by mero- and apocrine extrusion of its precursors) by cells rich in rough ER in a circular pouch of the anterior midgut which, in addition, contains many mitochondria-rich and presumably also endocrine cells (Fig. 117, 125)

The posterior gut is as the anterior one of the ectodermal origin. Its flat epithelium secretes a cuticle. Frequently this part of the gut is important for osmoregulation in insects. Endo- and epicuticle may be recognized but apparently are of different composition from that of the anterior gut. The muscular layer is composed of well developed inner and outer longitudinal components between which circularly arranged muscle cells occur. The Malpighian tubules open out into the anterior part of the posterior gut (see p. 303). which is termed the pylorus. The passage of the intestinal contents from midgut to posterior gut is controlled by a muscular circular fold (*valvula pylorica*), which is also said to play a role in the destruction of the peritrophic membrane. The terminal portion of the hindgut (the *rectum*), frequently is dilated and contains groups of voluminous tall cells constituting the rectal papillae. They reabsorb water and ions. Their plasma membrane exhibits countless deep and complex infoldings, especially in the lateral parts of the cells. The cytoplasm contains numerous mitochondria. Basally these cells are innervated by neurosecretory nerve fibres. Possibly these terminals extrude a factor similar to the vertebrate antidiuretic hormone. Further, this region is richly supplied by tracheae. These cells can also absorb water vapour (*Thermobia*); in water dwelling larvae of dipterans they constitute the anal papillae, which regulate the exchange of ions.

Finally, an important difference in comparison with the

vertebrate intestine should be mentioned: the insect intestine does not contain blood vessels. Oxygen is supplied by tracheae, the absorbed nutrients are transported through the matrix in the muscle

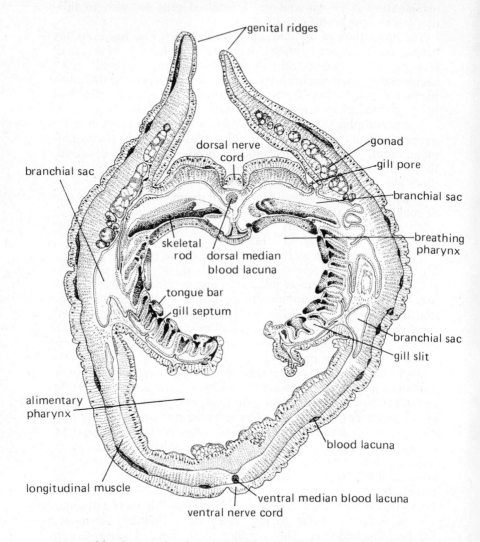

Figure 126. Cross-section through the gill region of *Ptychodera* (Enteropneusta). The pharynx is divided into a dorsal breathing and a ventral alimentary portion. The breathing pharynx is perforated by gill slits, which open into deep communicating pockets, the branchial sacs or gill chambers; these in turn open to the outside *via* the gill pores. After SCHNEIDER, 1908

layer into the haemolymph.

Hemichordates and lower chordates

The intestinal tract of tunicates, hemichordates (Fig. 126), and Acrania is characterized by a voluminous pharynx, the wall of which is perforated by numerous slits, which especially in ascidians can be of extremely complex structure. This pharynx serves for the capture of food and the drainage of surplus water, which is passed through the pharyngeal slits into the peribranchial space (= atrium) surrounding the pharynx. The cells lining the pharynx usually are columnar cells with tall cilia which frequently are innervated. Occasionally, especially in *Branchiostoma* groups of mucus-producing cells occur. In the ventral floor and the dorsal roof two epithelial furrows occur, ventrally the endostyle (see page 212 and Fig. 127) and dorsally the epibranchial groove. The epithelial cells of the latter are ciliated and produce mucoid substances. In *Branchiostoma* they are rich in certain enzymes, e.g. alkaline phosphatase. A peculiar feature of many of the epithelial cells in this area and other parts of the pharynx of *Branchiostoma* are huge basally located vacuoles.

In most ascidians the rest of the intestinal tract may be subdivided into a short oesophagus, a dilated stomach and a tubular intestine. The wall of all these parts is composed by columnar usually ciliated cells, a muscular layer is absent. Each of the above-mentioned sections is characterized by special cell types, the fine structure of which varies considerably in the individual species. In the oesophagus of *Styela, Polycarpa* and *Dendrodoa* endocrine cells have been found (Fig. 117).

In the stomach, the surface of which can be enlarged by circular and longitudinal folds, the epithelial cells are particularly tall and frequently contain pigment accumulations. In the majority of cells a well developed rough ER and Golgi apparatus, numerous mitochondria and apical secretory granules indicate secretory activity (enzymes and mucoid substances), apical microvilli, pinocytotic vesicles and abundant lysosome-like bodies indicate absorptive activity. In some species (e.g. *Botryllus*) specific protein producing cells have been described. In *Polycarpa, Dendrodoa* and *Styela* special mitochondria-rich cells with deep basal infoldings have been observed.

The stomach and often other parts of the intestinal tract of all ascidian species are surrounded by a network of fine tubules together forming the pyloric gland. The electron microscope has shown that the epithelial cells of these glands store vast amounts of glycogen, and in some genera, e.g. *Styela,* also lipid droplets.

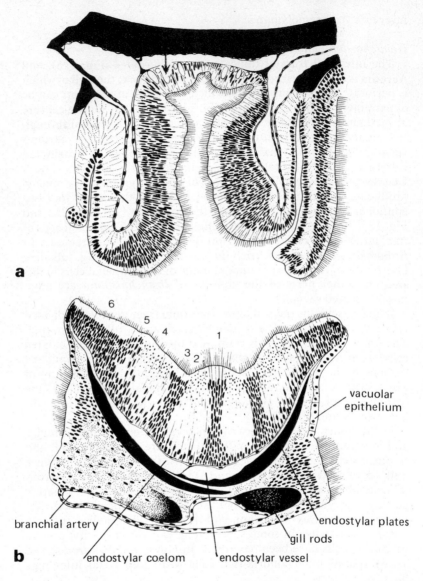

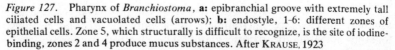

Figure 127.   Pharynx of *Branchiostoma*, **a:** epibranchial groove with extremely tall ciliated cells and vacuolated cells (arrows); **b:** endostyle, 1-6: different zones of epithelial cells. Zone 5, which structurally is difficult to recognize, is the site of iodine-binding, zones 2 and 4 produce mucus substances. After KRAUSE, 1923

The intestinal tract of *Branchiostoma* behind the pharynx is of a similar simple structure, being composed only of columnar ciliated cells (Fig. 121), among which endocrine cells occur. A peculiar structure is the intestinal caecum ('liver'), an anteriorly directed pouch of the midgut. It is composed of tall ciliated cells, which produce digestive enzymes and are rich in rough ER and secretory granules. They presumably also absorb digested food. Many of these cells contain fat droplets and basal accumulations of mitochondria.

Vertebrates

The vertebrate digestive tract consists of a number of sub-divisions, which may be classified in several ways. However, in lower vertebrates in particular it is often difficult to make clear distinctions between the individual parts of the system. Frequently it is simply divided into anterior-, mid-, and posterior gut (intestine). The anterior gut comprises the section from mouth to the end of the stomach and is composed of oral cavity, pharynx (in fishes bearing the gills, in air-breathing species the passage way for both respiratory and digestive systems behind the mouth), oesophagus (a tube leading to the stomach, in which ordinarily no digestion and absorption takes place) and stomach, an enlargement in which food can be stored and partly digested, the wall of which mostly contains glandular cells secreting hydrochloric acid, a few enzymes – normally for protein degradation – and mucus, and which is delimited against the midgut by a sphincter muscle, the pylorus. In fishes the area of the stomach may be indistinct and may even be absent as a separate organ. The midgut is that part, in which most of the food is digested and absorbed. It may also be termed the small intestine and often its anterior part is called duodenum.

It is frequently particularly difficult to draw a clear line separating mid and posterior gut. In many higher vertebrates (anurans, reptiles, birds, and mammals) a valve exists at this division. The chief function of the posterior gut is to reabsorb water. In mammals it is also called the large intestine.

Mucous membranes

The wet epithelial lining of the digestive tract (and of other organs opening out to the surface, Fig. 27) constitutes a barrier between the outside world and the cells and tissues of the body. It fulfils many important tasks and contains specialized cells among which mucus-secreting ones have been considered to be particularly important. Therefore this barrier membrane is called a mucous membrane. It comprises not only the epithelial lining but also a layer of underlying connective tissue, termed *lamina propria*; in its deepest part it usually contains a layer of smooth muscle cells, the *muscularis mucosae*. The mucous membranes ordinarily characterize the various parts of the intestinal tract particularly clearly. Therefore their description will be in the foreground of the following paragraphs.

Oral cavity.

The mucous membrane of the oral cavity of typically land-living tetrapodes is covered by a stratified non-keratinized squamous epithelium (Fig. 22). In fishes and amphibia this epithelium is relatively thin and contains mucous or ciliated cells. Most important structures of the oral cavity are teeth and tongue. The tongue normally bears chemoreceptor cells, frequently forming clusters (taste buds), they may be concentrated in certain areas, in which the surface of the tongue forms folds, grooves, or projections collectively called papillae. Besides taste buds, thermo-, pressure-, and pain receptors occur (Fig. 84).

The structure of teeth may best be understood by studying their embryonic development, for both ectoderm and mesoderm take part in their formation (Fig. 124). In mammals during embryogenesis an ectodermal epithelial shelf, called dental lamina and arising from the epithelium of the oral cavity grows into the underlying connective tissue. The outline of the dental lamina corresponds to that of the dental arch of adult animals. (In fishes, Amphibia and reptiles no typical dental lamina occurs, here teeth can arise in most parts of the oral cavity, especially in the roof.) From the lamina epithelial buds develop, which are termed tooth buds. They assume the shape of a thick walled bell and give rise to a tooth. Deciduous and permanent teeth of mammals arise in identical fashions. A bud which is differentiated into a bell-shaped structure is termed the enamel organ. Its outer wall is composed of a simple squamous or cuboidal epithelium (outer enamel epithelium). Attached to it from the outside are numerous capillaries. The inner wall of the enamel organ consists of tall columnar epithelial cells, termed ameloblasts (= ganoblasts). They are specialized cells producing tooth enamel. Between these two layers the epithelial cells become greatly loosened forming a stellate reticulum termed the enamel pulp. Those cells of it near the ameloblasts lie closely together and constitute the *stratum intermedium* rich in enzymes, in particular phosphatases. This group of cells is important for the production of enamel.

The mesodermal cells which are enclosed in the bell initially collectively constitute the dental papilla, later they usually form the dental pulp or pulp. They lie closely together and are richly supplied by blood vessels and nerve fibres.

Under the influence of the ameloblasts the outer layer of the pulp, which directly borders them, transforms into an epithelium-like layer, the individual cells of which are interconnected by apical junctional complexes, including tight junctions, and are termed odontoblasts; they become responsible for the production of dentin. Ameloblasts and odontoblasts at first.are only separated by a basement membrane, but soon hard intercellular substances are deposited by them which separate the two. The odontoblasts are usually the first to start with the production of their hard substance.

Odontoblasts consist of a cell body and a long branched apical cytoplasmic process (= Tomes' fibre), which extends to the dento-enamel junction. The perikaryon is characterized by a well developed granular ER and a large Golgi area near the nucleus. The odontoblastic process contains microtubules, microfilaments and light vesicles. The elongated apex of these cells at first secretes a soft ground substance and collagen fibres together forming the predentin, which becomes calcified by incorporation of apatite crystals. Thus dentin, also in fully developed teeth, is pervaded by countless small canaliculi, which house the living cytoplasmic processes of the odontoblasts (orthodentin). This situation is reminiscent of the osteocytes. If also perikarya of the odontoblasts are incorporated into the dentin, as can happen in teleosts, the dentin is termed osteodentin. If blood vessels enter the dentin, as may also occur e.g. in teleosts, we speak of vasodentin.

Also the tall ameloblasts possess an apical process, which, however, is shorter than that of the osteoblasts (Tomes' process). Only in marsupials is it relatively long and reaches the dentino-enamel junction. Therefore the enamel of these animals is also pervaded by tiny canaliculi, which however in the mature tooth do not contain living cell processes (see below). Neighbouring cells are interconnected by basal and apical junctional complexes. The basal cytoplasm contains dense accumulations of mitochondria, above which the elongated nucleus is located. Rough ER cisternae occur around the nucleus and in the apical half of the cell. An extensive Golgi apparatus is situated along the central axis of the apical half of the cell. Near it abundant electron-dense granules can be found, which are produced in the Golgi area. They seem to concentrate in the apical process, which further contains microtubules, microfilaments and elements of the smooth ER. The granules contain the soft matrix of the enamel, which is secreted at the apex of the cells. The matrix hardens by deposition of apatite crystals and finally the mature enamel contains about 95 per cent of mineral content, it is the hardest product of the vertebrate body. Enamel is secreted in the form of rods, which are interconnected by a matrix-like interrod substance, which also calcifies. When the enamel is deposited, the ameloblasts degenerate. In some animals, e.g. rodents, the enamel may contain iron salts, which render it yellow or brown.

In lower vertebrates it seems to be an open question, whether the teeth are covered by a true type of enamel or by a particularly hard type of dentin, termed vitrodentin. In all these animals ameloblasts occur, however uncertainty exists in regard to their secretory activity. In sharks the ultrastructure of the surface hard substance corresponds to that of true enamel, particularly important is the absence of collagen. However, in contrast to the higher vertebrates no basement lamina occurs between enamel and dentin.

From the oesophagus to the posterior gut the alimentary tract

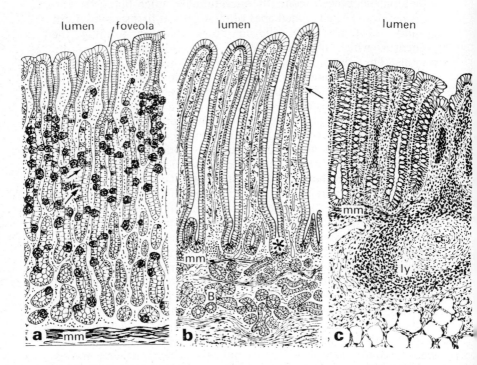

Figure 128. Mammalian gastrointestinal tract; **a:** stomach (fundus); mucous membrane with fundic glands; arrows point to the big mitochondria-rich parietal cells, mm: *muscularis mucosae;* **b:** duodenum with four tall villi at the bases of which the crypts (asterisk) extend down to the *muscularis mucosae* (mm), B: glands of Brunner in the submucosa, arrow points to goblet cell; **c:** colon, only crypts, rich in goblet cells, mm: *muscularis mucosae,* ly: lymph nodule. After KRAUSE, 1923; BARGMANN, 1967

ordinarily is composed of four layers: the (innermost) mucous membrane (= *tunica mucosa*), the submucosa (= *tunica submucosa*), the muscularis (= *tunica muscularis*) and the serosa. The general construction of the mucous membrane has already been briefly described (see page 247). The submucosa interconnects mucous membrane and muscularis and consists of loose connective tissue with collagen and elastic fibres. It contains larger blood vessels and lymph vessels and a vegetative nervous plexus (Meissner's plexus *Plexus submucosus*). The muscularis is composed of two main layers of smooth muscle cells, an inner layer of circularly disposed a..d an outer layer of longitudinally disposed fibres. In the oesophagus and anterior part of the stomach cross-striated muscle cells occur relatively often, in some fishes all of the muscularis consist of cross-striated muscle cells. Between inner and outer layer of muscle cells a second vegetative nerve plexus occurs (Auerbach's plexus = *plexus myentericus*).

The serosa (= adventitia) is the outermost coat of the intestinal tube. It consists of loose connective tissue and is covered in the free portions of the tract with a single layer of flat mesothelial cells.

Oesophagus

In the oesophagus the epithelium of the mucous membrane often contains mucous (fishes) and/or ciliated cells (amphibians, reptiles). Usually it is a stratified columnar epithelium. In birds and mammals it is a stratified squamous epithelium, which may be keratinized (many mammals). In mammals the *muscularis mucosae* is particularly well developed. The submucosa and the *lamina propria* can contain a few mucus secreting glands (amphibia, mammals).

Stomach

In the light microscope the surface of the stomach is characterized by small pits (foveolae) at the base of which densely packed tubular glands open out (Fig. 128). These glands constitute the vast majority of the tissue of the mucous membrane and extend down to the *muscularis mucosa*. The mucous membrane is covered by tall epithelial cells, which also line the pits, many or all of which produce a protective mucous film which is particularly thick over the glands in the muscular stomach of the birds. In some part of the stomach the epithelium can cornify, e.g. in some Xenarthra, Pholidota and ruminants.

In the lower vertebrates up to birds, the glands normally contain one type of exocrine glandular cell, the so-called principal cell, which produces both hydrochloric acid and pepsinogen, a digestive enzyme. In amphibians these large cells are characterized by basally located rough ER cisternae and secretory granules and apically located concentrations of mitochondria, smooth-surfaced vesicles, long microvilli and occasional tubular invaginations at the surface.

In mammals different regions of the stomach are characterized by different types of glands, in the anterior (cardia) and posterior (pyloric region) parts of the stomach the glands are composed of mucus-producing cells. In the middle region (fundus) different

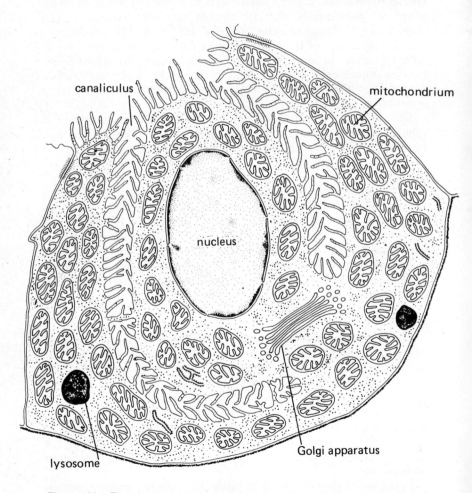

Figure 129. Fine structure of a parietal cell, note the abundant mitochondria and the extensions (canaliculi) of the apical plasma membrane. From REMANE, STORCH & WELSCH, 1974

glandular cell types occur. Predominantly at the bases of the glands the chief cells are to be found (Figs. 28, 128). They are rich in rough ER cisternae and large secretory granules and produce pepsinogen. The parietal cells tend to be concentrated in the middle parts of the glands. They are relatively large roundish elements unusually rich in mitochondria (Figs. 128, 129). The apical plasma membrane is invaginated by deep canaliculi lined by microvilli. Carbonic anhydrase is a characteristic enzyme of the plasma membrane of the canaliculi and plays a role in the formation of hydrochloric acid, the product of these cells. The neck region of the glands is chiefly made up of the mucous neck cells. They contain apically mucus and are relatively undifferentiated cells from which the renewal of the glandular cells takes place. Within the glandular epithelium of all stomach regions in all vertebrates individual endocrine cells occur, they usually are concentrated in the pyloric region, where a specific type of them, termed the G-cell, produces gastrin.

The stomach of teleosts is of a particularly variable structure. In many species it is characterized by finger-shaped appendages, the pyloric caeca which seem to produce mainly mucus substances.

Some teleosts and lampreys lack a distinct stomach.

Midgut

Usually the absorptive surface of the midgut is considerably increased by the formation of various folds, finger-shaped extensions termed villi (Fig. 128) and a brushborder on the free surface of the absorptive cells. One or several folds often take the shape of helically arranged shelves, e.g. in the lamprey, in sharks and some mammals, where they are termed *plicae circulares* or valves of Kerckring. At the base of the intestinal villi in birds and mammals tubular glands (crypts of Lieberkühn which are absent in the lower vertebrates) dip down into the *lamina propria* terminating at the *muscularis mucosae* (absent in e.g. lampreys and anurans). Villi and crypts are covered and lined respectively by a simple prismatic epithelium, which is composed of several cell types. The majority of cells are absorptive and termed enterocytes. They bear the brushborder mentioned above, which is particularly rich in enzymes and which is covered by a protective mucopolysaccharide surface coat. Below the brushborder a terminal web of microfilaments can be found in the enterocytes, which seems to anchor the microfilaments of the microvilli (Fig. 16).

The lateral parts of the terminal web are continuous with the apical junctional complexes. Below the terminal web a zone occurs with mitochondria, tubules of the smooth ER and lysosomes. Next follows the Golgi apparatus. Below the latter we find the nucleus, below and laterally of which cisternae of the rough ER and mitochondria are located. Ribosomes are scattered throughout the cells. Loosely distributed among the enterocytes mucus-producing goblet cells are to be found, which possess a distended apical half which is filled with mucus. In many mammals, in particular in herbivorous - and omnivorous species, the Paneth cells can be found at the base of the crypts. The ultrastructure of these cells corresponds to that of exocrine protein secreting cells (basally located rough ER, large supra-nuclear Golgi apparatus and apical secretory granules). In the rat the specific product of these cells has been found to be lysozyme, a bacteriolytic enzyme. In some insectivores and bats cell types intermediate between goblet and Paneth cells have been described. In the midgut epithelium of all vertebrates endocrine cells occur (Fig. 117). A further cell type has recently been detected in insectivores and rodents: the brush cell, which may represent a receptor cell. It is among others characterized by a slender apex bearing unusually long and thick microvilli. Only in Petromyzon ciliated cells occur in the intestinal epithelium.

The intestinal epithelium is constantly renewed - new cells are formed in the crypts, in which correspondingly many mitoses can be observed, old ones being extruded from the tips of the villi. In rats the lifespan of an intestinal epithelial cell is 2–3 days. The reticular connective tissue of the mucous membrane, which forms the core of the villi and is to be found between the crypts of Lieberkühn, contains a network of blood vessels and a rich supply of lymphatic vessels - both transport absorbed nutrients into the body. Further smooth muscle cells occur, which confer some mobility to the villi. In teleosts, in which a typical muscularis mucosae is absent, a layer of smooth muscle cells may frequently be found under the epithelium. Finally numerous free cells are located in this connective tissue (mast cells, plasma cells, lymphocytes, eosinophils, and histiocytes).

Only in the submucosa of the anterior part of the mammalian midgut mucus-secreting glands (Brunner's glands, Fig. 128) occur, which occasionally are to be found only in the course of the first millimetres (insectivores) but may extend to the middle of the midgut (horses, hares). The mucus of these glands is said to be important for the alkalization of the milieu in the lumen of the midgut.

Large intestine

The surface of the large intestine (= colon) frequently is smooth or bears only low folds or villi. In mammals the crypts are particularly well developed and contain abundant goblet cells (Fig. 128). The enterocytes are similar to those of the midgut but laterally are markedly interdigitated. Basally they may be separated by wide intercellular spaces into which microvilli project. These features are indicative of the main function of the terminal part of the gut: the absorption of water.

The intestine often bears 1-2 blindly ending evaginations, termed caeca. They usually are characterized by the same type of mucous membrane as the large intestine. Frequently, the typical structure of the mucosa is obscured by numerous lymph nodules, which, however, may also occur in other parts of the intestinal tract. In many birds the caeca also take part in digestion and absorption of nutrients. Their secretions hydrolyse starch, invert sugar and digest proteins. In various species of grouse, which during winter feed on the needles of conifers, a large part of the absorption of the food molecules obtained from this diet, occurs in the caeca.

Cyprinidae lack a stomach. In spite of this their intestine may be subdivided functionally and structurally into four regions. Absorption of lipids e.g. essentially occurs in the second, that of proteins in the third segment. Proteins are absorbed by pinocytosis due possibly to the absence of peptic secretion (gastric principal cells are lacking). The enterocytes performing this function are characterized by numerous pinocytotic vesicles and a complex tubulo-vesicular network in the apical cytoplasm. The tubules, at least in part, are deep invaginations of the apical plasma membrane. Many of the pinocytotic vesicles fuse to form a big supranuclear vacuole into which Golgi vesicles (primary lysosomes?) seem to empty their contents. These big vacuoles therefore seem to represent digestive vacuoles. They contain alkaline phosphatase.

Liver

The two most important glands originating from the intestine are the pancreas and liver. The structure of the pancreas is relatively simple (Fig. 29). The terminal secretory units are composed of enzyme and fluid-secreting cells the fine structure of which corresponds to the classical protein-secreting cells (Fig. 28). In mammals and teleosts the initial part of the duct system extends into the acini with the centroacinar cells (endocrine pancreas, see page 220).

The liver originally was also an exocrine tubular gland; as can still be seen in ammocoetes larvae and the adult hagfish. Its secretory product is the gall fluid important for the digestion of lipids, transported *via* the biliary ducts (absent in adult lampreys) into the intestine. It also seems to have acquired an excretory function at

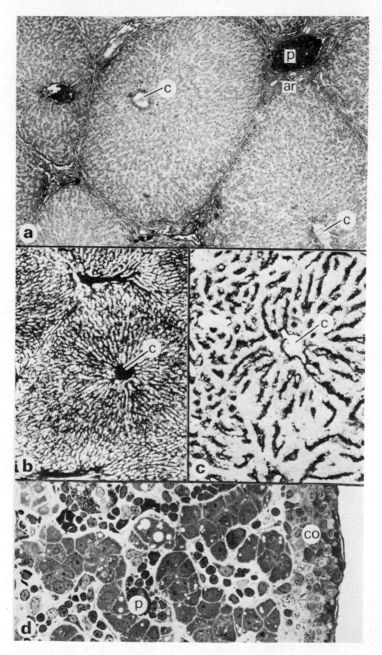

an early stage (excretion of endproducts of the haemoglobin metabolism).

The intimate association between this gland and blood vessels favours the acquisition of numerous additional functions, e.g. storage of energy-rich compounds (lipid and glycogen). Soon the classical glandular structure is replaced by a meshwork of cell cords intermingled with blood spaces (Fig. 130). The epithelial cells, termed hepatocytes, however, always retain their exocrine function and surround a narrow glandular lumen (bile canaliculi). The larger exocrine ducts (bile ducts) are surrounded by a cuboidal epithelium. In many species, e.g. teleosts, birds and in particular in mammals, the cell cords of the hepatocytes become radially arranged around a larger vein, termed the central vein and constitute small units called lobules. These may be clearly separated from each other by connective tissue, e.g. in the pig (Fig. 130) in other species they are less clearly recognized.

A demonstration of the blood capillaries, which run in parallel to the cell cords, however, usually visualizes the lobules (Fig. 130).

Liver lobule of mammals. In cross-sections the individual lobules ideally are of hexagonal outline and are more or less clearly separated from each other by loose connective tissue, which at least is always present in those corners of contact where three lobules meet, the portal fields. These can easily be recognized by the occurrence of at least one branch of the portal vein, the hepatic artery, a lymph vessel and a bile duct. The centre of the lobule is marked by the central vein, upon which anastomosing blood capillaries, termed hepatic sinusoids, radially converge from the periphery where they originate from the confluence of small branches of portal vein and hepatic arteries (Fig. 131). These sinusoids flank the hepatocyte cell cords, which also run radially from the periphery to the centre of the lobule. In the course of these rather long and wide capillaries an exchange of metabolites can take place between blood and hepatocytes, which usually are separated from the sinusoids only by a thin endothelium. Only in some ungulates a thin additional barrier, a basement lamina and some

Figure 130. Light microscopic preparations of the liver. **a:** pig, liver lobules surrounded by connective tissue, c: central vein, p: portal vein, ar: branch of the liver artery, x 50; **b:** rabbit, one liver lobule with central vein upon which numerous sinusoids converge, blood vessels outlined by injected ink, x 50; **c:** *Chromis* (teleost), demonstration of alkaline phosphatase, which in this animal outlines the sinusoids, c: central vein, x 100; **d:** *Ichthyophis* (Gymnophiona) example of the liver structure as found in the Urodelomorpha. The hepatocytes form cell cords in the centre of which runs a bile canaliculus, between the cords wide sinusoids with blood cells, p: pigment cell, co: cortical area of the liver in which white blood cells arise, x 310

reticular fibres, is present. Individual lysosome-rich cells of the endothelium, termed stellate cells of Kupffer, are characterized by their ability to phagocytize. They represent transformed monocytes and are part of the reticular endothelial system. The space between endothelium and hepatocytes is called space of Disse. In the electron microscope it can be seen to be filled by numerous microvilli extending from the hepatocytes. Occasionally it may contain peculiar lipid-storing cells.

The epithelial cell cords between the sinusoids consist of one cell type, the hepatocyte, which fulfils a multitude of tasks. This is partly reflected by differences in the finer details of the cytoplasmic

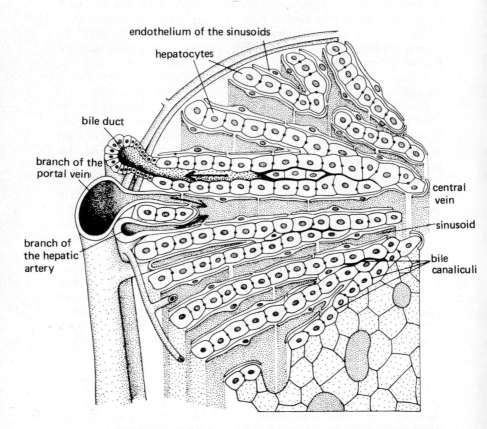

Figure 131. Diagrammatic representation of the radial disposition of the liver cell plates and sinusoids around a central vein, showing the centripetal flow of the blood and the centrifugal flow of the bile (arrows). After HAM, 1965, and BLOOM, FAWCETT, 1969

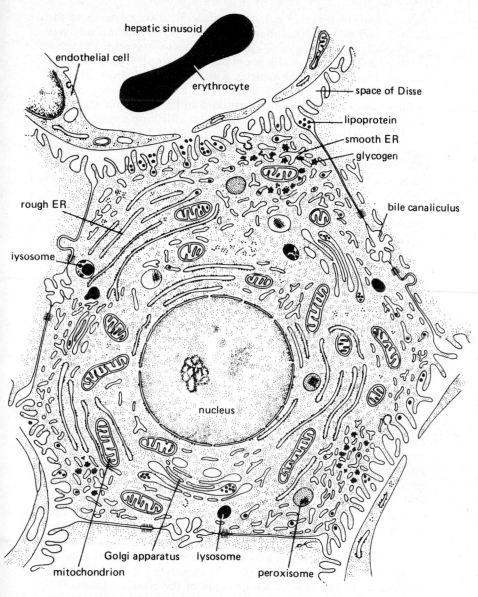

Figure 132. Fine structure of a mammalian liver cell and its relationships to other liver cells, the sinusoids and bile canaliculi. After BLOOM, FAWCETT, 1969

organization, as revealed e.g. by histochemical reactions or in the electron microscope. A number of functions varies rhythmically over a period of a day.

The cells (Fig. 132) usually are of polyhedral outline and contain a centrally located spherical nucleus, with much euchromatin and one or more big nucleoli. Occasionally a cell may contain two nuclei, about 15 per cent of the nuclei are said to be tetraploid and some exhibit an even higher degree of polyploidy. Striking components of the cytoplasm are stored materials: glycogen and fat. The amount of these substances varies according to different functional states of the cell. Rough ER cisternae and Golgi apparatus are well developed, mitochondria are frequent. The Golgi apparatus faces the bile canaliculus. Lysosomes, peroxisomes and smooth ER are also observed regularly, the amount of smooth ER is particularly variable; it plays among others a role in processes of detoxification and the formation of glycogen.

Between two neighbouring hepatocytes a minute tubular extracellular space can be found, termed bile canaliculus. It is separated from the remaining intercellular space and the space of Disse by junctional complexes including tight junctions. This system of canals drains the bile fluid from the lobule and leads it into the bile ducts of the portal field. In the electron microscope microvilli of the hepatocytes can be seen to project into the canaliculi. Because of their contents of specific enzymes, e.g. alkaline phosphatase and ATPase, the bile canaliculi can easily be demonstrated also in the light microscope.

Important for the function of the hepatocytes within the lobule is their supply with oxygen. Normally the periphery of the lobule obtains more oxygen than the centre, since the branches of the hepatic artery coming from the portal area open into the sinusoids already in the periphery. A functional zonation may therefore be recognized within the lobule, e.g. metabolic pathways critically dependent on oxygen are concentrated in the lobular periphery. During periods of low oxygen supply the centre degenerates first.

In the preceding paragraphs the lobule has been described as the functional unit of the mammalian liver. Recently another functional unit has found wide acceptance, the liver acinus. This is a unit whose centre is formed by a terminal branch of the portal vein, the hepatic artery and the bile duct. The vessels leave the portal area and run along one side of the hexagon of the classical lobule. The associated hepatic tissue, supplied by these branches, is termed the liver acinus. In ideal cross-sections it is of rhomboidal shape the pointed tips coinciding with the central veins of two classical lobules. According to this interpretation the classical lobule is not surrounded by a hexagon with six portal areas, but is of a more irregular shape and ideally has only three portal areas at its periphery.

Another attempt to define the functional unit puts the vessels of the portal area into the centre (portal lobule) all the tissue supplied by the vessels of this area belong to one portal lobule. The acinus mentioned above is a variant of this interpretation.

LITERATURE

ARNI, P. 'Zur Feinstruktur der Mitteldarmdrüse von *Lymnaea stagnalis* (Gastropoda, Pulmonata).' *Z. Morph. Tiere*, **77**, 1-18 (1974).

BECKER, G. L., CHEN, C. H., GREENAWALT, J. W., LEHNINGER, A. L. 'Calcium phosphate granules in the hepatopancreas of the blue crab *Callinectes sapidus*.' *J. Cell Biol.* **61**, 316-26 (1974).

BERRIDGE, M. J., GUPTA, B. L. 'Fine structural changes in relation to ion and water transport in the rectal papillae of the blowfly, *Calliphora*.' *J. Cell Sci.* **2**, 89-112 (1967).

BRUNSER, O., LUFT, J. H. 'Fine structure of the apex of absorptive cells from rat small intestine.' *J. Ultrastruct. Res.* **31**, 291-311 (1970).

DALES, R. P., PELL, J. S. 'The nature of the peritrophic membrane in the gut of the terebellid polychaete *Neoamphitrite figulus*.' *Comp. Biochem. Physiol.* **34**, 819-826 (1970).

FILSHIE, B. K., POULSON, D. F., WATERHOUSE, D. F. 'Ultrastructure of the copper-accumulating region of the *Drosophila* larval midgut.' *Tissue and Cell*, **3**, 77-102, (1971).

GARANT, P. R. 'An electron microscopic study of the crystal-matrix relationship in the teeth of the dogfish *Squalus acanthias* L. J.' *Ultrastruct. Res.* **30**, 441-449 (1970).

KUDO, S. 'Electron microscopic observations on avian esophageal epithelium.' *Arch. Histol. jap.* **33**, 1-30 (1971).

LEE, D. L. 'The fine structure of the excretory system in adult *Nippostrongylus brasiliensis* (Nematoda) and a suggested function for the excretory gland.' *Tissue and Cell*, **2**, 225-31 (1970).

LESTER, K. S. 'On the nature of "fibrils" and tubules in developing enamel of the opossum *Didelphis marsupialis*.' *J. Ultrastruct. Res.* **30**, 64-77 (1970).

LOIZZI, R. F. 'Interpretation of crayfish hepatopancreatic function based on fine structural analysis of epithelial cell lines and muscle network, *Z. Zellforsch.* **113**, 420-40 (1971).

MATUS, A. J. 'Fine structure of the posterior salivary gland of *Eledone cirrosa* and *Octopus vulgaris*.' *Z. Zellforsch.* **122**, 111-21 (1971).

MATTER, A., ORCI, L., ROUILLER, C. 'A study on the permeability barriers between Disse's space and the bile canaliculus.' *J. Ultrastruct. Res.* **11**, 1-71 (1969).

NÖRREVANG, A., WINGSTRAND, K. G. 'On the occurrence and structure of choanocyte-like cells in some echinoderms.' *Acta Zool.* **51**, 249-70 (1970).

PATZELT, V. 'Der Darm. In von Möllendorff, W. *Handbuch der mikroskopischen Anatomie des Menschen*.' *Bd.* 5. Teil 3. Springer Verlag. Berlin. 1-448 (1936).

PETERS, W. 'Zur Frage des Vorkommens und der Definition peritrophischer Membranen.' *Zool. Anz.* **30**. Suppl. 142-52 (1967).

PLENK, H. 'Der Magen. In von Möllendorff, W.: *Handbuch der mikroskopischen Anatomie des Menschen. Bd.* 5. Teil 2. Springer Verlag. Berlin. 1-234 (1932).

REITH, E. J. 'The stages of amelogenesis as observed in molar teeth of young rats.' *J. Ultrastruct. Res.* **30**, 111-51 (1970).

STORCH, V., WELSCH, U. 'Elektronenmikroskopische und enzymhistochemische Untersuchungen über die Mitteldarmdrüse von *Lingula unguis* L. (Branchiopoda). *Zool. Jb. Anat.* **94**, 441-452 (1975)

SUMNER, A. T. 'The cytology and histochemistry of the digestive gland cells of some freshwater lamellibranchs.' *J. roy. micr. Soc.* **85**, 201-211 (1966).

WALKER. G. 'The cytology, histochemistry, and ultrastructure of the cell types found in the digestive gland of the slug, *Agriolimax reticulatus.*' *Protoplasma*, **71**, 91-109 (1970).

WISSE, E. 'An electron microscopic study of the fenestrated endothelial lining of rat liver sinusoids.' *J. Ultrastruct. Res.* **31**, 125-150 (1970).

Chapter 8
RESPIRATORY ORGANS

Many small animal species do not possess any particular respiratory organs; in them the exchange of gases takes place *via* the body surface. In larger organisms special respiratory organs develop and integumentary respiration is of reduced importance. The respiratory organs are formed by various invaginations or evaginations of the epidermis or of the alimentary tract.

Tracheae
The tracheae are tubular ectodermal invaginations, which in insects originate from the lateral walls of the body, the pleura. They are lined by a cuticle, termed the intima. In land-living insects they open out on to the free surface of the body by small openings called spiracles (Fig. 133), two of which are to be found per body segment. In aquatic larvae, e.g. in Ephemerida and Odonata, the spiracles are usually closed. In these cases the tracheae form dense networks under the epidermis around the posterior gut or in different appendages (tracheal gills). The epithelium of the trichopteran tracheal gills is composed by a simple squamous epithelium covered by a thin cuticle and underlain by a basement lamina separating it from the haemolymph. Embedded into the epithelium are numerous tracheole containing extensions of tracheal end cells.

Normally the tracheae of the neighbouring segments are interconnected, frequently dilatations can be found, tracheal sacs, which store air.

Each trachea is composed of a simple epithelium (the invaginated epidermis) and the cuticular lining (Fig. 133). The wider the lumen of the trachea, the thicker the cuticle, in order to prevent a collapse of the trachea. The exocuticle frequently forms a helically arranged projecting ridge (taenidium); occasionally a surface relief composed of rings, nets or ladders, stiffens the tracheal wall. In larger tracheal branches a layer of epidermal cells surrounds the cuticle. In thin branches, the epidermal cells form rows, so that per cross-section only one cell pervaded by a cuticular tube is to be encountered. The

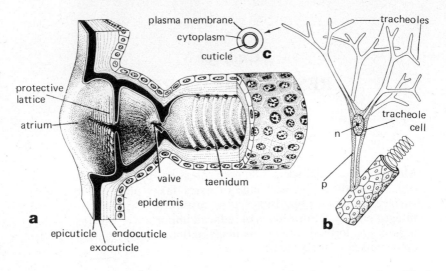

Figure 133. Tracheal system of insects. **a:** Diagrammatic representation of a spiracle, after SEIFERT, 1970; **b:** tracheal end cell, n: nucleus, p: cellular process connecting the end cell with a trachea; **c:** cross-section through a tracheole (electron microscopy). After SEIFERT, 1970, and WEBER & WEIDNER, 1974

cytoplasm of these cells contains a few rough ER cisternae, which synthesize a new cuticle after moulting, a few mitochondria, longitudinally arranged microtubules and fields of glycogen.

After repeated branchings, which are accompanied by a constant decrease in diameter of the cells, the tracheae terminate with a special tracheal end cell (tracheole cell), which corresponds to the site of gaseous exchange. This element is a particularly differentiated epithelial cell with long cytoplasmic extensions (Fig. 133). The cell body and its processes are invaginated by minute tubules, termed tracheoles or tracheal capillaries, these usually have a diameter of 0.2 μm and are in communication with the cuticle-lined tubes of the preceding sections of the trachea. The tracheoles are also lined by a thin cuticle (Fig. 136) , which however is not moulted. In many insects these terminal branches are filled with fluid, in others with air. The amount of fluid changes according to the composition of the surrounding haemolymph. If oxygen is needed, fluid is absorbed into the haemolymph and air is drawn into the tracheoles.

The transport of air in the wider sections of the tracheae is accomplished by alterations of the body shape (dorsoventral flattening or rhythmical shortening of the abdomen).

Tissues with a high demand of oxygen, e.g. flight muscles or luminescent organs, are richly supplied with tracheae and the association of tracheal end cells and the cells to be supplied with oxygen is so intimate, that in the light microscope it was believed that the tracheoles invaded these cells. In the the electron microscope can be seen that branches of the tracheal end cells containing tracheoles only project into the other cells without penetrating their plasma membrane. In flight muscle of the hornet tracheole containing fine extensions of the end cell even have been observed to project into mitochondria. The oxygen is thereby brought within a distance of 0.1 μm of some of the cristae. In some organs the tracheal end cells are modified. Near photocytes, e.g. they contain abundant mitochondria and are in contact with nerve endings.

Apart from insects, tracheae are also to be found in other land-living arthropods, e.g. in arachnids, and, modified rarely also in Crustacea (white bodies in the pleopods of land-living isopods). In Onychophora they are straight simple tubes.

Lungs

In air-breathing vertebrates the respiratory tract is divided into conducting and respiratory portions. The larger air-conducting pathways are lined by a pseudostratified ciliated epithelium, containing goblet cells and - in particular in the trachea - simple chemoreceptor cells (respiratory epithelium, Fig. 27). The section of the conducting part following the pharynx is a single wide tube, termed trachea (air pipe); it divides into two main branches, the primary bronchi, which lead into the lungs, where they give rise to the bronchial tree, which is of different construction in the tetrapods. In the trachea and bronchial tree the connective tissue layer below the epithelium contains numerous elastic fibres and smooth muscle cells. In the deeper parts of the wall mucus-producing mucous and serous glands and cartilage are to be found. In the trachea the cartilage forms rings (some reptiles, birds) or anastomosing branches (some reptiles) or horseshoe-shaped elements (some reptiles, mammals) in the bronchial tree irregularly shaped pieces.

The functional units of the respiratory portions are the alveoli, in mammals blind invaginations of the alveolar duct (Figs. 134, 135), the terminal sections of the bronchial tree. The wide opening of the alveoli is surrounded by a ring of smooth muscle cells. The alveoli are lined by a very thin uninterrupted epithelium in which in mammals two or three cell types can be distinguished. The typical pulmonary epithelial cells (pneumocyte I, alveolar cell I) are extremely thin squamous elements (particularly in birds). A second

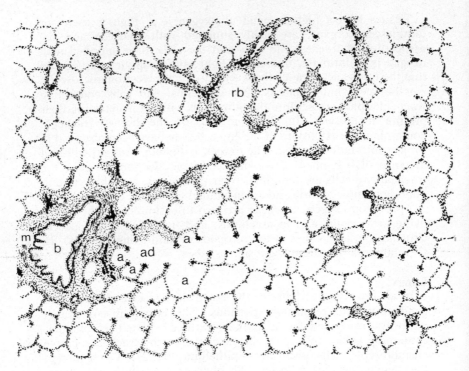

Figure 134. Low power survey of the light microscopical structure of the mammalian lung. ad: alveolar duct, a: alveole, b: bronchiole, m: smooth muscle cells, rb: respiratory bronchiole. After BARGMANN, 1967

epithelial cell type is of roundish shape; its perinuclear parts may be submerged into the thin connective tissue layer below the epithelium or they may bulge into the alveolar lumen (alveolar cell, septal cell, alveolar cell II, pneumocyte II). They are secretory cells with a well developed Golgi apparatus and secretory granules (lamellar bodies), the contents of which is believed to be phospholipid and to be released into the alveolar lumen, where it spreads on the epithelium and acts as a surfactant. It reduces the surface tension in the alveoli, which presumably would otherwise collapse at the end of expiration. A third cell type has been described in the alveolar epithelium of rodents; it may be a chemoreceptor cell and it is characterized by plump apical microvilli and abundant glycogen particles in the cytoplasm.

Below the alveolar epithelium reticular and above all elastic fibres occur. Embedded into this connective tissue are countless blood

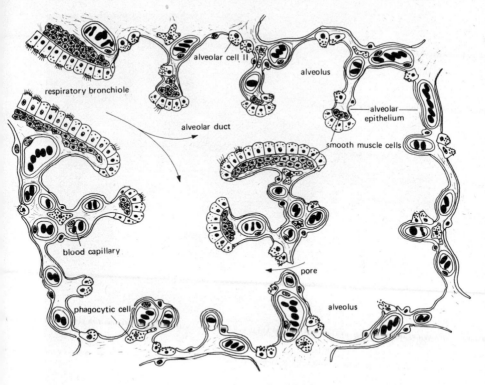

Figure 135. Schematic representation of the terminal portions of the air passages in the mammalian lung, arrows indicate flow of the air. After BLOOM, FAWCETT, 1969

capillaries which closely approach the alveolar epithelium. Fig. 136 shows the barrier the gases O_2 and CO_2 have to cross in the lung: the alveolar epithelium and its basement membrane, a narrow connective tissue space containing a few fibres, and the endothelium of the blood vessels with its basement membrane. In birds and mammals the connective tissue space may be absent in the areas of gaseous exchange and the basement membranes of the alveolus and capillary may fuse. In the connective tissue regularly macrophages occur, which presumably originate from the blood and correspond to transformed monocytes. They may be laden with phagocitized foreign particles and break through the alveolar epithelium into the alveolar lumen.

The term lung is also applied to various respiratory organs of invertebrates. They usually correspond to thin walled richly vascularized areas in the epidermis or in other places. The

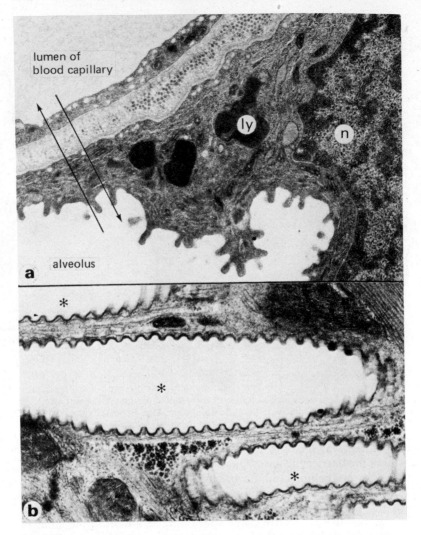

Figure 136. **a:** Fine structure of the air-blood barrier in the amphibian lung (*Ichthyophis*); arrows indicate the barrier, which is traversed by O_2 and CO_2: the endothelium of the blood capillary, a basement membrane, a narrow intercellular space containing connective tissue fibres, a second basement lamina and the alveolar epithelium. n: nucleus of alveolar epithelial cell, ly: lysosome. Both epithelia contain light pinocytotic vesicles. x 18 000. **b:** sections through tracheoles between muscle cells, *Chironomus* (Diptera) x 30 000

respiratory cavity of pulmonates, the holothurian water lungs, and the evaginations of the posterior intestine are examples. A peculiar situation is to be found in land-living crabs. In the land-living crab *Ocypode* the lung is characterized by a particularly thin cuticle (about 0.2 µm) which is secreted by an usually even thinner epithelium (Fig. 137). This is underlain by a blood space and a loose meshwork of cells. The epidermis with its cuticle is anchored in the underlying tissue by tall pillar-shaped cells containing abundant microtubules.

Gills

The respiratory organs of water-living animals usually are termed gills. In invertebrates they are thin-walled evaginations of the body surface receiving a rich supply of blood vessels. Frequently they occur in protected localities, e.g. under the carapace fold of Crustacea or in the mantle cavity of molluscs. This results in the necessity to produce a water current which supplies the gills with fresh water. It is produced by cilia on or beside the gills (molluscs, annelids, echinoderms) or by specialized parts of extremities (Crustacea). In Crustacea the epithelium of the gills is usually rich in mitochondria and exhibits deep basal infoldings. The apical surface bears microvilli or cytoplasmic folds, increasing the area of gaseous exchange, and is covered by a thin cuticle (Fig. 137).

The structure of epithelium on the gills of several invertebrates, e.g. numerous crustaceans, does not agree with an assumed respiratory function. The epithelium is relatively thick, largely filled by mitochondria and characterized by apical microvilli and basal infoldings. In the land-living crab *Ocypode* this surface epithelium furthermore is underlain by blood spaces which are delimited by podocytes (Fig. 137). Thus, these gills exhibit all ultrastructural characteristics of an organ of excretion, osmo- and ion regulation (see Chapter 10). Certainly they are not very effective respiratory organs.

The gills of the fishes are situated at clefts in the pharynx, which originally - e.g. in ascidians and Amphioxus - are a device for filtering food particles.

In teleosts the gill arches bear on their convex side two rows of filaments, each of which is supported by a cartilaginous rod. The surface of the filaments is studded on both sides with secondary lamellae. Into each lamella (Fig. 138) a branch of the branchial artery enters and forms here a dense net of capillaries. In the electron microscope this system simply corresponds to lacunae (blood spaces not lined by an endothelium) surrounded by lateral extensions of columnar contractile connective tissue cells. The cuboidal or squamous surface epithelium of the lamellae usually is composed of three cell types: simple supporting cells, rich in rough

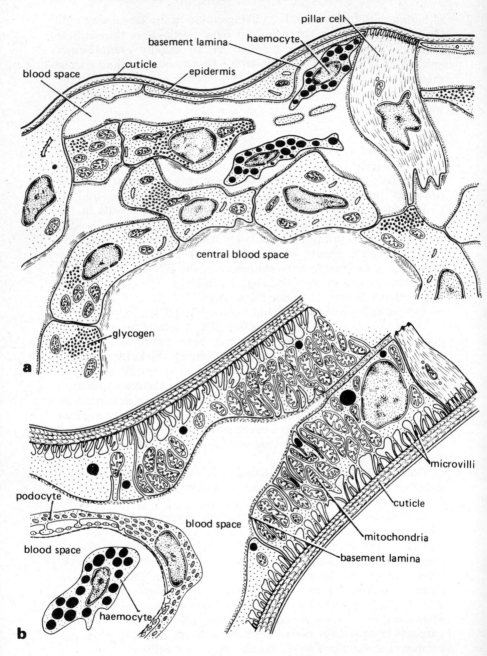

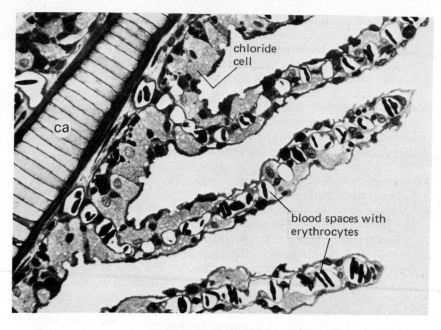

chloride
cell

ca

blood spaces with
erythrocytes

Figure 138. Gill of the teleost *Periophthalmus.* The lamellae contain an anastomosing system of blood spaces and are covered by an epithelium containing abundant pale chloride cells. ca: cartilage rod composed of disk-shaped cells. x 560

ER and microfilaments, mucus-producing cells and chloride cells. These are characterized by an apical cup-shaped invagination, a well-developed system of smooth ER tubules and mitochandria containing tubules of cristae (*Periophthalmus*) and mitochondrial granules. They presumably play a role in ion exchange.

The teleost pseudobranch is dorsally located in the transitory zone between oral cavity and pharynx, it is covered by the mucous membrane of the mouth and is composed of leaf-like structures, the surface of which is thrown into numerous folds. As in the gills each of these has a central axis consisting of capillaries and is covered by

Figure 137. Fine structure of lung (**a**) and gill (**b**) of the land-living crab *Ocypode.* The air-blood barrier in the lung(**a**) is about $0·2 - 0·3 \, \mu m$ in diameter. Below the thin epidermis a system of blood spaces occurs delimited by a meshwork of cells rich in glycogen. The epidermis of the gill (**b**) is usually composed of mitochondria-rich cells with apical microvilli and a basal labyrinth. Below the epidermis a blood space occurs. In the centre of this space blood vessels surrounded by podocytes occur. The fine structure of the gills indicates that they are organs of osmoregulation and excretion. After STORCH, WELSCH, 1975

an epithelium, the cells of which resemble the chloride cells.

This organ is richly supplied with nerve terminals and blood vessels and may correspond functionally to the *glomus caroticum* of mammals since it reacts to changes of O_2 and CO_2 in the blood; but it may also play a role in ion exchange.

In sharks the epithelium on the secondary lamellae usually is composed of one layer of squamous cells, but occasionally also stratified parts can be observed. The underlying connective tissue is composed of columnar cells rich in filaments between which blood containing lacunae occur. Lacunae also may be found in the gills of the lamprey, in which the lamellae are covered by a layer of voluminous cuboidal or columnar cells. The filaments are covered by two layers of epithelial cells.

In the electron microscope the epithelium covering shark gill filaments is composed of unspecialized supporting cells as well as individual mucus and chloride cells. The secondary lamellae are covered by a double layer of flattened unspecialized epithelial cells (mucus and chloride cells are rare). The connective tissue underlying the epithelium, as in teleosts, consists of widely spaced pillar cells, the flanges of which line an interconnecting network of blood spaces (lacunae). Attached to the outer surface each pillar cell is associated with several columns of collagen fibrils. The pillar cells presumably are contractile (also in teleosts).

LITERATURE

AFZELIUS, B. A., GONNERT, N. 'Intramitochondrial tracheoles in flight muscle from the hornet *Vespa crabro*'. *J. Submicr. Cytol.* **4**, 1-6 (1972).

BARETS, A., DUNEL, S., LAURENT, D. 'Infrastructure du plexus nerveux terminal de la pseudobranchie d'un téléostéen, *Sander lucioperca.*' *J. Microscopie.* **9**, 619-624 (1970).

BIELAWSKI, J. 'Ultrastructure and ion transport in gill epithelium of the crayfish, *Astacus leptodactylus* Esch.' *Protoplasma.* **73**, 177-190 (1971).

COPELAND, D. E., FITZJARRELL, A. T. 'The salt absorbing cells in the gills of the blue crab (*Callinectes sapidus* Rathbun) with notes on modified mitochondria.' *Z. Zellforsch.* **92**, 1-22 (1968).

DUNCKER, H.-R. 'Structure of avian lungs.' *Respir. Phys.* **14**, 44-63 (1972).

HATASA, K., NAKAMURA, T. 'Electron microscopic observations of lung alveolar epithelial cells of normal young mice with special reference to formation and secretion of osmiophilic lamellar bodies.' *Z. Zellforsch.* **68**, 266-277 (1965).

NEWSTEAD, J. D. 'Fine structure of the respiratory lamellae of teleostean gills.' *Z. Zellforsch.* **79**, 396-428 (1967).

RHODIN, J. A. G. 'Structure of the gills of the marine fish pollack *(Pollachius virens).*' *Anat. Rec.* **148**, 420-434 (1964).

SMITH, D. S. *Insect cells. Their structure and function.* Oliver and Boyd. Edinburgh. 372 S. 1968.

SKOBE, Z., GARANT, P. G., ALBRIGHT, J. T. 'Ultrastructure of a new cell in the gills of the air breathing fish *Helostoma temmincki.*' *J. Ultrastruct. Res.* **31**, 312-322 (1970).

STORCH, V., WELSCH, U. Über Bau und Funktion der Kiemen und Lugen von *Ocypode ceratophthalma* (Decapoda, Crustacea).' *Mar. Biol.* **29**, 363-371 (1975).

WEIBEL, E. R. 'The mystery of "non-nucleated plates" in the alveolar epithelium of the lung explained.' *Acta anat. (Basel).* **78**, 425-443 (1971).

WRIGHT, D. E. 'The structure of the gills of the elasmobranch *Scyliorhinus canicula* (L.).' *Z. Zellforsch.* **144**, 489-509 (1973).

Chapter 9

LYMPHATIC ORGANS, BLOOD CELLS, AND BLOOD VESSELS

Lymphatic organs are only to be found in vertebrates, although comparable tissues may occur also in invertebrates. Their chief function is to protect the organism against foreign agents, e.g. viruses and bacteria. They also play a role in the formation and destruction of blood cells.

The lymphatic system of mammals is relatively well known and consists of lymphoepithelial organs, lymph nodes, thymus, spleen. These organs have in common a frame work of reticular cells, in the interstices of which free cells are housed (page 80).

Lymphoepithelial organs

The lymphoepithelial system which can be found in most vertebrates, consists of numerous lymph nodules, which occur e.g. in the mucous membranes of the gut, the respiratory system and the urinary system. They are particularly prominent in the tonsils of the pharynx, where the epithelium forms deep pits. Below the epithelium the lymph nodules occur (Figs. 43, 139). The epithelium may be distorted and destroyed in the case of infections, if lymphocytes and plasma cells invade it.

Another characteristic lymphoepithelial organ is the *bursa fabricii* of birds. It corresponds to a pocket of the cloaca, the wall of which is thrown into numerous folds, which in young animals are covered by columnar epithelial cells. Below these, lymph nodules can be seen, which are composed of medulla and cortex, separated by a basal lamina, which is continuous with the basal lamina of the epithelium. The medulla is interconnected with the epithelium and corresponds to clumps of modified epithelial cells submerged into the underlying tissue. The medullary cells are of stellate shape; between their extensions lymphocytes occur, among which a peculiar type (light roundish nucleus with one to two nucleoli, irregular shape) occurs in the peripheral parts of the medulla (bursa lymphocytes), the same type of lymphocyte also constitutes the cortex. The bursa undergoes characteristic changes during ontogenetic development. In gallinaceous birds it begins to degenerate between the third and fifth month after hatching and finally is replaced by connective tissue containing fat, and smooth muscle cells.

Lymph nodes

Lymph nodes (Fig. 139) are only to be found in mammals. They are composed of accumulations of lymph nodules, and are surrounded by a connective tissue capsule. They are located along the course of the lymph vessels. Their main function is the production of antibodies.

One or several afferent lymphatics enter the node, one or rarely two efferent lymphatics leave it (Fig. 139). The capsule extends septa (trabecules) into the interior of the node, which is composed of reticular cells and lymphocytes and other free cells. The outer zone of the lymph node containing dense accumulations of cells is termed cortex, the inner loosely constructed part is termed medulla. Immediately below the capsule and near the trabeculae the reticular cells are separated by particularly wide intercellular spaces forming the subcapsular sinus (Fig. 139). This term here designates a coarse mesh which receives the lymph fluid from the afferent lymphatics which slowly filters through these spaces down to the efferent lymphatic. The reticular cells near it or traversing it are often loaded with foreign particles. The cortex contains the lymph nodules, which extend broad cell-rich anastomosing extensions into the medulla, termed medullary cords. These are mainly composed of plasma cells and lymphocytes.

The lymph nodules usually develop a germinal centre (page 81) in postnatal life, i.e. a light central area composed of larger cells with paler nuclei than in the cells in the peripheral parts of the nodules, which consist of densely packed typical lymphocytes. In these centres the lymphocytes transform into plasma cells, if antigens have entered the body fluids. The antigens possibly are at first incorporated into reticulum cells, which transfer them to lymphocytes. These undergo a development, characterized by an increase in size, loosening up of the nuclear structure, formation of ribosomes (immunoblasts) and the appearance of rough ER cisternae (plasmablasts). Finally, the mature plasma cell (Fig. 31) is characterized (1) by an eccentrically located spherical nucleus with heterochromatin often arranged like the spokes of a wheel or attached in coarse clumps to the inner surface of the nuclear membrane, (2) by abundant rough ER cisternae, (3) by a well developed large Golgi apparatus producing secretory granules. These cells synthesize γ-globulins (antibodies). Not all of the

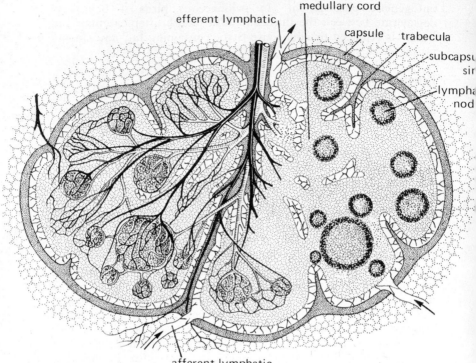

Figure 139. Schematic representation of a lymph node; left with, right without blood vessels; arteries black, veins annulated; arrows indicate flow of the lymph fluid. After KRÖLLING, GRAU, 1960

lymphocytes develop into plasma cells. Some are merely 'determined' by an antigen and rapidly develop into plasma cells during the next infection with the same antigen. Still others never transform into plasma cells (see below).

A zone between nodules and typical medullary cords is termed paracortical zone (thymus dependent zone). Structurally it is not clearly delimited; it never contains germinal centres. It houses those lymphocytes being determined by the thymus (see below) and mediating cellular immune reactions.

A lymph node is supplied with blood vessels. The artery enters it at the so-called hilus, which is also the site where the vein and efferent lymphatic leave the node.

A rich supply of capillaries may be found in the cortex. In the inner parts of the cortex, especially in the paracortical zone, typical small veins (venules) with a cuboidal endothelium may be observed. Through their walls lymphocytes migrate from the blood into the tissue of the node.

A few lymph nodes contain relatively wide sinusoidal channels, which partly contain lymph fluid and partly blood (haemal lymph nodes) or are entirely filled with blood (haemal nodes). Possibly they destroy blood cells.

Thymus

The thymus can be found in all vertebrates, in *Petromyzon* it may be demonstrated only in the larva. It is the first lymphatic organ to develop and function during ontogeny and seems to control the development of the other lymphatic organs. Its structure changes profoundly in the course of pre- and postnatal life. In mammals after maturation of the gonads it regresses (involutes) and is characterized by abundant fat cells; in other vertebrates cystic structures develop and few lymphocytes can be observed. Uniquely its reticular cells originate from entodermal cells of the pharynx. In young mammals the organ is lobulated. The individual lobules are composed by a pale staining medulla and a dense cortex (Fig. 140), composed of countless lymphocytes filling the interstices between the reticular cells (follicles do not occur in the thymus).

At the cortical surface the lymphocytes can form epithelium-like formations. In the medulla, the reticular cells are relatively densely packed, but lymphocytes are rather rare. The medulla reticular cells are interconnected by desmosomes and contain abundant microfilaments as well as lysosomes and smaller electron-dense granules, which are occasionally considered to be secretory granules with an endocrine function. These cells may become grouped concentrically around a central focus, where they produce keratin. Such structures are termed Hassall's corpuscles.

The blood vessels of the thymus are separated by a peculiar barrier from the specific thymic tissue. Each vessel is surrounded by a fibre containing perivascular space and an additional squamous epithelium. This barrier protects the thymic lymphocytes from the influence of antigenic macromolecules.

The lymphocytes of the thymus originate in the bone marrow, enter the thymus, multiply in the cortex, become specifically determined to fulfil tasks in the cellular defence reactions, leave the thymus and settle in the paracortical zone of the lymph nodes. These lymphocytes are termed T-cells (T=thymus).

In birds and reptiles the thymus tissue is also composed of cortex and medulla, which often, however, are less clearly separated. The

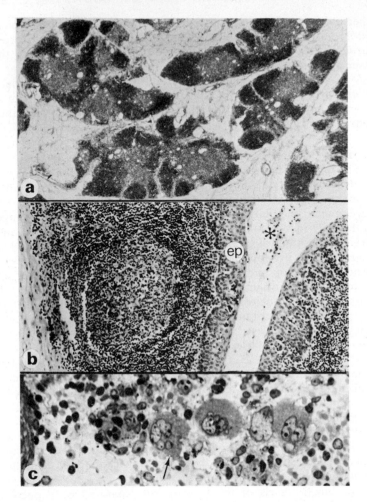

Figure 140.   Lymphatic organs. **a:**Thymus, *Galago* (prosimian), the thymus consists of numerous lobules with a dark cortical and a pale central zone. x 50; **b:** palatine tonsil, man, lymphatic nodule with pale germinal centre, in the epithelium of the pharyngeal cavity and in the lumen of the crypts (asterisk) individual lymphocytes occur. x 150. **c:** megakaryocytes in the spleen of the hedgehog (*Erinaceus*), note the big lobulated nucleus (arrow), x 450

medulla contains Hassall's corpuscles and myoid cells and in many places may be seen to extend projections to the surface of the organ. The myoid cells, which also occur in Amphibia and teleosts, contain cross-striated fibrils. In Amphibia the thymus medulla contains cysts, composed of cells or mucous substances. Mucous crystals also occur in the thymus of teleosts and sharks.

The thymus of teleosts is in direct continuation with the epithelium of the pharynx and is composed of a dense outer marginal, an intermediate cortical and a light inner medullary zone. In all of these zones mucus-producing cells occur. Lymphocytes are located both in the medullary and cortical zones.

Spleen

Mammals. Chief functions of the mammalian spleen are the production of antibodies, the destruction of erythrocytes, the redistribution of the end products of the haemoglobin decomposition, storage of blood. In those mammals in which the spleen is a blood reservoir, its capsule and trabeculae contain smooth muscle cells, which are responsible for the rapid expulsion of the blood.

In the light microscope the spleen may be seen to be surrounded by a connective tissue capsule extending septa (trabeculae) deep into the interior, which is composed of white (grey) and red pulp (Fig. 142). The white pulp corresponds to lymphatic nodules. In the red pulp abundant erythrocytes are to be found, which occupy various blood vessels and the interstitial spaces between the reticular cells. The spleen possesses characteristically distributed blood vessels.

The spleenic artery enters the organ at its hilus, courses through parts of the capsule into the trabeculae and enters the red pulp. Here it is partly or rarely also entirely surrounded by a sheath of lymphocytes, which occasionally becomes expanded to form lymphatic nodules, which may contain germinal centres. The nodules (also termed follicles) are supplied by an arterial branch of the follicular artery.

These sheaths of lymphocytes associated with the arteries of the red pulp constitute the white pulp, and the follicular artery emerges from the nodule to divide into 2–6 radiating branches termed penicillar arteries. These divide into small arterioles soon losing their muscular and elastic components and being surrounded by peculiar concentric sheaths of reticular cells and reticular fibres, termed ellipsoids. In the wall of these capillary blood vessels in some mammals, e.g. in the cat, slits have been described, which may be opened and closed and through which erythrocytes may escape. This section of the blood vessels is followed by the characteristic venous sinus = sinusoids (Fig. 141). Many observations show that the ellipsoidal capillaries open without interruption directly into the sinusoids. According to another interpretation the ellipsoidal capillaries freely terminate among reticular cells and the blood filters for a short distance through the interstitial space until it is

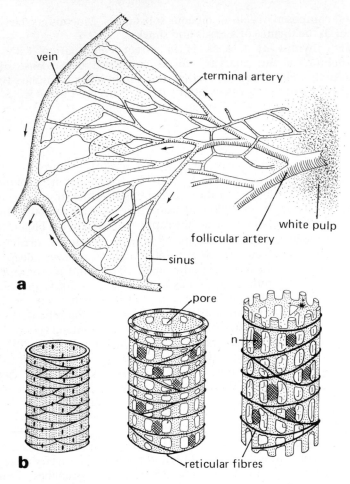

Figure 141. Mammalian spleen. **a:** Schematic representation of the terminal parts of the arteries, the sinuses and the initial parts of the veins, arrows indicate the direction of the blood flow, after KNISLEY: 1936; **b:** Schematic representation of the sinusoidal walls with variously wide pores; n: nucleus of a lining cell, after ROHR, 1960

collected in the sinusoids. The numerous sinusoids (which in the spleen are parts of the vascular system) are characterized by a wide lumen and a thin wall, which is composed of phagocytizing elongated reticulo-endothelial cells. Between them slits and pores exist, which may be passed by erythrocytes thus leaving the blood stream and being destroyed by the reticular cells. The sinusoids

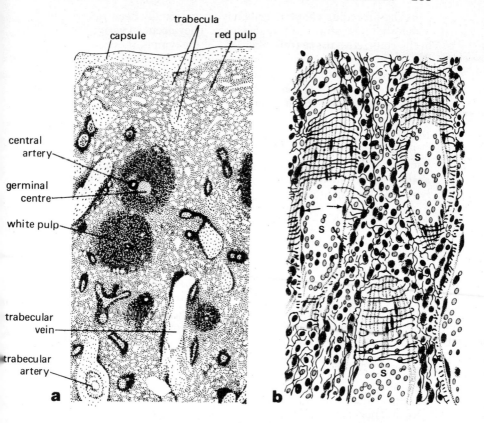

Figure 142. Mammalian spleen. **a:** Ordinary light microscopical preparation after MAXIMOW; **b:** silver impregnation to demonstrate the reticular fibres, which almost circularly surround the sinus (s); arrows point to nuclei of lining cells of the sinus, after BARGMANN, 1967

are surrounded by circularly arranged reticular fibres (Fig. 141).

The sinusoids may be opened and closed by sphincter muscles. Thus the passage of blood through them can be regulated. The sinusoids are continuous with veins, which finally leave the spleen at the hilus.

The red pulp of many mammals contains megakaryocytes (Fig. 140). A similar red and white pulp may also be distinguished in other vertebrates. In the light microscope the amphibian spleen seems to contain numerous blood-filled lacunae. The teleosts frequently contain particularly large ellipsoids. Agnathans lack a spleen.

In the preceding chapters cells have occasionally been referred to which share the ability of phagocytosis. They occur in various places in the connective tissue (reticular cells of the lymphatic system) or in the walls of particularly wide capillary or venous vessels, often termed sinusoids (e.g. in the liver (Kupffer cells), adrenal medulla, bone marrow and spleen). Together these cells constitute the reticulo-endothelial system (= macrophage system).

Blood cells

Blood cells are free, circulating cellular elements of the blood or haemolymph. Their structure is particularly variable and in many animal groups no agreement exists about the number of blood cell types and their definition.

Vertebrates

To begin with, the relatively well-known blood cells of the mammals will briefly be described. The following main cell types may be distinguished: red cells (erythrocytes) and white blood cells (leucocytes); in addition cell fragments, blood-platelets, occur. The mammalian erythrocytes (Fig. 143) are non-motile, highly specialized cells, which have lost their nucleus and organelles during maturation. They are usually biconcave disks filled with haemoglobin and a few microtubules at the outer edge of the disk. In some mammals they are oval and biconvex (camels).

Leucocytes. These cells contain a nucleus, usually of characteristic shape and structure, and cytoplasm with typical organelles, among which the granular elements are important for diagnosis. They are motile and under certain conditions can leave the blood stream and creep in amoeboid fashion through the connective tissue. Their functions are to protect the body against foreign invaders and to produce substances playing a role in the normal physiology of the vascular system, e.g. heparin. Two groups of leucocytes may be distinguished: granular and non-granular leucocytes (Fig. 143). Granular leucocytes (granulocytes) contain specific granules in their cytoplasm, which can be demonstrated by particular stains with the light microscope. According to their affinity for basic or acid dyes three types can be recognized: acidophilic (eosinophilic) granulocytes are selectively stained with acid dyes; basophilic granulocytes stain selectively with basic dyes, heterophilic (= neutrophilic) leucocytes usually have an affinity for both types of dyes, but differ from species to species in their staining reactions. The relatively rare acidophils contain a bi-lobed nucleus and oval to roundish granules, which correspond to lysosomes. In the electron microscope these granules contain in some species, e.g.

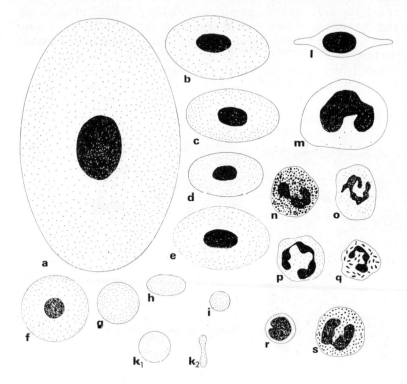

Figure 143.   Vertebrate blood cells, **a-k:** erythrocytes (a-f with g-k without nuclei) **l-s:** leucocytes. **a:** *Proteus* (Urodela); **b:** *Raja* (elasmobranch) **c:** *Testudo* (turtle); **d:** *Struthio* (ostrich); **e:** *Rana* (frog); **f:** *Petromyzon* (lamprey); **g:** elephant; **h:** lama; **i:** goat; **k:** man (disk-shaped); **k₁:** side view; **k₂:** section) **l:** thrombocyte of the frog *Rana,* **m:** monocyte (mammal); **n:** basophil (man); **o:** heterophil (rat); **p:** heterophil (man); **q:** heterophil (chicken); **r:** small lymphocyte (man); **s:** eosinophil (man)

in insectivores and rodents, a crystalline core, which may be due to the presence of heavy metals. The rare basophils contain an elongated twisted nucleus with one or two constrictions; their granules are relatively large and contain heparin and histamine, in some species they may also exhibit a crystalline substructure. In some mammals, e.g. cat, rat and mouse, they seem to be absent.

The hetero (= neutro-) phils are relatively abundant and contain a polymorphous nucleus, which may exhibit three to four constrictions and in females frequently bears the sex chromatin in the form of small appendages (drumsticks). They contain rather small granules of two types; (a) specific granules containing alkaline phosphatase and (b) lysosomes with acid phosphatase and peroxidase. In some species these granules are so small that they can hardly be seen in the light microscope (e.g. in the dog and rat), in the rabbit they are rather large. Heterophils ingest foreign particles, like bacteria, which have entered the body. Fig. 31 shows a heterophil of a frog

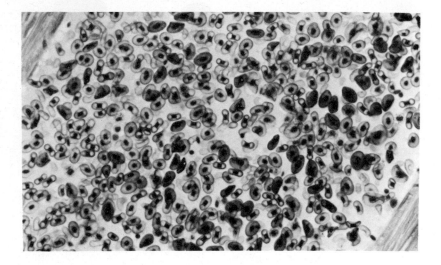

Figure 144.   Erythrocytes in a blood vessèl of the swimbladder of the eel. x 180

emigrating from the lumen of a blood vessel into the connective tissue.

Agranular leucocytes. Two types occur: Lymphocytes and monocytes (Fig. 143). Lymphocytes are relatively small and contain a dark staining nucleus, which is surrounded by a thin layer of cytoplasm. Usually the nucleus has an indentation on one side. The cytoplasm contains only a few organelles. The different types of lymphocytes (B-lymphocytes, which can transform into anti-body-producing plasma cells and T-lymphocytes taking part in

Figure 145.   Fine structure of blood cells and blood platelets. **a:** Erythrocytes containing haemerythrin of *Lingula* (Brachiopoda), note absence of organelles; n: nucleus. x 6000; **b:** amoebocytes of *Lingula*, x 6000; **c:** Erythrocytes of the teleost *Coryphopterus*, x 6000; **d:** accumulation of blood platelets, guinea pig; note the abundance of granular inclusions, x 18 000

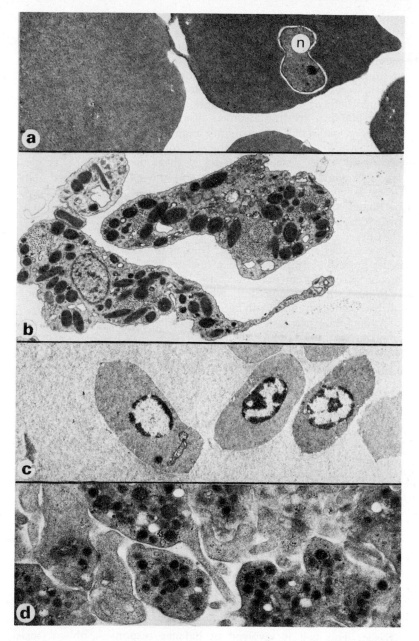

cellular immune reactions) as have been referred to on page 276 cannot be distinguished in the microscope. Monocytes are larger than lymphocytes and contain an oval or kidney shaped nucleus which is surrounded by a broad rim of cytoplasm containing a fair number of mitochondria and a few lysosomes. They transform into macrophages emigrating from the blood stream or settling down in the endothelia of some organs (Kupffer cells in the liver).

The platelets are tiny biconvex disks of roundish or oval shape. They correspond to cell fragments originating by pinching off from megakaryocytes (page 84). In the electron microscope (Fig. 145) a peripheral zone without organelles (hyalomere) and a central organelle containing area (granulomere) may be distinguished. The latter is composed of small roundish mitochondria, glycogen, lysosomes, microtubules and electron dense granules containing a 5-hydroxytryptamine-ATP-complex. Platelets play a role in blood clotting.

In the other vertebrates similar types of blood cells occur. The red cells, however, always contain a nucleus and often are rather big, biconvex, oval elements (Figs. 143, 144). The cytoplasm is also crammed with haemoglobin, which in the cod has a crystalline ultrastructure but ordinarily retains a few mitochondria (Fig. 145).

Among the leucocytes, lymphocytes and heterophils seem to occur in all species, eosinophils are probably absent in teleosts, basophils are of very irregular occurrence and have e.g. been described in frog. Platelets are replaced in non-mammalian vertebrates by spindle-shaped nucleated thrombocytes (Fig. 143), which also take part in blood clotting. In birds these cells are almost completely filled by the nucleus; in frogs they are smaller than erythrocytes and their nucleus exhibits a deep longitudinal indentation.

Invertebrates

In the invertebrates blood cells corresponding to erythrocytes and leucocytes also occur. Erythrocytes, however, are relatively rare and have been found in particular in animals with haemerythrin. Fig. 145 shows such a cell in *Lingula*, which closely resembles a vertebrate erythrocyte. *Magelona* (polychaete) is the only invertebrate the erythrocytes of which lack nucleus and organelles; these cells also contain haemerythrine. Usually the invertebrate blood cells are of the granular leucocyte type, also if they contain respiratory pigments, and are termed amoebocytes.

In pulmonate molluscs only one type of blood cell, the amoebocyte, occurs in the haemolymph and in the connective tissue. This cell is involved in defence responses, phagocytosis, and wound-healing. These cells are of irregular shape and extend numerous pseudopodia. Their cytoplasm contains lysosomes, glycogen and pinocytotic vesicles. These cells can transform into elements storing material in inflated rough ER cisternae. Some may also store lipids.

In the haemoglobin-containing haemolymph of oligochaetes two types of blood cells have been described: eleocytes and amoebocytes. The first store lipid, protein and inclusions typical for the chloragog tissue. They further can store haemoglobin-containing protein droplets and are usually considered to represent a motile portion of the chloragog tissue. In injured tissues the eleocytes can aggregate and play a role in regeneration. In polychaetes their number increases during the development of the gonads; possibly they have a function in the nourishment of the growing germinal cells. The amoebocytes are said to originate from the peritoneum and are highly motile cells. Their shape varies considerably, especially striking is a flower-shaped phagocytizing variant. Their cytoplasm contains ribosomes, glycogen and bundles of filaments.

According to studies in decapodes, crustacea are believed to possess only one type of blood cell, which, however, can appear in three different functional stages: (a) hyaline cells; develop a smooth endoplasmic reticulum and have a few small vesicles scattered in the cytoplasm, (b) half-granular haemocytes; these may be recognized by the presence of one or two Golgi apparatuses and by a fair number of electron-dense granules and lysosomes, (c) granulocytes; have electron-dense granules, which may contain a crystalline core and fill most of the cytoplasm. All three stages take part in haemolymph clotting. At first they form aggregations, then they release material. The granular inclusions of the granulocytes contain copper and may play a role in haemocyanin synthesis.

Also in *Limulus* only one type of blood cell occurs, the granules of which contain crystalline material presumably corresponding to haemocyanin.

In insects many different types of blood cell classifications exist, however; presumably also in these animals only one basic type of haemocyte is to be found, which, mainly according to light microscope studies, differentiates six developmental and/or functional stages: (a) prohaemocytes, small round to oval cells, the nucleus of which is surrounded by a thin rim of finely granular cytoplasm; (b) plasmatocytes, round, oval or spindle-shaped cells with a central nucleus and numerous cytoplasmic granules. These cells are motile and can extend pseudopodia; (c) granular cells, resembling round or oval cells with centrally located nucleus and cytoplasmic granules, they can extend fine protoplasmic extensions; (d) spherule cells, spindle-shaped or oval cells, filled with large granules; (e) cystocytes, round cells with granular material, which can be extruded forming isles of coagulation. This phenomenon results from a phenoloxidase, which causes the haemolymph to precipitate; (f) oenocytoids, large cells with a small eccentric nucleus and few granules and lamellar organelles, but abundant ribosomes and fine electron dense particular material in their cytoplasm. The ultrastructure of these cells resembles that of vertebrate erythrocytes.

Most of these cell types are interconnected by intermediate forms, which favours the concept of one basic cell type. In the electron microscope these cells usually contain various electron-dense granules, above all lysosomes.

The plasmatocytes usually contain abundant ribosomes and a few cisternae of the rough ER. Lysosomes are particularly frequent in granular cells. In the fly *Calliphora* an interesting additional type has been found, the thrombocytoid; these cells are characterized by a strong tendency to fragmentation (similar to the mammalian megakaryocytes) leading to the formation of 'naked nuclei', e.g. nuclei surrounded by an exceedingly thin layer of cytoplasm. The pinched-off fragments (resembling mammalian platelets) assume fusiform shape and form blood clots.

Echinoderms. The blood cells of the echinoderms are to be found in the coelomic cavities and in the lacunar system. Phagocytes and eleocytes have been described. Phagocytes originate from ciliated juvenile cells and may fuse to form plasmodia. Red and white eleocytes can be recognized. The red ones contain the pigment echinochrome, stored in electron-dense granules. The white ones correspond to melanocytes, in which the accumulation of pigment is suppressed as long as they remain in the haemolymph. They transform into melanophores on reaching the integument.

Blood vessels
Vertebrates
    The blood vessels ordinarily possess a wall which is composed of an inner layer of simple squamous epithelial cells (endothelium) and outer layers of smooth muscle cells and extracellular fibres.

    The wall of the smallest vessels, the capillaries, consists only of the endothelium, which is surrounded by a basement lamina (Fig. 146). The individual endothelial cells are interconnected by junctional complexes, including tight junctions (brain) and gap junctions (nexuses, muscle tissue). The cell organelles are concentrated in the area of the elongated nucleus, which often bulges into the capillary lumen. In many endothelial cells frequent light pinocytotic vesicles and microfilaments are to be found. Attached to the outer surface of

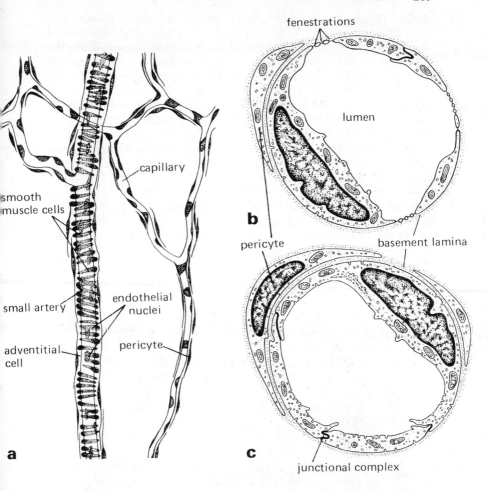

Figure 146. Mammalian blood capillaries and small arteries. **a:** Small artery and capillaries from the mesentery, whole mount preparation, endothelial nuclei: vertical; nuclei of smooth muscle cells: horizontal, after MAXIMOW; **b,c:** fine structure of the commonest types of capillaries in cross-section; **b:** fenestrated type; **c:** continuous or muscle type, after BLOOM, FAWCETT, 1970

the endothelium individual cells occur termed pericytes, characterized by numerous irregularly shaped cytoplasmic extensions, which at least in some species are able to contract; possibly they represent modified smooth muscle cells. The capillaries mentioned above are also termed continuous capillaries since their cytoplasm forms an uninterrupted border between blood and surrounding tissues. A second type of capillaries, fenestrated capillaries, has been demonstrated in endocrine organs. Here the cytoplasm of the endothelial cells exhibits local circular extremely attenuated areas (=fenestrae, 800-1000 Å in diameter), where the endothelial wall is thinner than a single unit membrane. The capillaries of the renal glomerula and the liver sinusoids of most mammals evidently have open pores in their endothelial cells.

In the pecten of avian eyes the capillaries are composed of relatively mitochondria-rich endothelial cells bearing numerous long apical and basal microvillus-like processes (Fig. 147), which in some birds have been shown to be thin cytoplasmic folds. The outer cytoplasmic extensions are separated from their basement lamina by a rather wide fibril-containing space. Although it is often difficult to detect capillaries in the light microscope, they may frequently be easily demonstrated by histochemical reactions, e.g. the demonstration of alkaline phosphatase often outlines them clearly (Fig. 147).

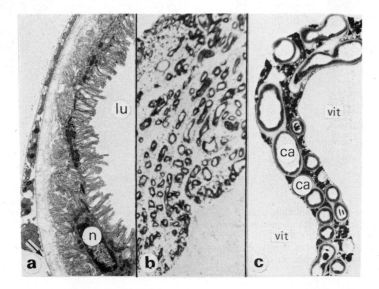

Figure 147. Details from the pecten in the eye of a gull (a,c) and a pigeon (b). The pecten contains abundant capillaries and pigment cells. a: Fine structure of the capillary wall; note the abundant apical and basal cytoplasmic folds. lu: lumen of capillary, n: nucleus; arrow points to the basal lamina; x 6000. b: Alkaline phosphatase in the capillary endothelium, x 105. c: Light microscope preparation; ca: capillaries in the pecten, vit: vitreous body, x 220

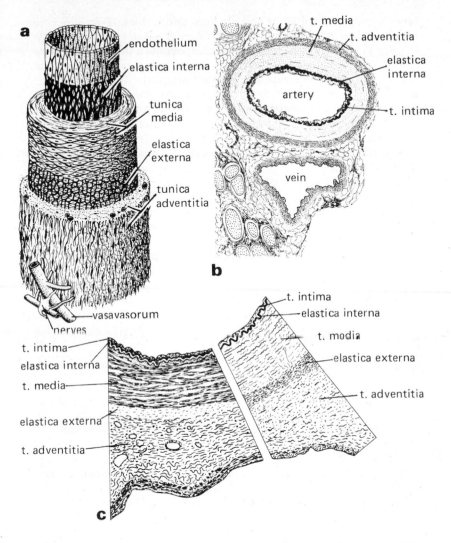

Figure 148. Structure of the wall of blood vessels; **a:** Artery, after LEONHARDT 1974; **b:** cross-section through artery and vein, stained with orcein to show elastic tissue, after LEONHARDT, 1974; **c:** part of the arterial wall, left: ordinary stain (hematoxylin, eosin), right: stained with orecin to show elastic tissue; note different appearance of the various layers, after STÖHR & V. MÖLLENDORFF, 1958

Veins and arteries are constructed according to the same plan (Fig. 148). Their walls are composed of three layers (1) *tunica intima*: consisting of inner endothelium and a thick layer of elastic fibres and/or membranes termed internal elastic membrane (= *elastica interna*). Between these two components a thin layer of loose connective tissue may be present, often basal processes of the endothelial cells penetrate the *elastica interna*; (2) *tunica media*: consisting of helically or circularly arranged smooth muscle cells, mucopolysaccharide matrix and a few collagen and elastic fibres; at its outer aspect, a concentration of elastic material can be present (external elastic membrane = *elastica externa*); (3) *tunica adventitia*, an outer coat, consisting of predominantly longitudinally oriented bundles of collagen fibres and fibroblasts; in larger vessels here also nerves and small blood vessels occur supplying the outer parts of the vessel wall.

In the large arteries near the heart, e.g. the aorta, the *tunica media* is composed mainly of elastic membranes.

In arteries these layers normally are clearly recognizable. In veins, however, the structure of the wall is less compact and regular, e.g. the *tunica media* is often relatively thin and loosely constructed or even may be absent, the *tunica adventitia* is often rather thick and may often contain bundles of longitudinally oriented smooth muscle cells. Some veins do not contain any muscle cells in their walls at all, e.g. in bones and the dura mater of mammals. Sharks always have non-muscular veins. In the neighbourhood of the heart veins may contain cardiac muscle cells. Frequently valves (folds of the *tunica intima*) are to be encountered in veins, preventing a back flow of the blood.

Lymphatic vessels (lymphatics). A system of closed lymphatic vessels with an own wall occurs only in birds and mammals. The lymphatic capillaries are relatively wide and of irregular outline; their walls are composed of a thin endothelium. The larger vessels additionally contain smooth muscle cells, which in the few large vessels may constitute a *tunica media* and *adventitia*. Valves frequently occur. In other vertebrates the system of lymphatic vessels is composed of lacunae and portions lined by an endothelium or by lacunae alone.

Invertebrates

Blood vessels are not of universal distribution and especially in small species may be completely absent or reduced to a central muscular heart. The blood then circulates in spaces between the organs and is identical with the fluids of the body cavities. If present, the vessels often correspond to tubular invaginations of the wall of coelomic spaces or channels and are lined by the basement lamina of the coelomic cells, which sometimes are epitheliomuscular cells (Fig. 149, page 123). Thus an own endothelium is normally absent. In *Branchiostoma,* however, a few irregularly distributed endothelial cells, widely separated from each other have been described in most vessels, under the epidermis even vessels completely lined by endothelial cells occur. In some species definite blood spaces exist which are simply delimited by collagen fibres and the ground substance of the surrounding connective tissue (e.g. many vessels of *echinoderms*). The contractile vessels of leeches are lined by a very thin uninterrupted endothelium (a transformed coelomic lining), which is partly fenestrated and surrounded by a basement lamina. The individual cells are interconnected by *zonulae adhaerentes,* and surrounded by an inner layer of longitudinally oriented and an outer layer of circularly oriented helically striated muscle cells.

layers: an inner endocardium composed of an endothelial lining, which is underlain by connective tissue, an intermediate thick myocardium composed of cardiac muscle cells, and an outer epicardium, consisting of connective tissue and a covering squamous epithelium.

The heart of tunicates corresponds to a tubular invagination into the pericardial space. Both the wall of the heart and the pericardium are composed of a single layer of cells. Those of the heart contain

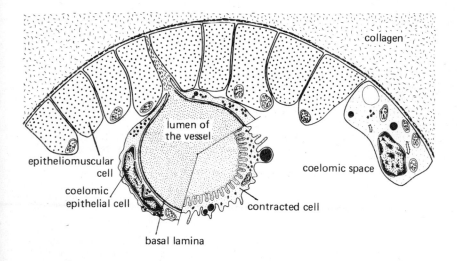

Figure 149. Fine structure of a typical invertebrate blood vessel, *Lingula* (Brachiopoda), which run outside, between or in infoldings of coelomic spaces. The lumen is surrounded by a basal lamina and contractile coelomic epithelial cells.

294   COMPARATIVE ANIMAL CYTOLOGY & HISTOLOGY

only a few myofibrils (in *Ciona* only one). No special pacemaker tissue has been detected so far. The heart of insects is not lined by an endocardial epithelium. Its wall is composed of circularly oriented striated muscle cells (rarely also longitudinally arranged elements occur) and an outer thin connective tissue layer (*adventitia*) (Fig. 34).

LITERATURE

BAUCHAU, A., DE BROUWER, M.-B. 'Etude ultrastructurale de la coagulation de l'hémolymphe chez les crustacés.' *J. Microscopie.* **19**, 37–46 (1974).
BOILLY, B. 'Ultrastructure des hématies anuclées de *Magelona papillicornis.' J. Microscopie.* **19**, 47–58 (1974).
CHARLEMAGNE, J. 'Aspects morphologiques de la différenciation des éléments sanguins chez l'Axolotl, *Ambystoma mexicanum* Shaw. *Z. Zellforsch.* **123**, 224–239 (1972).
DALES, R. P., PELL, J. S. 'Cytological aspects of haemoglobin and chlorocruorin synthesis in polychaete annelids.' *Z. Zellforsch,* **109**, 20–32 (1970).
GORDON, A. S. *Regulation of hematopoiesis.* Vol. I. 868 pp. Vol. 2. 1026 S. Appleton, Century, Crofts, New York (1970).
HAMMERSEN, F., STAUDTE, H.-W. 'Beiträge zum Feinbau der Blutgefäße von Invertebraten. I. Die Ultrastruktur des Sinus lateralis von *Hirudo medicinalis* L ' *Z. Zellforsch.* **100**, 215–250 (1969).
HOFFMANN-FEZER, G., LADE, R. 'Postembryonale Entwicklung und Involution der Bursa Fabricii beim Haushuhn (*Gallus domesticus*).' *Z Zellforsch.* **124**, 406–418 (1972).
HUHN, D., STICH, W. 'Fine structure of blood and bone marrow.' J. F. Lehmanns Verlag. München. 136 S., 1969.
HUMPHREY, J. H., WHITE, R. G. *Kurzes Lehrbuch der Immunologie.* G. Thieme Verlag. Stuttgart. 488 pp. 1971.
KALK, M. 'The organization of a tunicate heart'. *Tissue and Cell.* **2**, 99–118 (1970).
LUFT, J. H. 'The ultrastructural bases of capillary permeability.' In: Zweifach, B. W., Grant, L., McCluskey, R.T.: *The inflammatory process.* Academic Press. New York. 121–159. (1965).
PRICE, C. D., RATCLIFFE, N. A. 'A reappraisal of insect haemocyte classification by the examination of blood from fifteen insect orders.' *Cell Tiss. Research.* **147**, 537–549 (1974).
SNEDDON, J. M. 'Platelet microtubules and platelet function.' *Mem. Soc. endocrinol.* **19**, 793–802 (1971).
STANG-VOSS, CH. Über die Hämocyten von *Psammechinus miliaris* (Echinodermata).' *Z. Zellforsch.* **122**, 76–84 (1971).

Chapter 10
ORGANS OF EXCRETION, OSMO- AND ION-REGULATION

Pulsating vacuoles

Many limnic and marine protozoa and some sponges possess pulsating vacuoles functioning as excretory organelles and playing a role in the osmo-regulation of these animals. Usually they consist of a spherical vacuole, into which fluid is conducted *via* small tubules and which contracts rhythmically (Fig. 150). During the contractions (systole) it opens out to the free surface of the cell. During the expanding phase (diastole) the afferent tubules are in open connection with elements of the endoplasmic reticulum *via* small so-called nephridial tubules. This connection is interrupted during the systolic phase.

The following organs function in the vast majority of animals as excretory, osmo- or ion-regulatory elements, the protonephridia, Malpighian tubules, metanephridia (= nephridia). Confined to nematodes we find the H-cells (system of lateral channels), while cyrtopodocytes occur only in the Acrania.

Protonephridia

Protonephridia are tubular channels, with an opening at the free surface of the animal and a closed terminal portion extending into the body cavities. This closed ending is formed by a terminal cell (Fig. 151), which either bears a tuft of cilia extending into the protonephridial tube or a single long cilium (flagellum). In the latter case the terminal cell is termed a solenocyte. The wall of the tubular segment of the protonephridia in which the cilia exert their beats, may be perforated in different ways (Fig. 151). The terminal cells are also termed cyrtocytes or flame cells. They have been found in flatworms, round worms, Kamptozoa, molluscs and annelids.

In the miracidia of trematodes the flame cells are elongated elements with a terminal perikaryon extending numerous branched processes. In the tubular extension which forms the beginning of the protonephridial tube, the filtration apparatus is formed by two circles of rodlike cytoplasmic strands; the inner rods are located opposite the gaps between the outer rods (Fig. 151). The inner and outer rods are interconnected by delicate 'membranes', the exact nature of which is not yet known. This system of rods and interconnecting membrane separates the outer medium from the interior of the tube. In the lumen of the protonephridial canal a tuft of about 150 cilia may be found.

The terminal cell of *Stenostomum* (Turbellaria) is of different structure (Fig. 151). The nucleus is not in a terminal but in a lateral

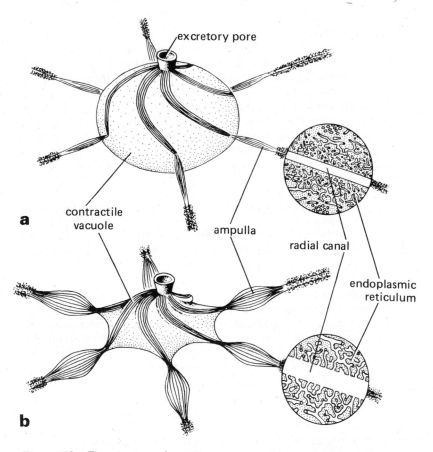

Figure 150. Fine structure of a protozoan contractile vacuole (*Paramecium*). **a:** diastole, **b:** systole (contracted). The vacuole can contract by means of contractile filaments on its surface; several radial canals lead into the vacuole. These canals during systole communicate with tubes of the endoplasmic reticulum. The fluid is expelled outwards *via* the excretory pore. After SCHNEIDER, 1957

position, the filtration apparatus is composed of inner and outer rods, at right angles towards each other; the inner ones are longitudinally oriented, the outer ones horizontally. Both types of

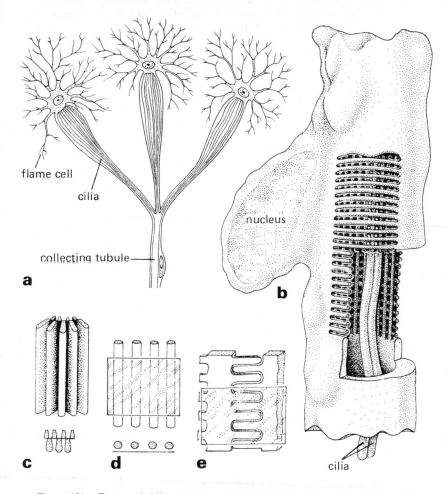

Figure 151. Protonephridia; **a:** protonephridium with three terminal cells (cestode, light microscopy); **b:** ultrastructure of a flame cell of *Stenostomum* (Turbellaria) with two cilia; filtration apparatus partly cut open; nucleus in lateral extension of the cell; **c-e:** Ultrastructure of different types of filtration devices; **c:** trematode (*Fasciola*); **d:** pulmonate snail (*Lymnaea*); **e:** kamptozoon (*Urnatella*); note differences in the arrangement of the cytoplasmic rodlets and the 'filtration membrane', in e: lateral cytoplasmic extensions of neighbouring cells and a filtration membrane form the filtration apparatus. After KÜMMEL, 1962, and BRANDENBURG, 1966

rods are interconnected by a 'membrane'. Inside the apparatus two united cilia occur.

According to another interpretation the flame cell of platy-helminths is a composite organ formed from two cells. One cell contains a large nucleus and bears the flagella which form the flame. The other cell which contributes the filtration device is the first tubule cell.

In adult polychaetes, e.g. nephtyids, the cyrtocytes form groups at the end of the protonephridial tube. They are solenocytes of peculiar structure (Fig. 152). The cells are composed of a collar-like part, which also contains the nucleus. This part extends a long stalk-like

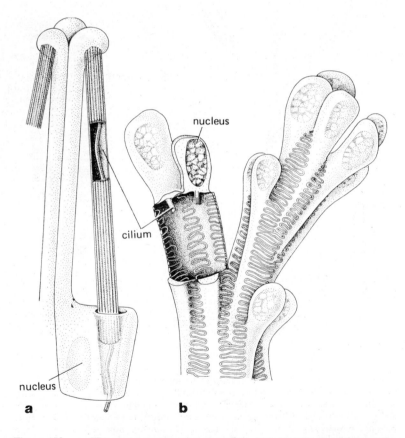

a   b

Figure 152.   **a:** Ultrastructure of solenocytes of *Nephtys* (Polychaeta) **b:** *Priapulus* (Priapulida); several flame cells form a common terminal protonephridial organ. The filtration area is partly cut open. After Kümmel, 1962, 1964

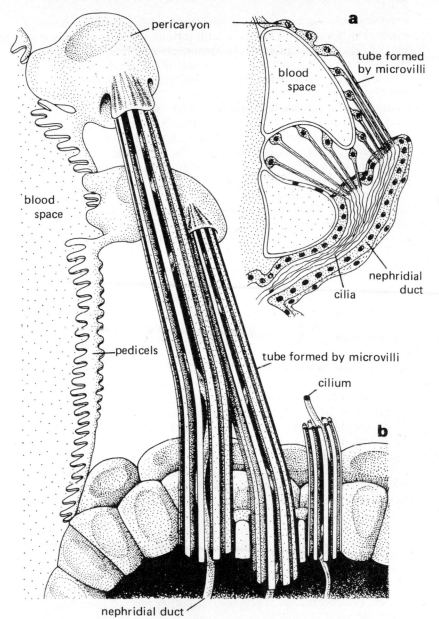

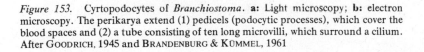

Figure 153. Cyrtopodocytes of *Branchiostoma*. **a:** Light microscopy; **b:** electron microscopy. The perikarya extend (1) pedicels (podocytic processes), which cover the blood spaces and (2) a tube consisting of ten long microvilli, which surround a cilium. After GOODRICH, 1945 and BRANDENBURG & KÜMMEL, 1961

extension into the body cavity, which terminally exhibits a spherical expansion, which gives rise to a long tubule, which is composed of longitudinal cytoplasmic rods interconnected by fine bridges and to the inner aspect of which a 'membrane' is attached. Inside of this tubule we find one flagellum. This tubule runs back to the collar and terminates here, but does not fuse with it.

In priapulids several terminal cells, with one cilium each, together form the terminal part of the protonephridial tube (Fig. 152). Each cell forms only one part of the tubular wall, which is surrounded by a basement lamina. Neighbouring cells are interconnected by numerous interdigitations. This type of filtration device is also found in Kamptozoa (Fig. 151).

The excretory organs of *Branchiostoma* contain a characteristic cell type (a modified epithelial cell of the coelomic lining), which in the light microscope was considered to be a solenocyte. In the electron microscope it was found that its fine structure markedly differs from that of the typical solenocyte (Fig. 153); it was termed cytopodocyte, since its perikaryon extends beside a tube of cytoplasmic rods, processes resembling those of podocytes (podocytic processes). These are branched and form an irregularly shaped system on the surface of the glomerular blood spaces of this animal. The podocytic processes of neighbouring cells are interdigitated and leave only narrow slits between them. Between these processes and the blood space a basement membrane and a few collagen fibres occur. The tube of long cytoplasmic rods mentioned above contains a cilium. The individual rods which might be considered as extremely long microvilli, are of triangular shape in cross-section and always occur in the number of ten. They are not interconnected by membranous material. They traverse the coelomic space and penetrate the epithelium of the nephridial tube, which opens into the pharynx.

In the protonephridia mentioned so far fluid is filtrated. The driving force is either a hydrostatic pressure gradient (filtration by pressure) or a concentration gradient (osmotic filtration). The fluid is filtered through the 'membrane' between the cytoplasmic rods of the filtration devices, through the basement lamina covering the intercellular spaces in priapulids and through basement lamina and fibrils under the pododytic processes in *Branchiostoma*. In this animal the ciliary beat possibly creates a negative pressure in the subchordal coelom, which draws fluid through the separating barrier. Possibly the blood pressure is another force of filtration.

H-shaped systems
In the nematodes long H-shaped cells exist, which are pervaded

by a tubule. The longitudinal parts of the 'H' run in the lateral epidermal ridges and are interconnected by one or several tubules in the short cross rod of the H-shaped system (Fig. 154). The tubule of the cross rod or of the left longitudinal extension opens out to the free surface of the body.

The fine structure of this system is known in *Ascaris*. In the centre e.g. of a longitudinal cytoplasmic process the lumen of the excretory

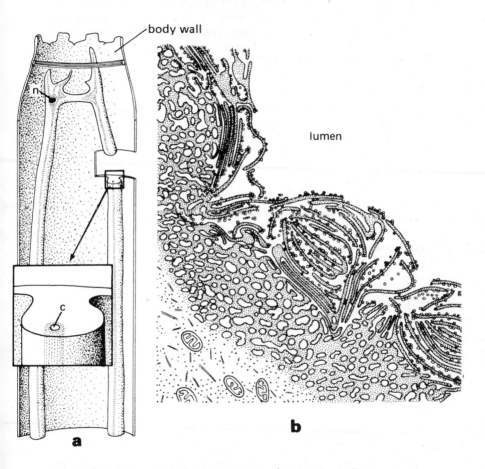

Figure 154. Tubular so-called excretory system of nematodes. **a:** H-shaped system, *Ascaris*; the system consists of a single H-shaped cell found on the inside of the body wall. Within the cell a canal exists, which opens out at an excretory pore; arrow points to inset, which shows a detail from a longitudinal cellular extension with the canal (c), n: nucleus; **b:** schematic representation of the ultrastructure of the cytoplasm lining the 'excretory' canal of an H-cell of *Ascaris*. After DANKWARTH, 1971

tubule is situated. This is surrounded by a cytoplasmic zone with numerous irregularly shaped foldings and projections (Fig. 154) (increase of the surface area). The outer part of the cytoplasm contains many microtubules and mitochondria with a dense matrix and few cristae; less frequent are free ribosomes, microfilaments, ER cisternae and Golgi apparatus. The outer plasma membrane exhibits infoldings, which however do not reach the central canal.

The function of these strange cells presumably does not relate to the excretion of end-products of protein metabolism; these are given off *via* epidermis or intestinal tract. They also do not seem to play a role in osmo-regulation, since the fluid they extrude usually is iso-osmotic or slightly hyper-osmotic with the body fluids. One function of them is the regulation of K^+ and Na^+ concentrations in the body

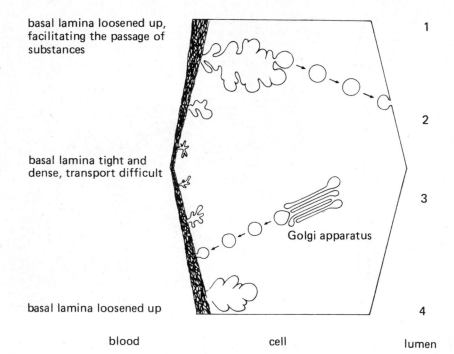

Figure 155.   *Drosophila* (fruit fly), shift of membranes in the initial segment of the Malpighian tubules during the trans-cellular passage of substances; 1: expanded basal infoldings of the plasma membrane, pinching off vesicles, which move to the apical plasma membrane; 2: This process comes to an end after the membranes of the basal infoldings are used up; 3: Cell becomes dehydrated with the aid of Golgi apparatuses; Golgi vesicles move to the basal plasma membrane; 4: Formation of new basal infoldings. After WESSING & EICHELBERG, 1969

fluid. The ventral gland of nematodes according to ultrastructural and histochemical observations plays a role in the digestive processes (see page 237).

Malpighian tubules

The Malpighian tubules are the excretory organs of arachnids and tracheates. They are terminally closed tubular appendages of the intestine, which in insects open into it at the beginning of the posterior gut. Their number is highly variable (coccids two, Lepidoptera usually six, many Orthoptera 150 and more). They also can be absent, e.g. in aphids. They extend into the body cavity and are surrounded by haemolymph. Occasionally they are fixed at cells of the fat body.

The epithelial wall of these tubules is composed of several cell types with different functions. The wall of the blind terminal segment consists of flat epithelial cells (Fig. 156) through which fluid of the body cavity is transported by means of small vesicles (Fig. 155). Passing through the cytoplasm, the contents of the vesicles is deprived of its water-component and finally extruded into the lumen of the tubule as a highly concentrated and mainly crystalline primary urine. The water contents of the cytoplasm correspondingly increases during the passage of the vesicles and must again be decreased. Hydration and dehydration alternate and each of these processes is characterized by changes of the cellular structure and the density of the basement lamina, which is considered as an ultrafilter (Fig. 155).

In the following sections of the Malpighian tubules different components of the primary urine are reabsorbed. The epithelial cells resemble those of the arthropod nephridial duct and those of proximal and distal tubule of the vertebrate kidney (see below). Their basal labyrinth is of unusally complex structure (Fig. 156); the apical microvilli contain mitochondria. Apical and basal plasma membranes contain ATP-ase.

Metanephridia

Metanephridia are tubules, which usually are open at both ends – one of them communicates with the body cavity, the other with the free body surface.

The metanephridium of *Lumbricus* begins with a funnel-shaped opening (nephrostome), located on a septum. It is followed by a repeatedly coiled tubule, which leads to the exterior of the animal. On its outside the nephridium is covered by coelomic epithelium. In the convoluted part of the tubule a number of specific sections can

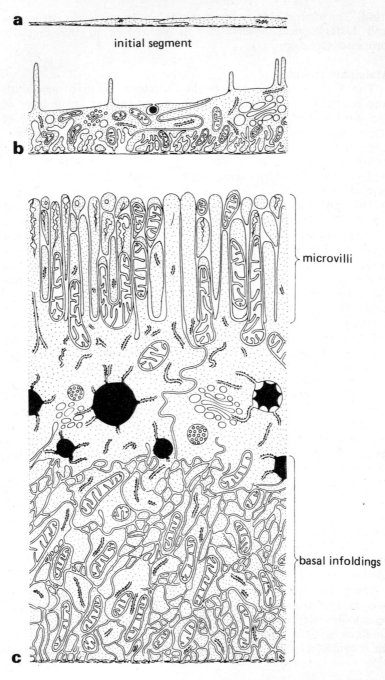

a

initial segment

b

microvilli

basal infoldings

c

Figure 156. Ultrastructure of epithelial cells of various segments of the Malpighian tubules in the larva of *Drosophila.* **a,b:** initial segment in various functional phases; **c:** proximal segment near the intestinal lumen, note the mitochondria within the microvilli. After WESSING & EICHELBERG, 1969

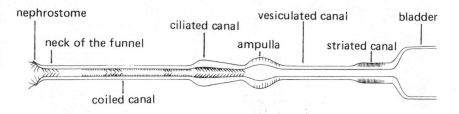

Figure 157. Schematic representation of a nephridium of *Lumbricus* (earth worm) with the distribution of cilia, microvilli and basal infoldings. After GRASZYNSKI, 1963

be recognized (Fig. 157), to which, however, different names are given. The nephrostome is followed by a ciliated neck piece, a long, 'coiled canal', a ciliated canal, an expanded ampulla, a 'vesiculated canal', a 'striated canal', and a bladder, which is followed by a duct leading to the outside.

(a) Neck piece: in cross-sections the lumen is surrounded by two or more cells, the apices of which bear short microvilli and cilia.
(b) 'Coiled canal': the longest part of the nephridium, relatively wide lumen, thin wall, in two areas cilia occur, in most parts apical microvilli.
(c) 'Ciliated canal': lumen at the beginning wider than of the looped canal, at its posterior parts relatively narrow; the ciliated epithelial cells contain brown pigments;
(d) Ampulla: epithelial wall relatively thick, containing numerous inclusions, no cilia, numerous bacteria in the lumen, a loose basal labyrinth.
(e) 'Vesiculated canal': thin-walled, a few microvilli, no basal labyrinth, numerous vacuoles in the cytoplasm of the epithelial cells.
(f) Striated canal: extensive basal labyrinth, characteristic fibrillar material in the cytoplasm.
(g) Bladder: wall composed of inner flat epithelium, a subepithelial layer of connective tissue fibres, muscle cells, coelomic epithelium.

In most leeches the nephrostome is closed. The nephridium of *Hirudo* is divided into several lobules, through which the nephridial

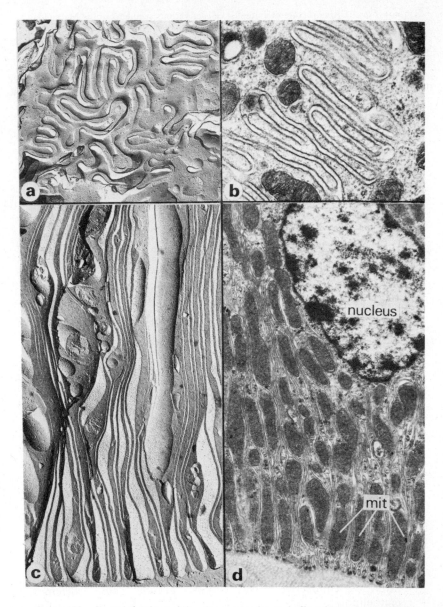

Figure 158.   Basal infoldings of the plasma membrane (**c,d**) and lateral cytoplasmic interdigitations (**a,b**); **a, c** freeze etched preparations. **a, c:** *Coenobita* (hermit crab), nephridium. **b** *Rana cancrivora,* kidney tubule, **d** blackheaded gull (*Larus*), salt gland. mit: mitochondrium. a, c, x 18 000, b x 24 000, d x 12 000

tubule is meandering. All epithelial cells are basically of the same structure: basal infoldings, numerous mitochondria, abundant glycogen particles and apical microvilli. It is assumed that the formation of the primary urine is achieved by secretory processes; pores in the capillaries supplying the nephridia indicate additional ultrafiltration. Substances to be secreted have to pass the following barrier: capillary endothelium, connective tissue space, epithelium of the nephridium.

Metanephridia also occur in most arthropods; in euarthropods, however, they are confined to certain regions of the body. They are in all arthropods of the same fundamental structure and consist of three sections:

(a) The initial segment (*sacculus*) is closed. It is derived from the coelom. The epithelial cells lining it are typical podocytes (see below). The saccule is surrounded by haemolymph. In *Scutigerella* (Symphyla) it is largely enclosed in an additional layer of muscle cells; also in this animal the haemolymph may reach the basement lamina of the podocytes. In *Polyxenus* (Diplopoda), fibrillar material is attached to the basement lamina, which in three areas is continuous with ligaments fixing the saccule in the head region. Occasionally the saccule is of a highly complicated structure. Into the lumen folds can extend, or it may form projections into the abdominal parts of the body.

(b) The saccule is followed by the nephridial duct (tubule, tubulus). In protarthropods (*Peripatus*) its mouthpart opening into the saccule still consists of a ciliated neckpiece, which in euarthropods is reduced to individual cells. The nephridial duct is lined by prismatic cells characterized by deep basal infoldings with associated long mitochondria (Fig. 158) and densely arranged apical microvilli. This duct may extend long projections into the body.

(c) The third section is formed by the urinary duct (ureter) the epithelium of which is similar to that of the nephridial duct. The basal infoldings are less deep. This duct opens at the base of extremities. Its distal portion may be formed by invaginations of the ectoderm; most parts of its wall, as is that of the complete organ, are of mesodermal origin.

Podocytes have already been referred to, which in many excretory organs occur at sites of ultrafiltration, and then allow only particles smaller than 30-50 Å to pass their barrier. Podocytes are stellate cells, resting on a basement lamina. They consist of a perikaryon and processes radiating into various directions and extending

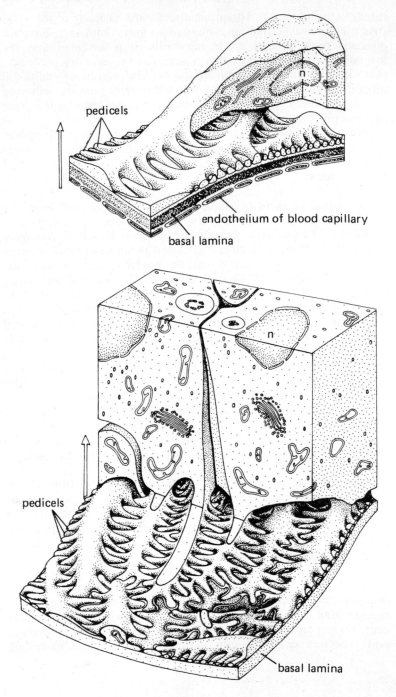

numerous small cytoplasmic projections (pedicels) (Fig. 159). The pedicels of neighbouring cells are intimately interdigitated. Between them narrow intercellular clefts may be seen in the electron microscope, which are closed by an electron-dense 'membrane'. This in mammals is composed of extracellular mucopolysaccharides. It plays an important role in the process of ultrafiltration.

Podocytes line the saccule of the arthropod metanephridia and occur in the glomerula of the vertebrate kidney. They also have been found in other animals, e.g. in cephalopods (branchial heart appendages) and polychaetes (*Sabella,* perioesophageal plexus).

Metanephridia also occur in adult molluscs, and these are in open communication with the pericardial cavity (coelom). The nephridium of gastropods consists of a nephridial sac (kidney sac) and a urinary duct (ureter) leading to the outside. The sac is connected with the pericardial cavity by the reno-pericardial duct.

It is assumed that in gastropods the production of the primary urine follows along similar lines to that in vertebrates. Ultrafiltration has been proven to take place in several species. In aquatic forms it presumably proceeds in the wall of the auricle of the heart, which is contained in the fluid-filled pericardial cavity. The primary urine is transported from the pericardial cavity via renopericardial canal into the kidney sac. In land-living species the epithelium of the kidney sac is considered to be the site of ultrafiltration, the renopericardial duct is very narrow in these species.

In the wall of the heart among others in *Poteria* (a land-living prosobranch) and in *Viviparus* (water-living prosobranch) podocytes have been found (Fig. 160). In *Poteria* they are present at the pericardial surface of the ventricle, in *Viviparus* they form a layer below the lining of the pericardial cavity (epicardium). The wall of the gastropod heart lacks an endothelium. Its inner lining is composed of muscle cells (in the ventricle more than in the auricle) and connective tissue fibres of variable amount, next follows a basement lamina, next - so far only in the *Viviparus* auricle - a layer of podocytes, which are attached to this lamina - next the pericardial epithelium, which in *Lymnaea* contains replacement cells. In *Poteria* the podocytes are included in the pericardial epithelium of the ventricle.

The renopericardial duct is lined by a ciliated columnar epithelium underlain by muscle cells between which, as in the heart,

Figure 159. Ultrastructure of podocytes. **a:** capillary endothelium, basal lamina and podocyte from a renal corpuscle of a mammalian kidney, n: nucleus, arrow: direction of filtration; **b:** podocytes from the saccule of the nephridium of *Orconectes* (Decapoda), arrow: direction of filtration. After KÜMMEL, 1965

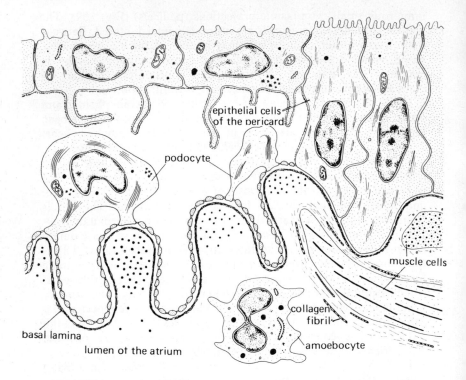

Figure 160.   Ultrastructure of the cardial atrium of *Viviparus*. After BOER, ALGERA & LOMMERSE, 1973

nerve terminals have been found.

The kidney sac is lined by cuboidal to columnar epithelial cells termed nephrocytes, characterized by moderately developed basal infoldings and densely arranged apical microvilli. The cells frequently contain a huge vacuole, filled with excretory concretions, many mitochondria, glycogen particles and peroxisomes. The contents of the vacuole is extruded into the lumen. The cells are surrounded by a plexus of capillaries, fenestrated and unfenestrated ones, both surrounded by a basement membrane, which is impermeable to haemocyanin. It is assumed that in species without podocytes fluid escapes through their wall; thus the nephrocytes of the kidney sac are presumably bathed basally by an ultrafiltrate of the blood; possibly this is transported through the pores in the septate junctions of the saccular epithelium into the lumen of the sac where it would correspond to the primary urine.

The epithelial cells of the ureter are prismatic and lack vacuoles with excretory concretions. Their basal labyrinth is elaborately folded and can extend into the cellular apex.

Vertebrate Kidney

The functional and structural unit of the vertebrate kidney is the nephron (*tubulus uriniferus*), presumably a modified metanephridium about one million of which are contained in each human kidney. The nephron is a tubular structure the wall of which is composed of a single layer of epithelial cells. One of its ends is closed, the other one is open and communicates with a common collecting duct, the ureter. The expanded closed end is invaginated by a tangle of blood capillaries – the glomerulus – and forms a two-layered capsule around it, termed Bowman's capsule. The whole complex glomerulus – Bowman's capsule is called renal corpuscle (Malpighian corpuscle). The nephron may be divided into several sections, for which, however, no uniform nomenclature exists. Only the terms proximal and distal tubule (see below) can be applied to most vertebrates. In Amphibia and reptiles, representative vertebrates, five sections follow the renal corpuscle: neckpiece, proximal tubule, transitory piece, distal tubule, connecting piece. The latter communicates with the collecting tubule, which because of its different embryonic development, is not considered to be part of the nephron, but the first part of the system of collecting ducts.

Proximal and distal tubule will be described in further detail. Neckpiece and transitory piece are ciliated and possess a cuboidal epithelium. In birds and mammals cilia are usually absent in the nephron, the neckpiece normally is also absent, the transitory piece is transformed into a thin-walled loop, connecting proximal and distal tubule (thin segment of the loop of Henle).

In lower vertebrates, e.g. in Amphibia, the nephron may communicate *via* a ciliated tubule with the coelomic cavity. This tubule, which opens into the nephron distal to the renal corpuscles, loses its connection with the nephron in anurans and opens into renal veins.

In birds and mammals the nephron is subdivided in the following way (Figs. 161, 162). The renal corpuscle is followed by (1) the proximal tubule, which consists of an initial convoluted part and a second straight portion, which descends into the medulla of the kidney (Fig. 162); (2) the thin segment (limb) of the loop of Henle; (3) the distal tubule, which again may be subdivided into a straight portion, which runs back into the cortex of the kidney, and a convoluted part, which makes contact with the afferent vessels of its glomerulus (*macula densa*, see below); (4) connecting piece, which is

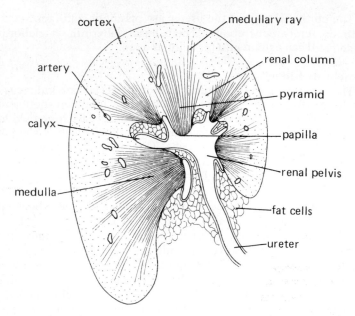

Figure 161. Schematic representation of a cross-section through a mammalian kidney. After LEONHARDT, 1971

poorly defined and more or less forms the terminal part of the distal tubule linking it with the collecting tubule. Straight portions of the proximal and distal tubules, and the thin-walled limb (transitory piece) together form the loop of Henle, which is of variable length in the individual species, but is particularly long in those of desert-dwelling mammals. The convoluted parts of neighbouring nephrons do not intermingle so that each nephron can be isolated by microsurgery. The straight and convoluted parts of the proximal and distal tubules are almost of the same structure, but differ functionally, e.g. by the possession of different enzymes. Transitory pieces (thin segments of the loop of Henle) may be absent in part of the nephrons of presumably all birds and mammals. The bend of the loop is often in the area of the transitory piece, but may also be in the area of the straight part of the proximal tubule. Each collecting tubule is in communication with about ten nephrons. The collecting tubules form bigger collecting ducts in very variable fashion.

Bowman's capsule resembles a double-walled cup. The inner wall, attached to the blood capillaries of the glomerulus, is also termed visceral layer, the outer wall is also termed the parietal layer. The

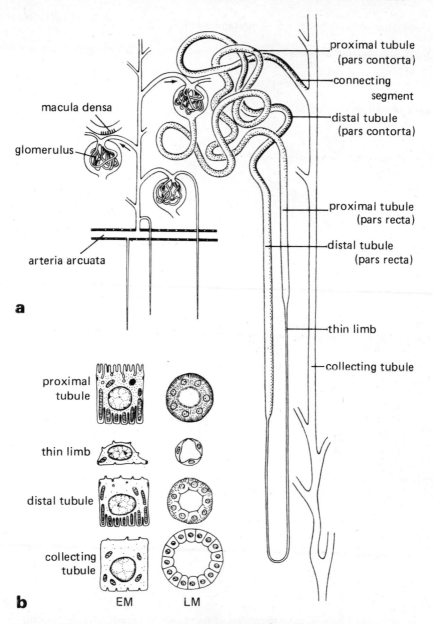

Figure 162. **a:** Schematic representation of a mammalian nephron (*pars contorta* = *pars convoluta*); **b:** epithelia of the individual segments of the nephron, EM: electron microscopy; LM: light microscopy. After BUCHER, 1966, LEONHARDT, 1974

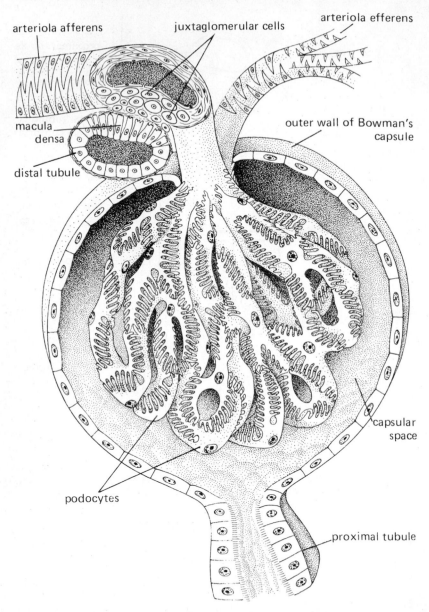

arteriola afferens

juxtaglomerular cells

arteriola efferens

macula densa

distal tubule

outer wall of Bowman's capsule

capsular space

podocytes

proximal tubule

Figure 163. Schematic representation of the mammalian renal corpuscle. Note the difference in diameter between *arteriola afferens* and *efferens*. The podocytes correspond to the transformed epithelial cells of the inner wall of Bowman's capsule. After v. MÖLLENDORFF, BARGMANN, GANONG, from REMANE, STORCH & WELSCH, 1974

cleft between them is termed the capsular (Bowman's) space (Fig. 164). Where the blood vessels enter the renal corpuscle (vascular pole) visceral and parietal layer may be seen to be continuous with each other. Both layers are underlain by an unusually thick basement lamina. The visceral layer is composed of podocytes (Fig. 163), which form a coat on the blood vessels and indicate the site of ultrafiltration in the vertebrate kidney. The barrier, which is passed by the primary urine consists (in all vertebrates) of the extremely thin capillary endothelium, which at least in mammals is perforated by circular pores, 50-100 nm in diameter, the thick basement lamina, which is a filter for very large molecules like ferritin, and the slits between the pedicels of the podocytes (filtration slits). The pedicels are interconnected by intercellular material, which seems to be the main filtration barrier, holding back all bigger molecules, but allowing molecules of a mol-wt 40,000 to pass.

Between endothelium and basement membrane connective tissue cells are occasionally to be found, and these are collectively called mesangial cells.

The epithelium of the parietal layer is usually squamous. In many vertebrates it contains bundles of microfilaments and is suspected to exert contractions.

The diameter of the renal corpuscle varies in the individual groups. Amphibia possess rather large birds rather small ones. In the adult *Petromyzon* a single elongated 9 cm long glomus exists, which arises by fusion of many glomeruli.

Proximal tubule. The epithelial cells of the proximal tubule (Figs. 162, 164) are usually columnar and are always characterized by their brush border. At the base of the microvilli numerous tubular invaginations extend into the apical cytoplasm (apical canaliculi). Similar to spined vesicles they are lined by fine filamentous material and at their cytoplasmic side bear short electron-dense 'spines'. Near these invaginations various vacuolar structures occur, which seem to concentrate reabsorbed protein and at least in part correspond to lysosomes. Peroxisomes are further typical constituents. Also the basal cell pole is of characteristic make up: attached to deep infoldings of the basal plasma membrane are numerous elongated mitochondria containing mitochondrial granules. The basement lamina is relatively thick. Laterally the cells are interconnected by numerous interdigitations.

The wall of the thin limb is composed of squamous epithelial cells with a few mitochondria and apical microvilli, which laterally exhibit deep interdigitations.

The epithelial cells of the distal tubule lack a brush border and

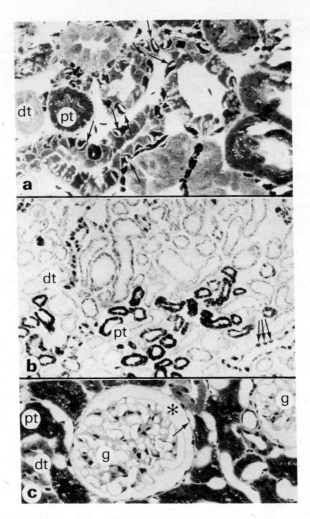

Figure 164. Light microscopical micrographs of the vertebrate kidney **a:** *Rana cancrivora* (saltwater frog), arrows point to cells with deep apical indentations in the connecting piece; pt: proximal tubule; dt: distal tubule; x 300. **b:** *Bufo* (toad), strong SDH- reaction in the proximal tubule (pt); arrows point to individual mitochondria-rich cells in the connecting piece, weak reaction in the distal tubules (dt) x 105. **c:** Rat, pt: proximal, dt: distal tubule, g: glomerulus (with wide open capillaries), asterisk, capsular space, arrow: outer wall of Bowman's capsule, x 200. a, c: Toluidine blue preparations

only possess a few individual microvilli. Their cytoplasm contains relatively abundant ribosomes and well-developed rough ER cisternae. The basal infoldings are deeper than in the proximal tubule and may almost reach the cellular apex. They are also associated with long mitochondria. At the *macula densa* the epithelial cells are tall and slender; their bases can be separated by rather wide intercellular spaces and are underlain by a relatively thin basal lamina. The location of the Golgi apparatus is also unusual, in contrast to the other epithelial cells of the nephron, where it is in supranuclear position, it is beside or below the nucleus. Under this epithelium the juxtaglomerular cells (see below) occur in the wall of the afferent vessels of the glomerulus. *Macula densa* and juxtaglomerular cells are termed together juxtaglomerular apparatus. It is assumed that the *macula densa* cells have a receptor function and influence the secretory activity (production of renin) of the juxtaglomerular cells.

The basal infoldings of the distal tubule can be absent in reptiles and caecilians. Such animals usually produce only iso-osmotic urine, whereas species with basal infoldings produce hypo- or hyperosmotic urine. Thus these infoldings are related to the ability of the kidney to build up osmotic gradients by active transport of ions. In some crocodiles and turtles the lateral cytoplasmic extensions seem to have taken over the function of the basal infoldings.

In many vertebrate groups individual segments of the nephron may exhibit certain peculiarities. In the connecting piece of amphibians particular cells regularly occur, e.g. in gymnophionans and toads and hylid and rhacophorid tree frogs mitochondria-rich cells with dark cytoplasm and apical brush border, in *Rana* species cells with deep branched apical invaginations extending almost down to the basal plasma membrane (canaliculated cells, Fig. 164) in *Xenopus* and *Hymenochirus* large flask-shaped cells with apical invagination and a perikaryon bulging into the underlying connective tissue. In the distal tubules of reptiles, glandular areas occur (Fig. 165). In male sticklebacks the majority of epithelial cells produce in spring a protein-rich secretory product, which is used for the construction of the nest.

Also the nephrons of other teleosts exhibit particularities. In many species the glomerulus is absent (aglomerular nephrons). In these species the nephron is composed of two parts: a brush-border segment and a collecting tubule. The first ones usually possesses a well developed basal labyrinth (*Nerophis, Syngnathus*), which in *Lophius,* however, is almost absent. Also in those marine teleosts with a glomerulus, a transitory piece and a distal tubule are absent. In the flounder the brush-border segment is composed of three subdivisions, differing in the high of their brushborder, the depth of

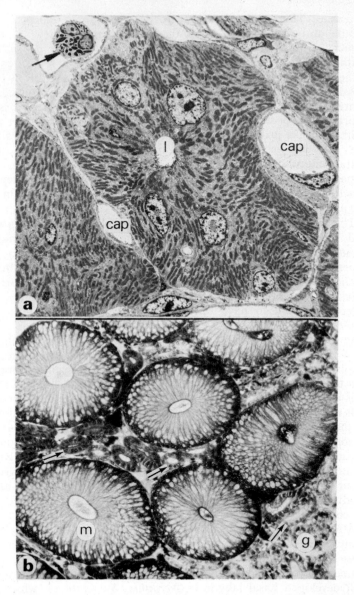

Figure 165.   **a:** Ultrastructure of the salt gland of the blackheaded gull (*Larus*). The glandular lumen (l) is surrounded by mitochondria-rich epithelial cells with deep basal infoldings, cap: blood capillary, arrow points to granulocyte. The epithelial cells are innervated by a well developed nerve plexus, x 2100. **b:** Light microscopical preparation of the kidney of a grass snake (*Natrix*), note the transformed mucus producing excretory tubules (m), between which ordinary tubules occur (arrows); g: glomerulus, x 140

the basal labyrinth and the contents of ribosomes.

The mammalian collecting tubules are dilmited by cuboidal epithelial cells, poor in organelles.

Juxtaglomerular cells. In the wall of the afferent vessels of the glomerulus transformed smooth muscle cells occur, which produce renin, an enzyme liberating the vasoactive substance angiotensin. These cells contain polymorphic electron-dense granules.

Salt glands

In many aquatic birds, predominantly in marine species (e.g. shearwaters, gulls), the kidney is supported by the osmoregulatory activity of the salt glands, which are located in a supraorbital position and open out by the external nasal opening. They secrete salts, above all NaCl, which is produced as a 5 per cent solution. Similar glands have been found in reptiles. Salt glands are branched tubular glands, the walls of which are composed of columnar pyramidal-shaped epithelial cells The ultrastructure of these cells resembles that of the kidney tubules, however, the basal labyrinth and the lateral extensions of the cells are still better developed (Figs. 158, 165). The cytoplasm is characterized by a wealth of mitochondria. Apical microvilli usually are absent. The glandular epithelium is innervated and surrounded by a dense network of blood capillaries.

Of basically the same structure are the rectal glands of elasmobranchs, which secrete a NaCl-rich fluid and open into the hindgut.

The epidermis may contain areas of active transport too; e.g. in the ventral tube of Collembola and in the cephalo-thoracic tergites of some syncarid crustaceans. Also the gills of crustaceans serve as organs of excretion, osmo- and ion regulation (see p. 269).

LITERATURE

ALBERTI, G., STORCH, V. Über Bau und Funktion der Prosoma-Drüsen von Spinnmilben (Tetranychidae, Trombidiformes).' Z. Morph. Tiere. **92**, 300-320 1974.

BOER, H. H., ALGERA, N. H., LOMMERSE, A. W. 'Ultrastructure of possible sites of ultrafiltration in some gastropoda, with particular reference to the auricle of the freshwater prosobranch Viviparus viviparus L.' Z. Zellforsch. **143**, 329-341 (1973).

BONGA, S. E. W., BOER, H. H. 'Ultrastructure of the reno-pericardial system in the pond snail Lymnaea stagnalis (L.).' Z. Zellforsch. **94**, 513-529 (1969).

BOROFFKA, I., ALTNER, H., HAUPT, J. 'Funktion und Ultrastruktur des Nephridiums von Hirudo medicinalis. I. Ort und Mechanismus der Primärharnbildung.' Z. vergl. Physiol. **66**, 421-438 (1970).

DANKWARTH, L. 'Funktionsmorphologie des Exkretionsorgans des Spulwurms Ascaris lumbricoides L.' Z. Zellforsch. **113**, 581-608 (1971).

DELHAYE, W. 'Histophysiologie compareé des organes excréteurs.' *Arch. Biol. (Bruxelles)* **85**, 235-262 (1974).

DIAMOND, J. M., BOSSERT, W. H. 'Functional consequences of ultrastructural geometry in "backwards" fluid-transporting epithelia.' *J. Cell Biol.* **37**, 694-702 (1968).

EISENBEIS, G. 'Licht- und electronenmikroskopische Untersuchungen zur Ultrastruktur des Transportepithels am Ventraltubus arthropleoner Collembolen (Insecta).' *Cytobiologie.* **9**, 180-202 (1974).

EL- HIFNAWI, E. S., SEIFERT, G. 'Über den Feinbau der Maxillarnephridien von *Polyxenus lagurus* (L.). (Diplopoda, Penicillata).' *Z. Zellforsch.* **113**, 518-530 (1971).

ERICSON, J. L., TRUMP, B. F. 'Electron microscopy of the uriniferous tubules.' In: *The kidney*, ed. by Ch. Roullier, A. F. Muller. Acad. Press. N.Y. 351-447 (1969).

HAUPT, J. 'Function and ultrastructure of the nephridium of *Hirudo medicinalis* L.' *Cell Tiss. Res.* **152**, 385-401 (1974).

KIRSCHNER, L. B. 'Comparative physiology: invertebrate excretory organs.' *Ann. Rev. Physiol.* **29**, 169-196 (1967).

KOECHLIN, N. 'Etude histochimique et ultrastructurale des pigments néphridiens et coelomiques d'une Annélide Polychété (sabelle).' *Ann. Histochim.* **17**, 27-54 (1972).

KÜMMEL, G. 'Die Podocyten.' *Zoolog. Beitr. N.F.* **13**, 245-263 (1967).

KURTZ, S. M. 'The kidney,' in: *Electron microscopic anatomy*, 239-265. Academic Press, N.Y. and London (1964).

LAKE, P. S., SWAIN, R., Ong, J. E. 'The ultrastructure of the fenestra dorsalis of the syncarid crustaceans *Allanaspides helonomus* and *Allanaspides hickmani.*' *Z. Zellforsch.* **147**, 335-351 (1974).

MÖLLENDORFF, W. v. 'Der Exkretionsapparat.' In: *Handbuch der mikroskopischen Anatomie des Menschen VII*, 1. Springer, Berlin, 1-328, (1930).

MIYOSHI, M., FUJITA, T., TOKUNAGA, J. 'The differentiation of renal podocytes. A combined scanning and transmission electron microscope study in rats.' *Arch. histol. jap.* **33**, 161-178 (1971).

POTTS, W. T. W. 'Excretion in the molluscs.' *Biol. Rev.* **42**, 1-41 (1967).

WESSING, A., EICHELBERG, D. 'Elektronenoptische Untersuchungen an den Nierentubuli von *Drosophila melanogaster*. I. Regionale Gliederung der Tubuli.' *Z. Zellforsch.* **101**, 285-322 (1969).

WILSON, R. A., WEBSTER, L. A. 'Protonephridia.' *Biol. Rev.* **49**, 127-160. (1974).

Chapter 11
REPRODUCTIVE ORGANS AND CELLS

Male animals

Two radically different types of male reproductive cells (sperms, spermatozoa) exist in the animal kingdom: those with and those without a flagellum. The flagellate type is the more primitive one, the aflagellate type is confined to a few groups (see below). The structure of spermatozoa is determined above all by the systematic position of the animal group and by the mode of fertilization.

Forms releasing their spermatozoa freely into the water retain a primitive type of spermatozoon. This primitive type is made up of a short roundish or conical head, a middle piece containing usually 4-5 spherical mitochondrial aggregates, and a tail consisting of a long flagellum (Figs. 166, 169). The head is mainly composed of the nucleus, but the tip usually contains an acrosome of variable morphology. The flagellum begins with a centriolar apparatus at the posterior part of the head, penetrates the middle piece, extends for about 50 μm, and terminates with a tiny end-piece. The middle piece contains the mitochondria, collected in usually 4-5 spherical or egg-shaped aggregates, the proximal part of the flagellum and the centriolar apparatus, which consists of two centrioles. The acrosome consists of an acrosomal vesicle, which is bounded by a membrane. Its ultrastructure may be very complex.

This primitive type of spermatozoon occurs in numerous and so widely separated phyla as the Porifera, Cnidaria, Ctenophora, Tentaculata (only Brachiopoda), Aschelminthes (only Priapulida), Nemertini, Sipunculida, Mollusca, Annelida, Enteropneusta, Tunicata (only a few species), and Acrania. It is retained in groups and species which have retained the primitive metazoan way for the discharge of spermatozoa freely into the water.

When internal fertilization takes place or the spermatozoa are released in the immediate proximity of the female genital opening, the morphology of the spermatozoa diverges to varying degrees from the primitive type. Differences from the primitive type are mainly confined to the head and the middle piece. These parts become more elongated. The mitochondrial mass is evenly distributed in the middle piece. This connection between the morphology of the spermatozoon and the method of sperm transmission is particularly evident in the phyla Nemertini, Annelida and Mollusca.

Unusually constructed flagellate spermatozoa e.g. are the biflagellate sperms of Platyhelminthes and the sperms of many tunicates. In the latter a middle piece with mitochondrial spheres is lacking; here the mitochondria are generally collected in a lateral body which is attached to the head region.

In some animal groups - in particular in gastropods - beside normal sperms atypical ones occur. These are characterized by an unusual increase in cytoplasm and a multiplication of centrioles. In the course of their development the chromatin dissolves to various degrees. In contrast to typical spermatozoa with a haploid set of chromosomes (eupyrene sperms) their chromatin is of reduced amounts (oligopyrene sperms) or absent (apyrene sperms). Typical (eupyrene) sperms attach after maturation to the atypical sperm, thus forming the very motile spermatozeugmata (Fig. 167). Also the nurse cells of *Littorina* must be considered to represent atypical sperms, which dissociate from the germinal epithelium and attract eupyrene sperms, the heads of which become embedded in the nurse cells.

In arthropods flagellate sperms are widely distributed. Prominent secondary fibres of the tail are present only in insects. Many unusual types of sperms are to be found mainly among crustaceans and arachnids.

Chelicerata. The primitive sperms with numerous unmodified mitochondria and a simple 9+2 axial tubular complex devoid of secondary fibres are conserved in Merostomata. In the arachnid group considerable differences in respect of the spermatozoan structure exist. In scorpions the mitochondria become fused to form large bodies in which the cristae are anastomosed. In Cheloneti the tail filament (9 + 2) is coiled around an annular single mitochondrial derivative. In Araneida the mitochondria which appear normal in spermatids fuse to form an opaque amorphous mass that disappears by the end of spermiogenesis; flagellum 9 + 3. The sperm usually is rolled up on itself and incysted in a 0.1 μm thick sheath formed by extracellular material. In Acarina usually

Figure 166. Spermatozoon of *Nausithoë* (Cnidaria), **a:** ultrastructure of the sperm head with the nucleus, which frontally is covered by a cap with acrosomal granules (enlarged in **b**) pc, dc: proximal, distal centriole. Arrows point to different cross-sections through the tail; **c:** complicated structure of the distal centriole; **d:** light microscopical appearance of the sperm. After AFZELIUS: 1971

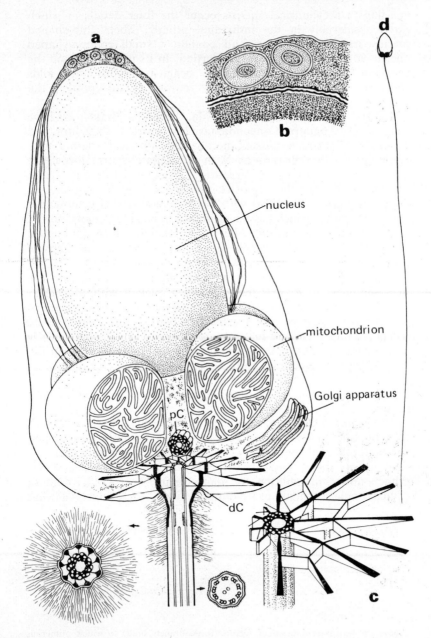

nucleus

mitochondrion

Golgi apparatus

pC

dC

non-flagellate cylindrical sperms occur the finer details of which vary considerably in the individual groups. Their club-shaped sperms are relatively large and contain a small comma-shaped nucleus in their slender terminal portion. In its neighbourhood the acrosome is located. The surface bears numerous thin folds arranged in parallel which are movable and propel the spermatozoon.

Crustacea: Sperms of Mystacocarida, Cirripedia, Branchiura have a tail with 9+2 pattern. Copepoda have lost centriole, flagellum, and acrosome. Anostraca possess non-motile spherical sperms with many arms. Further groups with aflagellate spermatozoa are Cephalocarida, Ostracoda, Peracarida, Decapoda. In the latter the acrosome possesses the explosive properties. The spermatozoa of decapods consist of a head with nucleus and several cytoplasmic extensions (arms) which have been shown to be able to move slowly. At the head a capsule may be differentiated, which contains a perforating organelle, which after explosion of the capsule penetrates the wall of the egg cell (explosive spermatozoa).

Amoeboid spermatozoa occur in Phyllopoda (*Crustacea*) and in Nematodes. In *Ascaris* they contain a nucleus without nuclear envelope. The cytoplasm is characterized by mitochondria, rich in mitochondrial matrix and a refractive body, which seems to be composed of protein and to originate from ribosomes. Temporarily it also contains lipids. An acrosome is absent. Pseudopodia in the anterior region come into contact with the egg cell and remove its surface coats.

Thus, in general, the crustacean spermatozoa are atypical and bizarre.

Tracheata: Chilopoda, Pauropoda, Symphyla have a 9 + 2 flagellum; in Diplopoda most genera produce unmotile disk-shaped spermatozoa, combined two by two in the same spermatophore.

In insects the sperms usually contain two elongated modified mitochondria; in addition to the ordinary 9 + 2 microtubules ('fibres') nine secondary outer doublet 'fibres' occur in the tail that

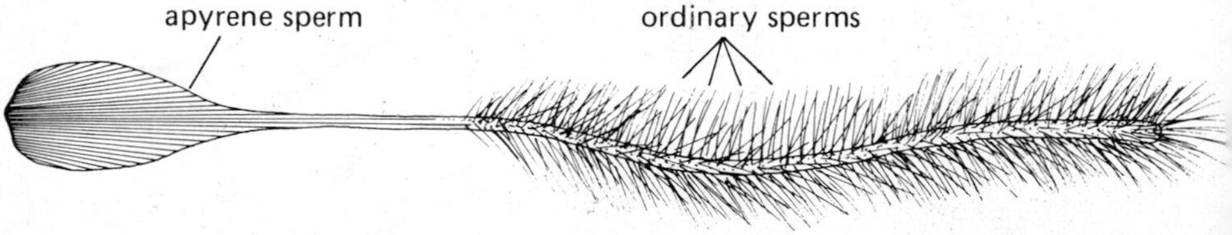

Figure 167. Apyrene sperm of *Opalia* (prosobranch snail) to which numerous ordinary spermatozoa are attached. After BULNHEIM, 1962

are rich in glycogen-like material, but otherwise similar to the central pair. Limiting the count to the principal elements only, the structure is now of the model '9 + 9 + 2'.

Vertebrates: The spermatozoa are almost all flagellate but display numerous differences. In many mammals they are of bilateral shape, in elasmobranchs and passerine birds they are of helical structure and rotate around their longitudinal axis.

The greatest variety of shape exists in fishes. Mormyridae are the only vertebrates with aflagellate sperms. In teleosts the acrosome is generally absent. This absence corresponds to the presence of micropyles in the egg envelopes.

The acrosomal region exhibits numerous peculiarities. It consists of acrosome (derived from the Golgi apparatus) and the subacrosomal material. This material is absent or scanty in frogs, passerine birds, and some mammals. It is of most complicated structure in lampreys, where it consists of a dense subacrosomal ring and a long, helical fibre running through the nucleus and far back into the tail surrounded by the membranes of the nuclear envelope. This structure plays a prominent role during fertilization (it is extruded to form the core of an acrosomal tubule during the acrosome reaction).

The mitochondrial collar can be flat (in teleosts if fertilization is external) or thick with many mitochondria in viviparous species. Spermtails in amphibians exhibit a variety of accessory structures, e.g. a so-called 'undulating membrane' in the plane of the central microtubules.

Reptiles and mammals have nine coarse peripheral fibres in their sperms (Fig. 169).

In many cases two or several sperms are enveloped by an extracellular sheath produced by special glands (spermatophores, Fig. 168).

Male reproductive cells originate in organs termed testes. The wall of these organs (the germinal epithelium) usually contains several developmental stages of the reproductive cells, which enable recognition of the typical maturation of these cells, which is characterized by mitotic and meiotic cell divisions and striking structural alterations. Very often the germinal epithelium contains supporting cells, in vertebrates termed Sertoli cells, which seem to play a role in the nourishment of the germinal cells.

The development of the spermatozoa will briefly be described in mammals. The testes contain the seminiferous tubules producing the spermatozoa and connective tissue the most important components of which are the Leydig cells (interstitial cells), which synthesize the male sex hormone testosterone (Fig. 170).

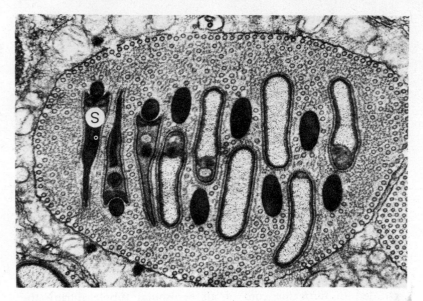

Figure 168. Porcellio (Isopoda); spermatophore, containing several (nine) spermatozoa (S), which are embedded into a matrix containing tubular structures. The spermatozoa are of unusual shape and possess three cytoplasmic extensions, one of which contains the electron dense nucleus. x 18 000

The wall of the seminiferous tubules is lined by a stratified epithelium containing supporting and spermatogenic cells. The supporting cells (Sertoli cells) rest upon the basement lamina of the epithelium and apically extend up to the lumen of the tubule (Fig. 171). Their shape is highly variable since they project numerous lateral processes between the spermatogenic cells, which however, ordinarily may be seen only in the electron microscope. Their cytoplasm is often darker than that of the germ cells. The ovoid light nucleus is located in the basal third of the cells and contains a prominent nucleolus with an acidophilic centre and two basophilic lateral components. The cytoplasm is characterized by longitudinally oriented microfilaments and microtubules, a rather well developed smooth ER, a few rough ER cisternae, annulated lamellae, elongated mitochondria with tubules and cristae, lipid inclusions and lysosomes. Animals with cyclical reproductive activities exhibit typical changes in respect of the contents of cell organelles. In resting periods the epithelium of the seminiferous tubules can predominantly consist of Sertoli cells.

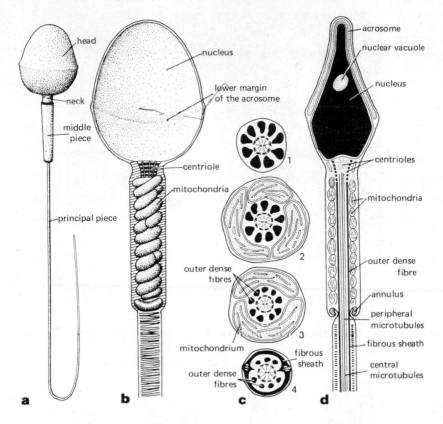

Figure 169. Human spermatozoon, **a:** light microscopy; **b:** fine structure, looked at from the outside; **c:** cross-sections (ultrastructure) through different levels of the tail, 1 neck, 2, 3 middle piece, 4 principal piece, centrally always the typical ciliary structure is to be seen, **d:** longitudinal section (ultrastructure), the annulus is composed of electron dense material and marks the end of the middle piece. After HORSTMANN, 1965, AUBERG, 1957, FAWCETT, 1958

The spermatogenic cells form layers of morphologically distinguishable types: spermatogonia, primary spermatocytes, secondary spermatocytes, spermatids and spermatozoa. All these cells represent distinguishable successive stages of the differentiation of the male germ cells (spermatogenesis). This process may be divided into several periods: (1) the spermatogonia proliferate by mitotic divisions and give rise to spermatocytes

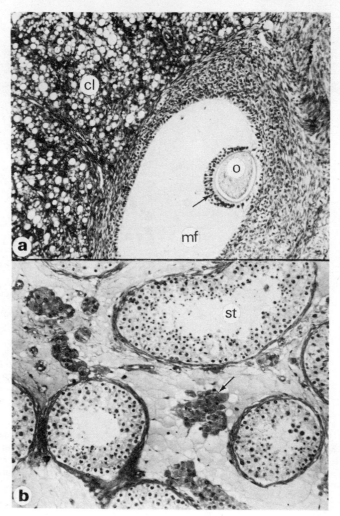

Figure 170. **a:** Ovary of a cat, o: ovum, surrounded by *corona radiata* (arrow) mf: mature follicle, cl: *corpus luteum* with lipid containing granulosa lutein cells (the lipid is marked by the light vacuoles), x 120; **b:** testis, man, st: seminiferous tubule, arrow points to group of interstitial cells of Leydig, x 110

(spermatocytogenesis) (2) the· spermatocytes undergo two matura-tion divisions, at the end of which haploid spermatids are present (meiosis); (3) the spermatids transform into spermatozoa (spermiogenesis).

The relatively small spermatogonia rest on the basement lamina and contain a light cytoplasm (Fig. 171). Their spherical or ellipsoid nucleus is usually rather pale and contains one or two peripheral nucleoli (type A) or a centrally located nucleolus (type B). Type A spermatogonia represent a dormant phase, type B give rise to spermatocytes. Before chromosome reduction these are termed primary spermatocytes, which are large pale cells with striking nuclear alterations, representing the various phases of meiosis; secondary spermatocytes are smaller.

All daughter cells arising from a type B spermatogonium remain connected by cytoplasmic bridges: Initially pairs of primary spermatocytes, then groups of four interconnected secondary spermatocytes and finally eight conjoined spermatids develop. The cytoplasmic bridges disintegrate during spermiogenesis.

Spermatids at first are small roundish cells. They soon develop small granules within their Golgi apparatus (in some species these occur already in the spermatocytes), which fuse and constitute the acrosomal granule, which is rich in carbohydrate and seems to represent a specialized lysosome. This granule becomes attached to the nucleus, flattens, spreads out and transforms into a cap covering about half of the nucleus (acrosomal cap, acrosome).

The final shape of this cap varies considerably in the different species.

During the transformations of the acrosomal granule, the nucleus of the spermatids exhibits alterations: its chromatin continuously becomes condensed, until finally the whole nucleus is filled by electron dense heterochromatin (Fig. 172). In the course of this process the nucleus generally assumes an elongated shape.

A further characteristic trait of spermiogenesis is the formation of a modified cilium, which builds up the tail. At first the centrioles move to the cell pole opposite the acrosome. The distal centriole forms a cilium, the proximal one is attached to the nuclear envelope. While the cilium is developing microtubules arise, which form a cylinder-like structure, the caudal sheath or manchette, which extends caudally from the posterior margin of the acrosome and surrounds the posterior part of the nucleus. The cilium initially is constructed according to the 9 + 2 pattern.

Its microtubules collectively are termed axoneme. Later it becomes altered, among others by the development of nine thick electron dense fibres running in parallel and outside of the nine doublets and by the formation of a sheath composed of fine-filamentous material (fibrous sheath) below the plasma membrane. Around the proximal part of the cilium a layer of mitochondria gathers around the nine thick fibres. At the end of spermatogenesis the manchette disappears and excess cytoplasm is cast off.

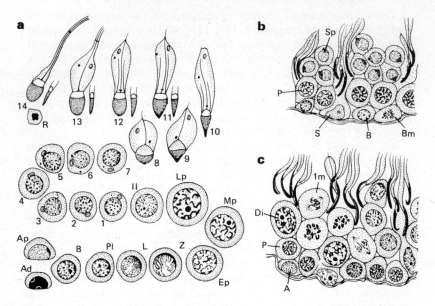

Figure 171. **a:** Spermatogenesis in the rhesus monkey. Ad: (dark spermatogonia), Ap: (pale spermatogonia), B: type B spermatogonium; Pl,L,Z,Mp,Lp: different stages of primary spermatocytes, the letters refer to stages of the prophase Pl: preleptotene, L: leptotene, Z: zygotene, Ep, Mp, Lp: early, mid-late pachytene; II: secondary spermatocytes. 1-14 stages of spermiogenesis. R: residual body. **b:** different stages of spermatozoan development in the seminiferous epithelium of the rat; P: pachytene of a primary spermatocyte, S: Sertoli cell with spermatids in its apical cytoplasm; B: type B spermatogonia; Bm: mitosis of a spermatogonium; **c:** 1 m: first meiotic division; Di: diplotene of primary spermatocyte; A: type A spermatogium; Sp: spermatid, After CLERMONT

The mature spermatozoon is differentiated into head and tail. The head contains the condensed nucleus and the acrosomal cap covering its anterior two thirds. The tail is further subdivided into neck, middle piece, principal piece and end-piece. The neck is a short section between head and middle piece. The middle piece contains the basis of the cilium, its microtubules and the thick fibres which are surrounded by the mitochondrial sheath, in the principal piece the ciliary microtubules and the thick fibres are surrounded by the fibrous sheath. The end piece only contains irregularly arranged microtubules.

The spermatozoa remain for some time with their heads enclosed in the Sertoli cells in the epithelium (Fig. 171). Then they leave it and gather in the efferent ductules (epithelium: tall ciliated cells and

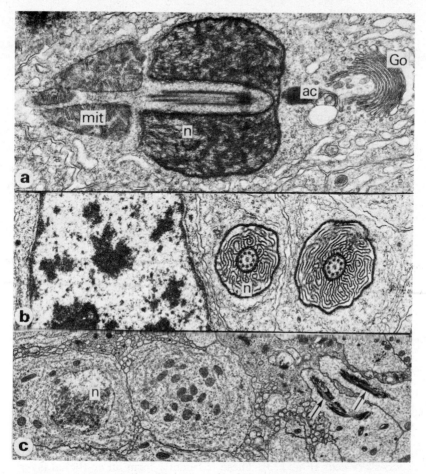

Figure 172. **a:** *Littorina* (prosobranch snail), spermatid, Go: Golgi apparatus, C: acrosome; n: nucleus, mit: mitochondrium x 18 000; **b:** *Littorina*, spermatids, left; cell with normal nucleus, right two cells with nuclei in which the chromatin is condensed to form filamentous structures, these nuclei (n) surround the cilium, x 18 000; a,b. Photo R. Kohnert, **c:** *Abrolophus* (mite), spermatids, left: cells with ordinary nucleus (n), right two cells with nuclei containing condensed fibrous chromatin (arrow) not surrounded by a nuclear membrane, x 18 000

lower cuboidal ones with secretory activity and also often bearing an apical cilium) and finally in the *ductus epididymidis*, where they can be stored and where they become fully maturated. Cross-sections through this duct show its regular construction. Its wall consists of a pseudostratified columnar epithelium with small basal and tall columnar cells. These bear an apical tuft of long and slender microvilli (stereocilia). Their cytoplasm is characterized by a very large Golgi apparatus, a well-developed smooth ER system, lysosomes and various vesicular elements. Possibly this epithelium is both of secretory and absorptive function. In other vertebrates, e.g. in lizards, this epithelium does not bear apical sterocilia and is filled with large amounts of secretory granules.

The testes of the other vertebrates are basically of the same structure as those of the mammals. In the frog the spermatogenic cells form clusters (spermatocysts) along the seminiferous tubules, which project into the tubular lumen and often are surrounded by a flattened epithelium (follicular membrane). The spermatogonia are (also in fishes) relatively large cells.

In most groups of animals sperms are formed in testes, which occasionally however structurally disintegrate at an early stage of development. Spermatogenesis in this case takes place in the body cavity. In sponges spermatozoa arise diffusively in the body.

It has already been mentioned that in most testes supporting cells are to be found. Their function is not well known. They may protect, nourish and liberate the spermatozoa. In many invertebrates cytophores occur, these are cytoplasmic bodies with or without a nucleus to which numerous spermatozoa are attached. They e.g. have been found in turbellaria, annelids, molluscs, arthropods and arrow worms. A peculiar mechanism for nourishment and transport of sperms is represented by the spermiozeugmata of some prosobranchs (see above).

Female animals

Female germ cells – egg cells, eggs – also usually differentiate in their own organs, the ovaries, and in connection with supporting or accessory cells (Fig. 173). These frequently form an epithelial layer around the egg cell and are termed follicular cells. The whole complex consisting of the egg cell and follicular cells is termed a follicle. Follicular cells seem to be absent in some groups, e.g. nematodes. They function presumably mainly as nutritive cells, in some insects they have been observed to transfer cell organelles into the cytoplasm of the egg cell. However, especially the follicular cells of many insects do not exhibit fine structural characteristics in indicating a nutritive function. If such a function has been demonstrated these cells are also termed trophocytes. The interrelations of such cells and the egg cells are manifold, in sponges and Cnidaria they can be phagocytized by the egg cells, in some insects they are located in special so-called nutritive chambers of the

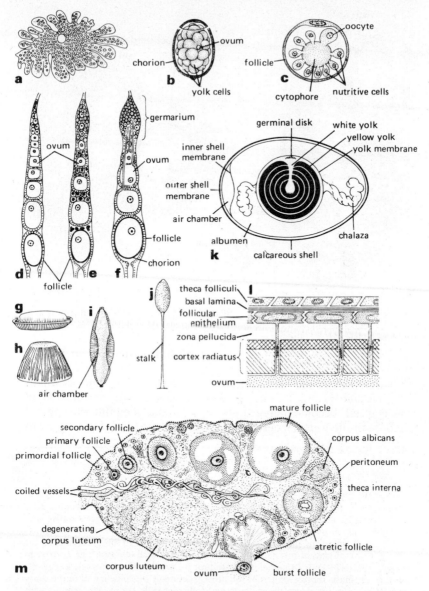

Figure 173. Egg cells and ovaries; **a:** ovum of *Chlorohydra* (Hydrozoa) with pseudopodial processes; **b:** composite egg of a cestode (*Diphyllobothrium*); the egg-shell (chorion) has a lid; **c:** composite egg of a leech (*Piscicola*), one oogonium forms an envelope (follicle), the other divides repeatedly; all daughter cells, one of which becomes the ovum, remain interconnected by the central cytophore; **d-f:** ovarioles of

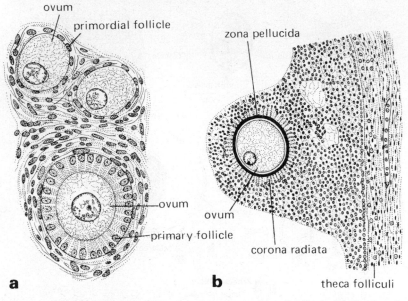

Figure 174. Follicles from the ovary of a cat, **a:** primordial (low epithelium) and primary (cuboidal to low prismatic epithelium) follicles; **b:** *cumulus oophorus* from a mature follicle. After SCHNEIDER, 1908

ovarioles and are in contact with cytoplasmic extensions of the egg cells.

The follicular cells surrounding the egg cells of some ascidians (e.g. *Molgula* and *Ciona*), in later stages of the maturation of the egg cell, become increasingly vacuolated and enable the egg cell to float in the water. These transformations are absent in viviparous

insects, **d:** panoistic ovariole, at the distal end only germinative cells occur (germarium), the germinative cells move proximally and become surrounded by follicular cells: **e, f:** meroistic ovariole, the germarium contains germinative and nutritive cells, **e:** polytroph ovariole; nutritive cells form layers between the ova. **f:** telotroph ovariole. The nutritive cells in the germarium extend long processes to the ova; **g-j:** several eggs of insects with different types of shell (chorion); **g:** *Tortrix;* **h:** *Panolis* (butterflies); **i:** (*Anopheles* (mosquito); **j:** *Chrysopa* (Neuroptera); **k:** egg of a bird; **l:** schematic representation of the ultrastructure of the follicle wall in the ovary of a teleost fish; the microvilli of ovum and follicular cells are in close contact with each other, **m:** longitudinal section through the female ovary; in the upper half: maturation of the follicle; right: regressive (atretic) follicle with well developed theca interna (producing oestrogens); below: ovulation, *corpus luteum* and regression of *corpus luteum*; the *corpus albicans* is a terminal stage of the *corpus luteum*. After various authors. From REMANE, STORCH & WELSCH, 1974

species, in which the follicular cells are very flat. In the ovary of echinoderms supportive cells are only in loose contact with the egg cells. In *Branchiostoma* the follicular cells of the ovary form an epithelial layer only around relatively mature eggs, their nuclei disappear in mature follicles.

Between follicular and egg cells in many species layers of extra-cellular material can be found. They are particularly well differentiated in vertebrates and many terms exist to designate them. According to electron microscope studies, however, there are far-reaching similarities in respect of their structure. All non-cellular (extracellular) layers between egg cell and follicular epithelium are termed *zona pellucida*. This may be further sub-divided. Directly below the follicular cells a clear space, containing mucopolysaccharides, can be distinguished in the electron microscope: the *zona pellucida sensu str.*, which is possibly formed by the follicular cells (Figs. 173, 174); next follows the *cortex radiatus*, which consists of electron-dense material, which presumably is secreted by the egg cell. This part can be of homogeneous and uniform structure (Amphibia) or exhibits further sublayers, e.g. in teleosts.

Particularly striking structures are the filament bundles of the *cortex radiatus internus* of many teleosts. Here the filaments are arranged basically in the same way as in the insect cuticle. They form the immediate surface layer of the egg cell. Both egg- and follicular cell extend microvilli between which temporarily even desmosomes can be observed. The microvilli penetrate the *zona pellucida*. Their radial arrangement may be just recognized in the light microscope and is responsible for the term *zona radiata*, which is also used to designate the extracellular layer around the egg cell. (In mammals the term *corona radiata* exists; it designates a layer of follicular cells around the egg cell in mature follicles, (Fig. 174).

In mammals the follicular cells are separated by a basement lamina from the connective tissue of the ovary. The layer of connective tissue cells surrounding the follicle or in its neighbourhood transforms into steroid hormone producing cells (*theca interna*).

In the vertebrate ovary various stages of the follicle development can be recognized. In mammals this process is of particularly high differentiation: the consecutive stages are termed primordial, primary, secondary and mature (Graafian, tertiary) follicles (Fig. 173).

In primordial follicles which represent an inactive stage, the large egg cell is enveloped by a single layer of flattened follicular cells (which are also termed granulosa cells). The big light nucleus of the egg cell is in eccentrical position, its cytoplasm contains an extended Golgi apparatus, annulated lamellae, numerous mitochondria and multivesicular bodies. The ER system is of relatively poor development.

In the primary follicles the follicular epithelium is cuboidal or low columnar (Fig. 174). In later stages of its development it transforms into a stratified epithelium, at first composed of two cell layers (secondary follicle). The size of the egg cell increases, the Golgi apparatus divides into several Golgi areas, at first to be found scattered throughout the cytoplasm but later concentrating below the plasma membrane. The rough ER increases in volume, the number of ribosomes and multivesicular bodies increases. Occasionally direct connections between mitochondria and rough ER may be observed; in such cases the lumen of the ER cisternae communicates with the intracrista space of the mitochondria. This close relation is possibly an expression of the transport of proteins into the mitochondria. In addition lipid or yolk-containing granular inclusions as well as stacks of proteinaceous lamellae with attached glycogen particles occur in many species.

In later stages of the secondary follicles (two or more layers of follicular cells around the egg cell) a clear space forms around the egg cell, the zona pellucida into which microvilli of egg and follicular cells extend. The zona pellucida of mammals is of a simple rather homogeneous structure.

In the mature follicle fluid-filled spaces appear between the follicular cells. They fuse and form a large vacuole, the anthrum. The egg cell does not further increase in size, however, but the follicle continues to grow until it reaches its maximal size. The follicular wall then is relatively thin and is composed of several layers of granulosa cells. The egg cell is located in a local thickening of the follicular epithelium, the cumulus oophorus (Figs. 173, 174). In terminal stages the cumulus loosens up and the corona radiata becomes clearly recognizable. Briefly before ovulation the follicular cells actively secrete fluid so that the follicular wall is under considerable pressure. The egg cell with the corona radiata leaves the epithelial lining of the follicle, which finally ruptures. The egg cell escapes into the oviduct, the follicular epithelium transforms into the corpus luteum.

The ovary of mammals, birds and reptiles is a compact organ composed of follicles and connective tissue (stroma) with blood vessels, lymph vessels, nerves and steroid hormone-producing cells. In birds and reptiles no fluid filled spaces occur in the follicles, the egg cells are very much larger than in mammals and contain abundant yolk inclusions. The follicular epithelium of birds usually is composed of one layer of cells only; in lizards it is composed of several layers of small and large granulosa cells. In Amphibia the ovary consists of several fluid-filled chambers in the thin walls of which the yolk-rich egg cells develop which are only surrounded by a thin layer of follicular cells. Also, in teleosts the yolk-rich egg cells develop in thin septa of the ovary extending into its fluid-filled lumen and are surrounded by one layer of follicular cells. In sharks the ovary is again of a compact structure, the follicles develop within a connective tissue (stroma). The follicular wall may be pseudo-stratified, the egg cells become unusually large (2-3 cm). In the compact ovary of *Petromyzon* the egg cells temporarily seem to dissolve their nucleus, it becomes reorganized during fertilization.

The maturation of the female germ cells differs in some respects from that of the male ones. The differences are particularly obvious during the meiotic cell divisions. In many primary oocytes these are dependent on the penetration of the spermatozoon into the cytoplasm of the egg cell. In *Branchiostoma* and many vertebrates the second maturation division is caused by the contact between sperm and egg cell. In sea urchins both divisions occur before the entry of the sperm. The primary oocyte gives rise to two secondary oocytes, one of which is of the size of its mother cell, the other being very small and only containing nuclear material and a narrow rim of cytoplasm (first polar body). The second meiotic division of the normal secondary oocyte again gives rise to two cells of unequal size: the large mature ovum retaining most of the cytoplasm and the small second polar body. The first polar body also may divide; so that one primary oocyte can give rise to an ovum and three polar bodies.

In contrast to the male germ cells, in the female ones a tendency to increase their cytoplasmic volume can be observed.

In summary the cytoplasmic differentiation of the female germ cells is characterized by the following features: formation of fat-, protein, and carbohydrate stores (deutoplasm), development of a morphogenetic organization in the cytoplasm, which cannot be demonstrated structurally, formation of surrounding extracellular and cellular layers.

LITERATURE

BACCETTI, B. ed. *Comparative Spermatology.* Academic Press, New York, London (1970). 573 pp.
——, DALLAI, R., FRATELLO, B. 'The spermatozoon of Arthropoda.' XXII. *J. Cell Sci.* **13**, 321-335 (1973).

BREUCKER, H., HORSTMANN, E. 'Die Spermatogenese der Zecke *Ornithodorus moubata* (Murr).' *Z. Zellforsch.* **123**, 18–46 (1972).

BROWN, G. G. 'Some comparative aspects of selected crustacean spermatozoa and crustacean phylogeny.' *Proc. 1st. int. Symp. comp. spermatology.* Rome-Siena. 183–203 (1970).

FAWCETT, D. W. 'The topographical relationship between the plane of the central pair of flagellar fibrils and the transverse axis of the head in guinea-pig spermatozoa.' *J. Cell Sci.* **3**, 187–198 (1968).

——, ANDERSON, W. A., PHILIPPS, D. M. 'Morphogenetic factors influencing the shape of the sperm head.' *Developmental Biol.* **26**, 220–251 (1971).

FOOR, W. E. 'Zygote formation in *Ascaris lumbricoides* (Nematoda). *J. Cell Biol.* **39**, 119–134 (1968).

FRANZÉN, A. 'On spermiogenesis, morphology of the spermatozoon, and biology of fertilization among invertebrates.' *Zool. Bidr. Uppsala.* **31**, 355–482 (1956).

GIESE, A. C., PEARSE, J. S. ed. 'Reproduction of marine invertebrates,' vol. I. Acad. Press, New York (1974), 546 pp.

GÖTTING, K.-J. 'Der Follikel und die peripheren Strukturen der Oocyten der Teleosteer und Amphibien.' *Z. Zellforsch.* **79**, 481–491 (1967).

HOLLAND, N. D. 'The fine structure of the ovary of the feather star *Nemaster rubiginosa* (Echinodermata, Crinoidea).' *Tissue and Cell.* **3**, 161–175 (1971).

HOPKINS, C. R., KING, P. E. 'An electron microscopical and histochemical study of the oocyte periphery in *Bombus terrestris* during vitellogenesis.' *J. Cell Sci.* **1**, 201–216 (1966).

HORSTMANN, E. 'Structures of caryoplasm during the differentiation of spermatids.' *Morphol. Aspects of Andrology.* **1**, 24–28 (1970).

KESSEL, R. G. 'The origin and fate of secretion in the follicle cells of tunicates.' *Z. Zellforsch.* **76**, 21–30 (1967).

JOHNSON, A. D., GOMES, W. R., VANDEMARK, N. L. *The Testis*, vol. 1. Academic Press, New York, London. 668 S. (1970).

LAVIOLETTE, P., GRASSÉ, P.-P. 'Fortpflanzung und Sexualität.' *Allgemeine Biologie,* Bd. 2. G. Fischer Verlag. Stuttgart. 256 S. (1971).

LEE, D. L., ANYA, A. O. 'The structure and development of the spermatozoon of *Aspicularis tetraptera* (Nematoda).' *J. Cell Sci.* **2**, 537–544 (1967).

MATTEI, X., MATTEI, C., REIZER, C., CHEVALIER, J. H. 'Ultrastructure des spermatozoides aflagellés des Mormyres (Poissons Téléostéens).' *J. Microsc.* **15**, 67–78 (1972).

REGER, J. F., FAIN-MAUREL, M.-A. 'A comparative study on the origin, distribution, and fine structure of extracellular tubules in the male reproductive system of species of Isopods, Amphipods, Schizopods, Copepods, and Cumacea.' *J. Ultrastruct. Res.* **44**, 235–252 (1973).

SILVEIRA, M. 'Intraaxonal glycogen in "9+1" flagella of flatworms.' *J. Ultrastruct. Res.* **44**, 253–264 (1973).

YASUZUMI, G., SUGIOKA, T. 'Spermatogenesis in animals as revealed by electron microscopy.' XXVI. *J. submicr. Cytol.* **3**, 297–307 (1971).